T0314219

Many Ways to Be Deaf

Many Ways to Be Deaf

INTERNATIONAL VARIATION IN DEAF COMMUNITIES

Leila Monaghan,
Constanze Schmaling,
Karen Nakamura,
and Graham H. Turner,
Editors

Gallaudet University Press
Washington, D.C.

Gallaudet University Press
Washington, DC 20002

http://gupress.gallaudet.edu

Printed in the United States of America

Library of Congress Cataloging-in-Publication Data

Many ways to be deaf / Leila Monaghan . . . [et al.], editors.
  p. cm.
Includes bibliographical references and index.
ISBN 1-56368-135-8 (alk. paper)
  1. Deaf—Cross-cultural studies.   2. Sign language—Cross-cultural studies.
3. Identity (Psychology)—Cross-cultural studies.   4. Social adjustment—Cross-cultural
studies.   5. Intercultural communication.   6. Culture conflict. I. Monaghan, Leila
Frances, 1960–

HV2395.M36 2003
305.9′08162—dc21   2002192872

∞ The paper used in this publication meets the minimum requirements of American
National Standard for Information Sciences—Permanence of Paper for Printed Library Materials, ANSI Z39.48-1984.

Contents

Preface

The core arguments of this book's chapters were written before September 11, 2001. This preface was written shortly afterwards. For us, the tragedy of 9–11 makes an international perspective even more important than before, and that perspective is exactly what this book provides. Deaf communities, like all communities, have commonalities and differences. Deaf people in Austria, Japan, and Nigeria are not only Deaf but also Austrian, Japanese, or Nigerian. They live in worlds of sight and gesture within specific national, social, political, and economic systems and, yet, are also part of an international world of Deaf people.

One of the most remarkable aspects of the writings here is how the authors bear witness to the massive changes that have happened in Deaf communities everywhere. Starting in 1880, the dominant mode of education of deaf people was "oralism." (Notable exceptions include some places in the United States and Ireland.) Deaf children were expected to learn to speak and to understand speech despite the fact that they had little access to spoken language. Although schools for deaf children focused on training children to fit into a hearing world, Deaf adults gathered in cities and towns where they formed their own communities, often based on school ties from childhood, and communicated freely with one another, usually in sign language. In 1960, however, academic views began to change. Research on American Sign Language showed that signed languages' linguistic properties similar to other languages. Systematic studies of signed languages around the world have shown how every language is both unique and complex and how new languages spring up wherever deaf people have been cut off from other signing groups.

The growing awareness of the uniqueness and complexity of language has evolved in tandem with the growing political self-determination of Deaf people (such as the March 1988 Deaf President Now [DPN] protests at Gallaudet University) and the recognition that signed languages are just one aspect of rich cultures. The title of this volume, *Many Ways to Be Deaf*, is an allusion to the groundbreaking international conferences and celebrations, Deaf Way and Deaf Way II, sponsored in 1989 and 2002 by Gallaudet University, that followed on the success of these DPN protests. The title has been recast, however, to emphasize the variation that exists everywhere. The challenges faced by deaf people in Sweden are quite different from those in Nicaragua and are set on a common global stage.

The Deaf world is not only changing rapidly but also, as this book shows, changing in many different ways. These chapters on communities in Europe,

Asia, Africa, Latin America, and the United States are a product of both a growing international consensus on the issues that need to be examined and a strong belief that variation and change are at the heart of what we need to consider.

Key themes of this volume include how Deaf communities have survived despite opposition by those who thought and think that Deaf people should not be allowed to have their own separate communities outside of hearing cultures, how forms of education interact with and are reflections of larger sociocultural processes, and how signed languages are crucial parts of Deaf communities everywhere. Examples of repression include the genocidal policies of the Austrian Nazi government against deaf and other disabled people, and an international history of widespread and active denial of natural signed languages. Development of schools for the deaf has closely followed the rise of nationalism around the world, and in turn these schools have often been the seeds of signing Deaf communities. Even when schools have been oralist in nature, children's desire to communicate has led to the repeated reinvention of signed languages.

Commonalities among the authors include that we all work within a Stokoean linguistic paradigm, see signed languages as natural languages with the same kind of variation found in spoken languages, and value the roles that culture and history play in the formation of Deaf cultures and sign languages. On the other hand, the authors come from a wide range of disciplines, from socio- and historical linguistics to linguistic anthropology, sociology, history, education, and literature. Although all the authors have in-depth knowledge of at least one Deaf community, some are natives of the cultures they are describing, including being Deaf, hard of hearing, a child of a Deaf parent, or are a member of the larger hearing culture of a particular society. Others have worked completely outside their first cultures. Many of these papers are collaborative efforts, so researchers combine different strengths. One of the most positive developments to occur while editing this book is that the book's authors and a number of other scholars have joined in a wide-ranging discussion about linguistic and sociocultural variation in Deaf communities. That is, we not only study communities but also have become part of a community ourselves.

Authors vary on whether they use the terms *deaf*, *Deaf*, or *d/Deaf* and also on the terms *hearing* or *Hearing*. The upper case *D* in the term *Deaf* is a convention that has been used in the United States since the early 1970s to connote a "socially constructed visual culture" whereas the lower case *d* in *deaf* refers to "the audiological condition of hearing impairment" (Erting 1994, xxix). The term *d/Deaf* is used by Wrigley (1996) and LeMaster (chapter 8) among others to indicate complex situations that fall between these two choices. The uses of these terms range widely. Nancy Frishberg, during a discussion in the "Deaf Ethnicity" session at the American Anthropological Association, November 1997, argued for the careful use of *bigD-Deaf*, particularly when referring to deaf education. "Even those institutions which inculcate Deaf values cannot be called Deaf schools, because they are organized for the purposes of the State, not for the promotion of the ethnicity or identity." The usage in this preface and the introduction is mixed. In the summaries, *bigD-Deaf* has been used to refer to organizations that are self-consciously related to Deaf identity whereas *deaf* has been used with reference to most individuals and education. On occasion, the phrase *deaf or Deaf* has been used, usually in places where *d/Deaf* would also be used. Although the distinctions made by these terms can be useful, they are also often arbitrary, reflecting the fuzzy line between audiological and social deafness or Deafness.

Let us now turn to a more personal account of how this book came to be. Graham H. Turner, Karen Nakamura, and Leila Monaghan started this process. Although all the papers contributed for this book have been considerably revised, the majority of them were originally part of two panels at larger conferences, one organized by Graham at the Sociolinguistic Symposium II in Cardiff in September 1996 and the other organized by Karen and Leila at the annual meeting of the American Anthropological Association (AAA) in Washington, D.C., in November 1997. Berenz's work on Brazil and Ann's work on Taiwan were solicited at other meetings. Karen started assembling papers from the AAA session for publication in early 1998, and Leila combined these with papers from the Cardiff meeting and took over general editorial duties in spring 1998. Graham obtained our contract with our first publishing company at about the same time.

Leila then oversaw the extensive revisions of all these papers and shepherded manuscripts from computer to computer as she moved. She would particularly like to thank UCLA's Departments of Anthropology and Linguistics and Temple University's Department of Anthropology for computer space, office space, and intellectual companionship, as well as her partner-teacher, Maria Hosein, who helped make it possible to finish this book while Leila was teaching elementary school. Charles Monaghan carefully copyedited almost every manuscript, E. Jennifer Monaghan also chipped in with proofreading, and both provided Leila with invaluable moral support and shining examples of authorship and editing.

Leila thinks Constanze Schmaling walks on water. Constanze is the reason that this book got finished, taking on the enormous task of readying the manuscript for publication with Gallaudet University Press, including checking all references and doing a final proofreading. When this book was orphaned after our break from our first press, William Webber of Erlbaum Press showed us great courtesy and we are grateful for it. We would also like to thank the anonymous reviewers for Erlbaum and Gallaudet University Press for their insightful and helpful suggestions. Last but absolutely not least, we would like to thank John Vickrey Van Cleve, Ivey Pittle Wallace, and Deirdre Mullervy of Gallaudet University Press. Vic showed an uncommon and very helpful interest in the book even when we were committed elsewhere. Ivey was a model of what an acquisitions editor should be—responsive to questions and always cheerful, and Deirdre did the mighty work of helping wrestle the manuscript into final, ready to be published form with great grace and good spirits.

Leila Monaghan and Constanze Schmaling

REFERENCES

Erting, Carol J. 1994. Introduction. In *The Deaf Way: Perspectives from the International Conference on Deaf Culture*, ed. C. J. Erting, R. C. Johnson, D. L. Smith, and B. D. Snider, xxiii–xxxi. Washington, D.C.: Gallaudet University Press.

Senghas, Richard J., and Leila Monaghan. 2002. Signs of their times: Deaf communities and the culture of language. *Annual Review of Anthropology* 31: 69–97.

Wrigley, Owen. 1996. *The politics of deafness*. Washington, D.C.: Gallaudet University Press.

1 | A World's Eye View: Deaf Cultures in Global Perspective

Leila Monaghan

> *The world of humankind constitutes a manifold, a totality of interconnected processes, and inquiries that disassemble this totality of interconnected processes into bits and then fail to reassemble it falsify reality.* (Wolf 1997, 3)

There are myriad beginnings to deaf history, such as in 16th-century Spain where a hearing monk named Pedro Ponce de León taught two deaf brothers to speak, read, and write. Their tale, like many other beginnings discussed in this book, embodies the themes of education and literacy. As the recording of past events, history often connotes literacy (Eric Wolf invoked this usage in his ironic title *Europe and the People without History*, the source of my opening quotation). De León is remembered not only because he trained the Velasco brothers to speak but also because people wrote about his work.

The beginnings of deaf history are not only varied but also are deeply rooted in local politics and culture. For example, oralism, the teaching of speech to deaf children, was known as the *German method* and manualism, teaching deaf children through signing, as the *French method*. The fate of these methods in the 19th century reflected the ongoing battles between these two European powers. When European influence spread to North and South America, Africa, and Asia, so did deaf education. Fascism, postcolonialism, and civil rights movements have all had their impact, for worse or better, on the lives of deaf people.

EARLY WRITINGS

Pedro Ponce de León's achievement of teaching speech to Francisco and Pedro Fernandez de Velasco y Tovar "directly challenged the conventional wisdom of the day, which held that deaf people were uneducable, could not learn to speak,

1

and could not achieve salvation" (Plann 1997, 13). He did not, however, develop his revolutionary techniques out of thin air. Susan Plann (1997) hypothesizes that he combined the systematic signs of his sometimes silent Benedictine order with what would be known today as home signs, the personal and idiosyncratic signs, of the young brothers.

I begin with the story of the Velasco brothers, however, because it has elements that will reappear throughout this chapter and in the rest of the book. One of these elements is the importance of education. As mentioned earlier, while history in general is the recording of events in the past, it carries with it connotations of literacy. Historical events are more often recognized in times and places where literacy and, therefore, records exist.

In the 17th century, teaching moved out of the monastery and into the hands of private tutors. The idea of teaching speech to Deaf people also spread throughout Europe. This achievement was possible because Spanish wealth—land and revenues from wool and American silver—was concentrated in the hands of a few families (Wolf 1997) who could support first the monasteries and later private tutors. Teaching speech was necessary because of inheritance laws: Mute sons could not be legal heirs to property. The powerful Catholic Church also taught that speaking was necessary to know God and thus achieve salvation. Closely connected with this was being able to read the Bible. By the 1500s, life for the deaf children of the Spanish aristocracy was complex enough that simply learning by seeing would not have enabled them to take full part in the society; teaching speech partly solved this dilemma.

European society, however, had no one standard way of teaching deaf children. Rachel Sutton-Spence (chapter 2) looks at the variety of forms that fingerspelling (creating letters of the alphabet on the hands) took during this period and the different roles played by fingerspelling in British deaf education. As in Spain, tutors were the first teachers of the deaf. From the 1640s on, fingerspelling alphabets and techniques for teaching deaf students were major intellectual topics in Britain. John Wilkins presented an arthrological fingerspelling alphabet in 1641 (which also was useful as a secret code on the eve of the British Civil War). Spanish tutor Juan Pablo Bonet's teaching methods, originally published in 1620, were described by exiled English Royalist Kenelm Digby in 1644. By the second half of the 17th century, both William Holder (1669) and John Wallis (in 1674; see Conrad and Weiskrantz 1984) published accounts of teaching deaf students how to speak. As Sutton-Spence points out, although both men were interested in teaching speech, no clear distinctions were made at this time between this oralist goal and manual methods. For these teachers and, from 1760 on, for those in the private schools run by Thomas Braidwood and his family, teaching methods involved a combination of signing and speech teaching. All these methods were used also in individual or small group settings with students from families wealthy enough to afford private instruction, an approach that, as Harlan Lane (1984) argues, certainly improves the chances of success with the imperfect art of teaching speech.

MANUALISM AND THE INSTITUTIONALIZATION OF DEAF EDUCATION

The first person to teach large numbers of deaf children was l'Abbé de l'Epée, a Frenchman who was inspired by meeting two deaf sisters. Lane's imaginative account, based on Epée's writings, describes them as two young deaf women, sisters in misfortune. Understand what this meant: the deaf cannot go to school; cannot read or write; have few friends. With hearing parents, conversation is sparse, kept to essentials. These women cannot have a real trade but neither can they marry; they are useless to themselves and a heavy burden to indigent parents. . . . When the father dies the family becomes poorer still; the two young women do needlepoint to put bread on the table. (1984, 57)

A priest had instructed these girls in the lives of saints using engravings, but he had died, leaving them without any access to the teachings of the Catholic Church. Epée volunteered to take his place: "Believing these two children would live and die in ignorance of their religion if I did not attempt some means of instructing them, I told . . . the mother she might send them daily to my house" (Epée 1776 in Lane 1984, 58).

Epée developed a number of approaches that were fundamentally different from those of previous instructors. First, as alluded to above, he was interested in reaching as many students as possible, unlike most who limited the number of pupils to achieve their goal of teaching their students to speak. Supporting himself and his pupils on a modest inheritance, Epée opened the French National Institute of Deaf-Mutes, the first public school for the deaf, sometime between 1759 and 1771, accepting children of humble origins (Plann 1997, 80). The school received royal sponsorship from Louis XVI in 1778. Epée publicized his methods (unlike the oralists who often publicized their achievements but kept key components of their methods to themselves) and lobbied for the creation of other deaf schools, 21 of which were founded during his lifetime. The most important difference, however, was that Epée recognized that his deaf students already had a language of sorts, albeit one he saw as having no grammar. This problem he solved with "methodical signing" whereby he added French grammar to his students' signs. It was Epée's acceptance of signing that led manualism to be known as the French method (Lane 1984, 60–62; Fischer 1993).

Epée's major nemesis was Samuel Heinicke, inheritor of Bonet's oralist methods. After a career as a private tutor, Heinicke started the first oral public school for the deaf in Leipzig in 1778 under the sponsorship of the prince of Saxony. Although Heinicke published on deafness that same year, he kept the greater part of his methods secret during his lifetime. As Sutton-Spence (chapter 2) points out, however, pure oralism, with no signing or gestures of any kind, did not start until later. So although Heinicke was an ardent oralist, among the techniques he used was fingerspelling. He was also very influential in the German-speaking states and trained many of the teachers for other schools, which led to oralism being known as the "German method" (Lane 1984).

The third European country to have a school for the deaf was Austria. The school opened in Vienna in 1779 after the Holy Roman Emperor Joseph II visited Epée's school in Paris (Joseph would have been visiting his sister and brother-in-law, Marie Antoinette and Louis XVI). Franz Dotter and Ingeborg Okorn (chapter 3) describe the method used by the Viennese school as mixed, using both the French signing and German oral methods (not surprisingly, given the royal ties to France but the linguistic commonalties with the German states).

Dozens of schools based on the ideas of Epée were founded throughout the

world. These included a school started in 1795 in Madrid by José Fernandez Navarrette (Plann 1997); a school in St. Petersburg supported by the Dowager Em-
press Feodorovna in 1806 (Williams 1993); Manillaskolan, founded by Per Avon
Borg in Sweden in 1809 (chapter 4; Piroux 1842–1843; Lane 1984, 64); various
schools in Switzerland founded between 1811 and 1838 (chapter 5); the Connecticut Asylum for the Education of the Deaf and Dumb Persons, started by Thomas
Gallaudet and Laurent Clerc in 1817 (chapter 6); St. Mary's, an Irish girls school,
in 1846 and St. Joseph's, an Irish boys school, in 1857 (the break perhaps related to
the aftermath of the Irish potato famine, 1845–1851) (chapter 8); and the Imperial
Institute of Deaf-Mutes, founded by Padre Huet in Brazil in 1857 (chapter 9). The
influence of Epée's methods was also felt in Britain when de Puget, a pupil of
Epée's successor Sicard, succeeded the second Thomas Braidwood at the Birmingham school in 1825 and his protégé opened the Doncaster school in 1829
(chapter 2).

During the first half of the 19th century, government and religious groups,
particularly the Catholic Church, were the main educators of deaf students. This
is a change from the previous practice of wealthy families supporting individual
tutors. As Douglas Baynton argues, in the United States, "deafness was most often
described as an affliction that isolated the individual from the Christian community" (1996, 15). The French National Institute of Deaf-Mutes continued to be
heavily Catholic. Navarrette, who started the Spanish school, was a Piarist father.
Catholic priests and Protestant missionaries founded the schools in Switzerland.
Gallaudet was a Congregational minister. Two separate orders founded the Irish
schools: Dominican nuns (St. Mary's) and the Christian Brothers (St. Joseph's).[1]

The Dominicans went on to found numerous other deaf schools, including
the first South African deaf school in 1863 (chapter 10) and schools in Australia,
Germany, New Zealand, and the United States. The French National Institute's
graduates also played key roles in establishing these new schools, including Clerc
in the United States and Huet in Brazil. Huet also went on to found the first
Mexican school in 1865 (Lane 1984, 251) and Clerc trained a large number of deaf
teachers and administrators throughout America.

Given the relative rarity of deafness, the sparsity of the general population
compared to today, and the slow systems of transportation, most of these early
deaf institutions were residential boarding schools. Children who spent 24 hours
a day together often developed strong friendships. Adding to these friendships
were family connections. In the United States, the Connecticut Asylum and other
schools for the deaf drew from communities with high rates of genetic deafness,
like Martha's Vineyard in Massachusetts. These communities sometimes had
their own indigenous sign languages and the language of the students from these
areas often became incorporated into the languages used at these boarding
schools. Certain families had generation-spanning relationships with specific
schools.

These ties of friendship and family eventually became the basis for a number
of robust adult Deaf communities. Starting in 1834, the Parisian Deaf community's elite held banquets honoring Epée's birthday (Mottez 1993). Vienna was the
center of Austrian Deaf culture with 10 clubs and an active café life (chapter 3).
In 1854, alumni from the Connecticut Asylum, by this time known as the American School for the Deaf, officially started the first U.S. Deaf club (Van Cleve and

Crouch 1989, 89). The founding of Gallaudet College in 1864 showed that, with vigorous lobbying, the greatly expanding possibilities for higher education in the United States also could include deaf people (Monaghan 1993).

These communities developed in part as a defense against the incursion of oralism into schools for the deaf. The formation of the Deaf-Mute Committee that organized the Parisian banquets was prompted in part by the growing oralist policies of the National French Institute's governing board. Between 1822 (the death of the Abbé Roch-Ambroise Sicard, Epée's pro-signing successor) and 1838, the Institute's governing board and its director, Desiré Ordinaire, questioned the importance of sign language and the role of deaf teachers. However, in 1838, the appointment of Adolphe de Lanneau, who had good relations with the adult Parisian Deaf community, restored the Institute as the center of manualism (Mottez 1993). Even when oralism was the official policy, as in Switzerland and at New York's Lexington School for the Deaf, Deaf communities could flourish (chapter 5; Van Cleve and Crouch 1989). Students of oral deaf schools, like their signing school counterparts, would band together in clubs after graduation.

THE RESURRECTION OF ORALISM

The influence of oralism in two centers of the Deaf community, France and the United States, reflects the oralist paradigm in the 19th century, particularly in the latter half. Because signing was known as the French method and oralism as the German method, it is useful to look at the relationship between France (despite its vacillation with respect to teaching methods) and Germany, particularly at how issues such as the rise of nationalism and educational reform played out. The shifts in political power between these countries and the general movement toward centralized states affected the international balance between signing and oralism.

Ironically, France's most famous leader, Napoleon Bonaparte, started many of the reforms, such as standardized and general education, that led to the success of oralism, the German method, at the Milan Conference of 1880, where delegates declared the "incontestable superiority of speech over signs" (in Lane 1984, 394). Though the repression of spoken languages other than French also began under his reign (Schiffman 1996), he was quite supportive of the National Institute, reappointing Sicard as director in 1799. Sicard, like many other priests, had been caught in the Reign of Terror in 1792, barely escaped execution, and eventually ended up fleeing into exile before being granted amnesty by Napoleon (Lane 1984).

Napoleon's brother and King of Spain, Joseph Bonaparte, was also an important supporter of the French method. Manual education in Spain at the school founded by Navarrette was one of the first casualties of Napoleon's defeat. Navarrette's protégé and successor, José Miguel Alea Abadia, a supporter of Joseph, had to flee the country after France's defeat at the battle of Vittoria in 1813, and an oralist, Tiburcio Hernandez, was appointed as his successor (Plann 1997).

Any influence that French methods had in the German states (not including the Austro-Hungarian Empire with its mixed method) disappeared after Napoleon's final defeat in 1815. "Whereas sign language had been flourishing in the school Heinicke founded at Leipzig, with the oralist resurgence, his son-in-law

Carl Reich took charge and banned both sign and, for good measure, fingerspell-ing" (Lane 1984, 299). In the meantime, German-speaking states were developing international reputations for scientific research, particularly linguistic research, and for advanced educational methods.

On the education front, the German-speaking Swiss Johann Pestalozzi preached a Rousseau-influenced creed of children's "inner dignity," which led to the curriculum's widespread liberalization (Silber 1965). Saxony, the Leipzig school's location, and its neighbors Prussia and Bavaria were known for high literacy rates among their populations. In 1850, 81% of Prussian and 83% of Bavar-ian male children ages 6 to 14 were enrolled in school, compared with 60% of French and 66% of English boys (Maynes 1985, 134). Oralism benefited from the high esteem of the general German educational system and well-organized teacher training courses. As Horace Mann wrote in his report on his 1843 Euro-pean tour, the Germans "stand pre-eminent among the nations of Europe in re-gard to the quantity and quality of education." It was on this tour that Mann first saw German oral schools and with, as Lane points out, little background in deaf education, declared German schools "decidedly superior" to American signing schools (in Lane 1984, 298).

German-speaking states were the first to be influenced by the German oralist fervor. In chapter 5, Penny Boyes Braem, Benno Caramore, Roland Hermann, and Patricia Shores Hermann describe how, around 1840, schools in the German-speaking part of Switzerland switched from Epée-influenced methods to strict oralism, allowing no signing at all. Because Switzerland had no training programs for teachers of the deaf, the schools imported German school directors along with their oral methods. Sign language was not the only language under fire at this time. Boyes Braem et al. also describe how a local Swiss language, Rhaeto-Romansh, was under attack.

It is important, however, to see nationalist ideas not only as part of an abstract political philosophy but also as the ideological component of the warfare that gripped Europe throughout the 19th century. Napoleon's ideas lived on in the form of rebellions against traditional royal leaders: an 1830 uprising against the King of Saxony; an 1848 rebellion against Louis Phillipe of France, who abdicated and was eventually replaced by Louis Napoleon, Napoleon's nephew; unification movements in Germany and Italy; and a dramatic reduction in the clergy's power, particularly the Catholic Church (Pearson 1994). These unification movements spawned numerous wars, but despite this, the German states grew in economic power, eventually replacing France as the economic center of Europe.

Milan makes an interesting case study for examining the interrelationships among nationalism, signing, and oralism as well as the complex relations among France, Austria, and Germany. A disciple of the Abbé Ottavio Assarotti, founder of the Genoa school, started Milan's first school for the deaf. Assarotti had been a student of Sicard and introduced a version of methodical signing. He had also had his school officially sanctioned by Napoleon in 1805 (Lane 1984; Radutsky 1993). Between 1815 and 1859, Milan's region, Lombardy (part of what is today northern Italy), was part of the Austro-Hungarian Empire and so was influenced by the Viennese mixed-teaching methods. By 1861, after wars between France, Piedmont, and Austria and after uprisings in Sicily and Naples, most Italian states, including Milan, declared themselves part of the Kingdom of Italy (Pearson

1994). As had happened elsewhere, this drive to create unified, supposedly homo-geneous nations affected the acceptance of minority languages, including sign language.

> Pressure to unify was naturally accompanied by an attempt to suppress minorities. When regional spoken dialects were being suppressed in favor of a single national language and culture, it is not difficult to imagine the fate of the language and culture of the deaf community, even more dis-tant, impenetrable. (Radutsky 1993, 249)

In 1854, a second school for the deaf was started in Milan. Its director was Father Giulio Tarra, who was eventually converted to a pure oralist view by Abbé Serafino Balestra of the Como institute. Como is even farther north than Milan, just three miles from the Swiss border. Oralism, therefore, entered from the German-influenced north and traveled south. In Germany, its prestige was en-hanced by other German advances in education, linguistics, and biology (Radut-sky 1993). The French had no comparable scientific backing for their methods, and Louis Napoleon did not look favorably on instruction in sign language as his uncle had done. France also lost its role as Italy's "Great Power sponsor" after 1859 (Pearson 1994, 11). The landscape of deaf education across Europe was changing. In 1867, Austria gave up its mixed method for oralism. In 1869, a decree from Milan's minister of public instruction banished all sign language in the prov-ince.

Balestra, Tarra, and colleagues planned the infamous 1880 Milan Conference as part of their campaign to spread oralist teaching philosophies. This convention was held only 11 years after the banning of signs from Milan; a relatively new regional philosophy was being exported throughout the world.

One reason for the rapid spread of oralism was the growing professionaliza-tion of deaf education. Just as new governments and ways of organizing nations were being installed across Europe, the instruction of teachers of the deaf also was being organized. The resolutions passed at the Milan Conference were carried out relatively easily in many places because of teaching's growing bureaucratization. France's national education system, for example, changed to oralism after the convention, phasing out signing over a seven-year period. In 1887, the Parisian National Institute published a farewell to all the "deaf professors who were leav-ing their posts at the school since as of this date it will no longer have students taught by the old method" (in Lane 1984, 397).

In chapter 4, Sangeeta Bagga-Gupta and Lars-Åke Domfors provide an inter-esting example of this process to formalize teacher training. In 1874, Sweden's first college for teachers of the deaf was established at Manillaskolan, also home to the country's first deaf school. The school had been founded on French princi-ples but was influenced also by Germany, just across the Baltic Sea. During the 19th century's last decades, the school had reached no agreement about which method should be used. While education within the school was moving toward an oral model, contemporary laws were pushing education back toward signing. In 1889, Sweden's government passed a compulsory education law and statutes relating to the training of teachers of the deaf. Mandated subjects included "man-ual communication . . . its origins, development, and use in education" (in chapter

4, 70). By the turn of the century, however, Sweden had changed to oralism, aided by German literature and teaching methods.

As Sutton-Spence (chapter 2) points out, the situation in England was quite different. In 1889, the government, in the form of a Royal Commission, recommended oralism for all children. Even so, the combined method, including fingerspelling, continued to be used in many schools. The decentralized British education system, with schools run by a wide number of different agencies, was affected differently from centralized systems like that of France, which gave up its manual methods under Louis Napoleon, and from Sweden, whose teacher training program affected all the schools in the country.

The rise of European national states was connected with other trends, such as a decrease in the influence of the church. This pattern was also true in the United States. In his book on the history of signing and oralism in the United States, Douglas Baynton argues that, before the Civil War, a key goal of schooling was religious education. After the war, however, "deafness was redefined as a condition that isolated people from the national community" (1996, 15). A priority became ensuring a common language, which was defined by oralists as teaching children how to speak.

A common language, however, is not the only marker of a nation. As Blommaert and Verschueren (1992) argue, it is just "one identity marker among others" (359). Another marker is an imagined common genetic heritage. In the United States, the same people who promoted German oralist programs, Samuel Gridley Howe and Alexander Graham Bell, saw heredity as a key part of deafness. They argued for ways to limit Deaf people from having children and, by doing so, prevent the "formation of a deaf variety of the human race" (Gardiner Greene Hubbard in Winzer 1993, 288). With his prestige from the invention of the telephone and other devices and his involvement in the late 19th-century eugenics movement, Bell's efforts, in particular, had the aura of science about them. The term *eugenics* was coined by Francis Galton (1883) to describe the study of heredity's role in mental abilities.[2] Under the mantle of eugenics, Bell argued for limiting marriage between two deaf partners. Despite a widely distributed newspaper article connecting him with a bill limiting deaf marriages, Bell did not see limited marriage as a matter for government intervention but as a moral responsibility.

> It is the duty of every good man and every good woman to remember that children follow marriage, and I am sure that there is no one among the deaf who desires to have his affliction handed down to his children. (Bell 1891 in Winefield 1987, 94)

This view was one of the aspects of Bell that made him profoundly unpopular with the signing Deaf community of his day. Compared to other eugenicists of the time, however, his was a relatively mild stance. Others in the United States, Germany, and Scandinavia favored sterilization, particularly to prevent traits thought to lead to criminality, including sexual immorality and feeblemindedness (Carlson 2000; Witkowski 2000, 6).[3]

With this increased emphasis on being able to speak and the biological roots of deafness also came an increased emphasis on different kinds of hearing loss. Donald Grushkin (chapter 6) discusses the ramifications of being neither deaf nor hearing but hard of hearing. Before the 1860s, any pupil (whether deaf or hard of hearing) with enough hearing loss to attend a special school received a similar manual education whereas, after oralism swept the United States, hard of hearing or "semi-mute" children were held up as the ideal students (as they had been under European oralist programs for years).

The influence of oralism increased well into the 20th century. By the end of World War I, 80% of deaf students in American schools were taught by exclusively oral methods (Baynton 1996, 5). Despite this trend, what is now known as American Sign Language (ASL) continued to be used unofficially in schools for the deaf throughout the United States. As Ceil Lucas and Susan Schatz argue (chapter 7), most deaf people learn the language of their signing peers rather than the spoken language of their usually hearing parents.

Just as the specter of oralism had pushed the Parisian community to found its Deaf-Mute Committee in 1834, numerous Deaf organizations started just after the Milan Convention of 1880. The first meeting of the American National Association of the Deaf was also held in 1880. International deaf congresses followed a few years later, first in Paris in 1889, then in Chicago in 1893 and Geneva in 1896. These congresses all lobbied for the combined method of teaching, emphasizing that both signing and speech were necessary (Lane 1984). Other reactions to the spread of oralism included the creation of films and a dictionary (Long 1909) to record ASL (see Van Cleve and Crouch 1989).

AWAY FROM THE EUROPEAN CENTER

The rising oralist ideology of the European mainland and the United States had varying effects elsewhere. The Catholic Church maintained its influence in Ireland, and girls and boys were educated in sign language by silent orders until after World War II (chapter 8). The result was a highly literate but not particularly organized Deaf community. In populous and sprawling Brazil (chapter 9), only a minority of deaf people were educated and only recently have national deaf organizations been established. The education policy was manualist, following Huet's Parisian practices, but switched to a "pragmatic oralism" after Brazilian educators toured Europe at the end of the 19th century. By the time Norine Berenz visited Brazilian schools in the mid-1980s and 1990s, most of the classrooms were oralist but varied according to the pedagogical philosophy of teachers and schools.

In chapter 10, Debra Aarons and Louise Reynolds point out that, in South Africa, deaf education during the late 19th century was for European students only. The teaching methods that were used depended on who started the school. St. Mary's, founded by Irish Dominican nuns in 1863, and the Worcester School for the Deaf and Blind, started by the Dutch reform church in 1881, both used sign language. On the other hand, German Dominican nuns started a school on the Eastern Cape, and their methods were strictly oral. A pattern similar to that found in early 19th-century Europe and the United States, emphasizing the importance of getting God's word across, seems to be key to understanding the use of sign language in the first two cases whereas the influence of German oralism explains the third.

The influence of both the interest in government-sponsored education and the Milan Conference can also be seen in New Zealand during this period. New Zealand's Education Act of 1877 had a compulsory attendance clause, and three years later the Parliament established Sumner, New Zealand's first school for the deaf. The head of the committee selecting the first principal argued for oralism, saying that with the manual method

> there is a far greater danger . . . that deaf mutes should shun the society of those who are not deaf, and thus by congregating together, should in many cases increase the natural and inevitable disadvantages arising from their affliction. (Vogel 1879 in Allen 1980, 11)

As in South Africa, the first students were white, but after another compulsory education act specifically applying to Sumner was passed in 1902, the first Maori name appears on the rolls (Allen 1980; Monaghan 1996).

As part of a much larger set of educational reforms, the first school for the deaf in Japan was a signing school founded in Kyoto in 1878. Unlike the broad-reaching education system of Japanese general public and missionary education schools established at this time, the Kyoto school and the Tokyo school founded shortly after were private, like many of the early schools in Europe, and served only the children of the wealthy. Another small school was also started in Osaka but did not last. Not until after World War II was education for the deaf in Japan made compulsory (chapter 11; Nakamura 2001).

Just as the manual method had spread across Europe in the wake of Napoleon's armies, colonial powers in Asia also spread their specific brand of deaf education. A school system based on French sign language was introduced into Viet Nam during French colonial rule sometime after 1858 (chapter 15). In the middle of the 19th century, Japan was the lesser partner in a number of "unequal treaties" with the United States and European nations; by 1911, all these treaties were withdrawn and Japan was itself occupying a range of Asian territories. However, Japan was not immune to the same tide of nationalism and expansionism that had swept Europe. Japan won Taiwan (then Formosa) from the Chinese during the Sino-Japanese War and occupied Taiwan from 1895 to 1945 (Miller et al. 1995). One result of this occupation was the introduction of Japanese-style deaf education to Taiwan. The Tainan school, established in 1915, was staffed with teachers from Tokyo. The Taipei school was set up two years later and staffed with teachers from Osaka. The dialects these teachers brought with them became the basis for what is now known as Taiwanese Sign Language (chapter 12; Chao, Chu, and Liu 1988, 9; Smith 1999).

Not only were countries expanding, the international Deaf community was expanding as well. The international congresses continued, although the attending organizations were somewhat reluctant to formalize ties by creating an international association. At the 1912 International Deaf Congress in Paris, Austrian delegates proposed a world deaf association, which the congress rejected because not enough countries had strong national associations (chapter 3). The first deaf association in New Zealand, for example, was not started until 1926 (Monaghan 1996). In 1924, however, the first World Games for the Deaf were held. Six nations gathered in Paris to compete in events modeled after those in the Olympics (Stewart 1991; Lane, Hoffmeister, and Bahan 1996).

Other deaf institutions were also expanding. By the 1930s, the All Russian Federation for the Deaf (the VOG), a bureaucratic organization based closely on other Soviet-era government agencies, was the key social structure for Russian deaf people. It concerned itself with issues such as the standards of instruction in the mostly oral Russian school system and employment after graduation (Williams 1993; chapter 13). Schooling for the deaf also was spreading. For example, various religious organizations started schools for nonwhite children in South Africa (chapter 10), and in the 1940s, a few small, oral private schools were set up in Nicaragua. As Richard Senghas (chapter 14) argues, small schools such as these, unlike larger schools, do not necessarily become the basis for strong communities.

DEADLY ENEMIES OF DEAFNESS

Despite a growing international Deaf community, the foes of Deaf culture and sign language were very strong during the first part of the 20th century. Between 1907 and 1958, the sterilization of mentally retarded people was legal in 30 states in the United States, but none of these laws was specifically directed toward deaf people. The general discussion did create an environment, however, in which deaf partners were considered "undesirable" by themselves and others, with the result that deaf people were less likely to marry than the population at large (Winzer 1993).

The situation was worse elsewhere. A 1911 German law on the schooling of blind and deaf children included a sample questionnaire to be given to students about issues such as hereditary deafness. The law and its questionnaire reflect the two main routes taken by oralists for integrating deaf children into hearing society—first, educating them to fit into the hearing world and, second, preventing deafness from occurring at all. The movement gained more ground in the 1920s. Professional education journals contained discussions such as "Should deaf-mutes marry?" (Biesold 1999, 16). Similar discussions also took place in Switzerland (chapter 5). In 1926, a detailed survey was sent out concerning hearing loss, designed to give researchers information that would help "stem the tide of deafness" (Hepp and Nager 1926, 11). Boyes Braem et al. describe how this survey effort was the beginning of a drive to prevent Swiss deaf women from having children that included forbidding marriage between deaf people, sterilizations (usually voluntary), and abortions. This drive lasted until at least the end of the 1950s. Nakamura (chapter 11) describes similar pressures in Japan.

In chapter 3, Dotter and Okorn describe the most drastic and deadly example of the effects of eugenics, the Nazi *Rassenhygiene* program's effects on the Austrian Deaf community. Hitler sought the "purity of the Aryan race" by his genocidal program to rid the world not only of Jews and Romanies but also of disabled people. Soon after coming to power in 1933, he promulgated a "sterilization law for persons suffering from a variety of mental and physical difficulties" (Biesold 1999, 4). Under this law, approximately 15,000 hereditarily deaf people were sterilized and another unknown number were victims of the "euthanasia" program for disabled people in Germany and Austria during the World War II era. Horst Biesold describes how, in Germany, these programs included "moving residents of medical or psychiatric institutions to 'primitive lodgings' where 'mortality will naturally be substantially greater'" (1999, 160–61); killing handicapped children by lethal injections and starvation; and through the T4 program, murdering at least 70,000 disabled adults in "gas chambers disguised as shower rooms" between 1939 and 1941 (1999, 163).

Despite this systematic genocide of disabled people, there was also organized support in Austrian and German Deaf communities for the Nazis. Dotter and Okorn (chapter 3) show that deaf people were active in the Austrian Hitler Youth Movement. Biesold (1999) describes how members of the Reich Union of the Deaf of Germany were incorporated into the Nazi Party. Some passively supported the Nazis in an attempt to avoid the sterilization program, while a few actively supported the Nazi regime, denouncing Jewish community members (many of whom got caught in death camps with fellow hearing Jews) and the "hereditarily diseased" (1999, 100).

NEW WORLD ORDER

The end of World War II in 1945 brought changes everywhere. The appeal of the eugenics movement faded in response to the horrifying abuses committed by the Nazis. B. F. Skinner's behaviorist research and Franz Boas's ideas of cultural relativity in which nurture rather than nature was the key to understanding human actions began to gain acceptance (Winzer 1993). A number of other trends are apparent in this postwar period: the growth of internationalism; the rise of the United States to become the leading nation in scientific research and economic might; the rise of newly independent nation-states around the world; and technological advances, particularly the hearing aid, which allowed different forms of deaf education, including mainstreaming in hearing schools.

Despite the failure of some earlier international movements such as the League of Nations, the formalization of international relationships grew. Although the League of Nations lost any influence it had during World War II, it was succeeded in 1945 by the United Nations. In 1951 at a meeting in Rome, the Deaf world followed suit and created its own international organization. The World Federation of the Deaf (WFD) solidified the ties fostered by the international congresses begun in Paris in 1889. Today, the WFD is the official voice of deaf people in organizations such as UNESCO (the United Nations Educational, Scientific, and Cultural Organization) and the World Health Organization (WHO).

The United States was a dominant force in the new postwar world order. When it occupied Japan after World War II, it helped establish a nationwide oral deaf education system. In 1948, schooling for Japanese deaf children became compulsory (chapter 11). Japan, in turn, lost Taiwan after World War II. Jean Ann, writing about the third major deaf school in Taiwan (chapter 12), describes how Chiang Ssu Nung, a deaf refugee from mainland China, started the Chiying School in Kaohsiung. To this day, deaf people from Kaohsiung use a Chinese-influenced sign language that is different from the Japanese-influenced Taiwanese Sign Language of Taipei and Tainan.

In 1952, when members of the Thai royal family were interested in establishing schools, they turned to then Gallaudet College in the United States for training and introduced American Sign Language into Thailand. This move ignored the already existing sign languages of the cities like Bangkok and Chiangmai and the isolated rural villages with high degrees of deafness such as Bhan Khor (Woodward 2000; chapter 15). By the late 1950s, the postwar changes had also spread to Africa. The first deaf school, run by British Methodists, was opened in Lagos, Nigeria, in 1958. In 1960, the same year as Nigerian independence, Andrew Foster, a missionary from Gallaudet, opened a second school in Ibadan. Other schools followed (chapter 16).

These countries are the forerunners of a huge boom in the development of deaf schools after World War II. Just as deaf education had expanded in Europe in the 1800s with the development of European nation-states, growth in deaf schools worldwide has reflected the growing number of independent nations around the globe. The world saw a tremendous burst of nation building in the 1960s and 1970s. We can look at U.N. membership as a rough indicator of this trend. Dozens of new countries—often ex-colonies of England, France, and other states—entered the United Nations between 1960 and 1979, including 36 African, 11 Caribbean, 7 Middle Eastern, 6 Asian, and 6 Pacific Island nations. Some of the many education programs started during this period include programs in Saudi Arabia in 1964, Nepal in 1966, Dominican Republic in 1967, Namibia in 1970, and Nicaragua in 1978 (Erting et al. 1994). Of these nations, only Saudi Arabia could afford the latest technical equipment like powerful hearing aids and inductor loops. Other nations continued to expand their programs. In Nigeria, for example, 43 schools either specifically for the deaf or for a general disabled student population opened between 1958 and 1985 (Ojile 1994).

Changes also occurred in countries with previously established education systems. Barbara LeMaster (chapter 8) describes how, after more than 100 years of producing signing, literate students, Irish schools changed to oralism. When Irish deaf people went to England looking for work, they were frustrated by the fact that they were expected to speak like their English counterparts, so they requested that speech be taught at the schools. Signing was banned in St. Mary's after Irish Dominican sisters turned to Holland for techniques for teaching speech in 1946 and brought back with them a complete oralist philosophy. St. Joseph's followed 11 years later.

Pre–World War II, wartime, and postwar international epidemics (particularly, rubella and reactions to streptomycin and other new antibiotics) and the general postwar baby boom also caused a major jump in the number of deaf children worldwide. In Japan, for example, children deafened by ototoxic doses of streptomycin filled the new compulsory schools (chapter 11; Nakamura 2001) while in New Zealand, rubella caused a deaf population boom and forced the creation of two new deaf schools. There was an average of 46 students a year entering the New Zealand deaf public education system between 1942 and 1959, a huge leap from the 27 (many of whom were part of a deaf population spike just after World War I and the 1917 Spanish flu epidemic) before 1942 (Monaghan 1996).

Although hearing aids were invented at the beginning of the 20th century and brought with them distinctions among different degrees of hearing loss (chapter 6), they became small enough for easy personal use only after World War II and became a key tool in the fight to "fix" deaf children. Hearing aids, however, were affordable only in places with considerable economic resources such as the United States, Europe, and New Zealand.

Opponents of signing long recognized the importance of residential schools in developing Deaf communities—A. G. Bell started arguing for day schools in 1877. With the technological tool of hearing aids as well as the ideas of desegregation that followed the 1954 *Brown vs. Board of Education* and the American civil rights movement, the idea of mainstreaming entered the discourse (Winzer 1993, 376). In many ways, mainstreaming deaf children is a natural extension of the educational philosophy that tries to change the child to fit in with hearing society.

In New Zealand, for example, a network of itinerant teachers and advisors to support mainstreaming was created in 1957 when a British visiting specialist trained four New Zealand teachers. Starting in 1959, even students who were acknowledged to be too deaf to be appropriately mainstreamed were moved out of the three centralized residential schools for the deaf into small deaf units around the country. Units continued to be established through the 1980s. In the mid-1960s, Kelston School for the Deaf in Auckland faced possible closing because not enough children were attending, but another rubella bulge (90 students in 1968, Kelston's largest entering class ever) interfered with this outcome. By 1992, however, 80% of deaf students were being mainstreamed (Aspden et al. 1992; Monaghan 1996).

Extensive mainstreaming in Japan began in 1970 (chapter 11) while, in the United States, the key event was the passage of Public Law 94–142 in 1975, requiring "least restrictive" environments for all students considered as disabled. Because "least restrictive" was usually defined as being in regular hearing classrooms, enrollment in U.S. residential schools for the deaf has declined. Before the 1960s, almost 80% of deaf children attended residential schools, but by the mid-1990s, only 30% did (Winzer 1993; Lane, Hoffmeister, and Bahan 1996; chapter 6). This trend toward mainstreaming continues. In 1993, Austria passed a law providing for the possibility of mainstreaming, and extensive mainstreaming also started in Switzerland in the 1990s (chapter 3; chapter 5). In contrast, active schools for the deaf in areas without access to expensive hearing aids, including schools in Nigeria and the African areas of South Africa, are producing strong signing communities.

RECOGNITION OF SIGN LANGUAGE AND THE GROWTH OF AN INTERNATIONAL DEAF COMMUNITY

Despite this trend toward mainstreaming in the wealthier countries, a major revival of signing has taken place in the last 40 years that includes international academic support for sign languages and the growing politicization of Deaf communities worldwide. In 1960, William Stokoe published *Sign Language Structure*, which applied the principles used in understanding spoken language to sign languages. Stokoe described the location, handshape, and movement of signs and argued that these distinctions were the equivalents of phonological forms used to describe parts of spoken sounds. Changes in any one of these three variables could create a new sign. In American Sign Language, for example, if a bent index finger is twisted at the cheek, it is the sign APPLE; however, if the same handshape is made but the location is moved to the side of the eye, it is the sign ONION (Stokoe 1960; Stokoe, Croneberg, and Casterline 1976).

The first major change in educational policy arising from this legitimization of signing led to the classroom use not of natural sign languages like ASL but of a variety of Total Communication (TC) approaches. TC is the modern version of Epée's methodical signs, a way to encode spoken (or written) English on the hands. In 1965, no programs in the United States were using TC, but by 1976, 107 deaf programs out of 122 (87.7%) that were surveyed used it (Garretson 1976, 94). Gerilee Gustason, one developer of Signing Exact English (SEE 2), a key TC approach, said her method "appealed to people because it was still English . . . not a different language like ASL. So things kind of went BOOM overnight" (in Ramsey 1989, 128).

The "boom" in TC programs was an international one. Australian educators, for example, developed a signed English system based on Australian Sign Language called Australasian Sign English, and New Zealand introduced this system into Kelston School for the Deaf in 1975. Most of the students who might have attended Kelston had been mainstreamed into hearing schools, particularly those who had some hearing or who were academically advanced, leaving a multihandicapped population that was very badly served by the oral teaching methods used at the deaf school. A coalition of teachers, parents, and Deaf community leaders lobbied for the national acceptance of this system (Aspden et al. 1992; Monaghan 1996).

In Austria since the 1970s, a few hours of teacher training each week have been devoted to "cultivating signs," including both Austrian Sign Language and Signed German (chapter 3). In Switzerland, one school in Zurich accepted TC in the 1980s (chapter 5). Signed spoken language or TC systems are also used today in Britain (chapter 2), Thailand (Wrigley 1996; Woodward 2000), Taiwan (chapter 12), and elsewhere.

Sweden, however, went far beyond introducing a signed spoken language system into its classrooms. As Bagga-Gupta and Domfors show (chapter 4), Stokoe's work as well as Brita Bergman and Inger Ahlgren's work on Swedish Sign Language led to a radically pro-signing policy. In 1981, the Swedish parliament recognized sign language, *teckenspråk*, as the first language of deaf people. The legislation followed a 1977 "home language reform" measure allowing minority and immigrant children to receive instruction in their native language. The legislation has been so far-reaching that even children with cochlear implants receive education in sign language (Fjord 1999–2000, 2001).

Despite the reforms that have resulted from this policy, other issues still need to be resolved. Bagga-Gupta and Domfors look particularly at the "paradox of bilingualism," contradictions raised by trying to teach a minority language within the hearing majority culture. Issues include how teaching and testing deaf children with materials geared toward white, middle-class, hearing children in fact create a situation where deaf children are disabled by being compared to this norm. This dynamic has occurred despite concerted attempts to create a system with a level playing field. One of the major advantages for Deaf community members, however, is that individuals have acquired access to a wide range of services in sign language.

The relationship between research undertaken by scholars from the United States and the recognition of sign language in other countries was even more direct. Richard Senghas (chapter 14) was part of a loosely affiliated group of researchers including Judy Kegl, Ann Senghas, and Laura Polich who studied linguistic and cultural aspects of Nicaraguan Sign Language. Although a few small schools opened in Nicaragua in the 1940s, these schools did not lead to an organized Deaf community. In 1978, however, the Nicaraguan Ministry of Education opened a number of special deaf schools, including one in Managua. Although schooling was originally conducted by oral methods, a signed language and a distinct Deaf culture have emerged among the school's students and graduates. This language was legitimized starting in the mid-1980s by the presence of Kegl, Senghas, Polich, and other North American researchers. One of the effects has been to expand the Nicaraguan deaf education system from exclusive use of oral methods to include signing methods. The Swedish Deaf community has also played a role in developing the Nicaraguan Deaf community, contributing money and personnel to building a national Deaf organization.

As Constanze Schmaling (chapter 16) points out when describing the situation in northern Nigeria, influence from abroad is not always benign. An ASL-based Signed English system was introduced into Tudun Maliki school in Kano when it opened in 1977. The American system is quite different from the local Hausa Sign Language used by Kano's active and informal urban Deaf community. The "A for Apple" in her title refers to the fact that, although fingerspelling lessons start with the word *apple*, referring to a fruit until recently not easily available in Kano, ASL has no sign for the indigenous guava fruit. There are numerous other problems with the introduction of foreign-influenced sign forms, particularly when they are used by teachers who barely know them. Some African countries, including Botswana, Ethiopia, Mali, and Tanzania, have been exposed to multiple foreign sign languages including ASL, Danish, German, Swedish, Finnish, and French Sign Languages. Just as local African spoken languages were derided for not being developed enough for various purposes during colonialism, local sign languages are sometimes ignored in favor of foreign, well-documented languages from richer nations.

Back in the United States, Stokoe's work was the first of many steps toward the widespread recognition of both natural sign languages and Deaf culture. As reflected in the first meeting of the National Association of the Deaf in 1880, sign language and Deaf culture have long been seen as inextricably linked. In Carol Padden's (1989) definition of Deaf culture, for example, she cites valuing American Sign Language as a key component. By the time of the "Deaf President Now" (DPN) protest of March 1988, however, a clear sense had developed of Deaf culture being more than just ASL. Gallaudet University, the university in Washington, D.C., for deaf and hard of hearing people, erupted when Elisabeth Zinser, a hearing person with no background in Deaf culture and no knowledge of sign language, was appointed president. As Christine Multra wrote in Gallaudet's *Buff and Blue* newspaper, "Who cannot help but laugh ironically at . . . [the] statement that Zinser 'fit all the criteria with the exception . . . of understanding deafness and deaf culture?'" (in Jankowski 1997, 129).

There are numerous parallels among Gallaudet's DPN protests and other U.S. civil rights movements, both conscious—one banner at the protest read "WE STILL HAVE A DREAM" (Sacks 1989, 154)—and unconscious. Katherine Jankowski, for example, characterizes the DPN Protest as the "'enthusiastic mobilization' stage" (1997, 137) of a larger cultural movement.

In the United States, ethnicity is a profoundly salient cultural category. As a result, the Deaf community is often compared to an ethnic group. Robert Johnson and Carol Erting (1989) look at ethnicity and socialization in a preschool for deaf children, while Tricia Leakey (1993) compares deaf and African American vocational education. Grushkin (chapter 6) picks up this theme in his analysis of hard of hearing people by discussing how this group is of "mixed ethnicity," neither Deaf nor hearing yet sharing traits of both. American Norine Berenz also uses an ethnicity model when she compares the nascent Brazilian Deaf community to the African American community, particularly how each succeeded by "vigorously rejecting long-standing negative imputations imposed on the community from outside" (chapter 9, 175).

Several authors in this volume also look at the Deaf rights movements and find a number of contrasts between the countries they are examining and the United States. Boyes Braem et al. (chapter 5), for example, look at Deaf Swiss Germans as a minority language group rather than an ethnicity and compare reactions to Swiss German Sign Language to reactions to another minority language, Rhaeto-Romansh. These authors focus on issues such as the romanticized views of both these languages and compare these notions to the sociolinguistic realities.

Karen Nakamura (chapter 11) shows how there is no one common definition of deafness in Japan. Groups from different generations and political perspectives have radically different definitions. The older generation, just pre- and post–World War II, tend to have a very broad, encompassing definition of deafness that includes people who in the United States would be considered hard of hearing. The younger generation (particularly the recent post-mainstreaming generation) views deafness in a number of different ways, varying from a Deaf culture (*defu karucha*) model that consciously copies the U.S. example to a view that expresses desire for assimilation. Nakamura also connects these intergenerational differences with the shallow roots of the Japanese Deaf community that is, at most, only three or four generations deep.

The formal aspects of Brazilian Deaf culture are even younger. As Berenz (chapter 9) describes, although the first deaf school was founded in 1857, the first national deaf organization run by deaf people was established only in 1987. Two deaf delegates to a national conference on disabilities, Ana Regina de Souza e Campelo and João Carlos Carreira Alves, were given a mandate to start a national organization. This group, Federação Nacional para a Educação e Integração dos Surdos (FENEIS), has led the fight for recognition of sign language in Brazil, including a well-attended march in September 1994 that demanded sign language be recognized and taught in schools for the deaf. With the rise of FENEIS and the introduction of sign language classes at the Universidade Federal do Rio de Janeiro, there has been a major shift in what is expected of Brazilian deaf people. Previously, people were judged on their Portuguese language skills whereas now they are judged on their ability in Língua de Sinais Brasileira.

The Irish community (chapter 8) offers one of the most striking contrasts to the United States. LeMaster, who had wide experience with the American Deaf community before doing research in Ireland, found that the people she expected to be most aware of their Deaf identities, the older, nonvoicing signers who attended school when education was strictly manual, were in fact less aware of their deafness than the younger, more oral generation. The older generation come from

a time when signing was considered normal, have excellent literacy skills, and
seem to feel more integrated into general Irish society. The younger generation,
in contrast, are expected to deal with hearing society without the benefit of sign
language and are made more responsible for bearing the communicative load in
conversations. Thus, they often feel their deafness more sharply than the older
generation. This younger, oral generation, therefore, shares the American notion
of Deaf ethnic identity despite the fact that sign language is not a key part of their
self-definition.

More broad-reaching social changes can also have radical impact on the lives
of deaf people. The end of the Soviet Union and the introduction of perestroika
in the late 1980s and early 1990s as well as the legacy of apartheid in South Africa
have both had huge effects on those Deaf communities.

One focus of Michael Pursglove and Anna Komarova's work (chapter 13) is
the changing role of the VOG in Russia's Deaf community. During Soviet times,
the VOG was the key deaf organization. It both provided a wide range of services
and imposed an official ideology of oralism on local communities. Since perestroika, local branches of VOG have been much more independent but have also
stopped receiving automatic government funding. Instead, branches receive tax
breaks for their business ventures, part of a wider program of tax-based incentives
for the disabled. The Moscow branch of the VOG made use of the new openness
to publish a small book on Russian signs as well as to establish a bilingual school
and a Deaf studies center. Sign language has gradually been gaining recognition.
The Deaf community, however, has also suffered from the dark side of perestroika. Igor Abramov, the author of Moscow's introduction to signs, was murdered outside his home, presumably by gangsters who wanted the VOG's tax
breaks for themselves.

Although educational policy in South Africa began to change after the end of
apartheid and the 1994 election of Nelson Mandela as president, the legacy of
apartheid has left its marks on the structure of the local Deaf communities. As
Aarons and Reynolds show in chapter 10, racial and economic lines divide both
the education system and the resulting Deaf communities: White children and
mixed-race children were educated in oral English or Afrikaans; Indian and black
children (despite being from nine different spoken language groups) were educated in oral English. The oralist policies were particularly unsuccessful in the
black schools, leading to the development of a number of strong signing communities. Before the new constitution of 1996, however, deaf education was not compulsory and the majority of deaf black children did not attend any sort of school.
Different groups were encouraged to think of themselves as using different sign
languages. The *Dictionary of South African Signs* (Penn 1992–1994) lists English
words with sign equivalents from 11 different racial and geographical groups.
Despite this variation, most Deaf signers in South Africa understand each other,
and, since the end of apartheid, different deaf groups have been trying to work
together. The constitution of 1996 ended formal racial segregation in classrooms
and recognized the right of deaf children to use sign language in school, but by
1999, these reforms had not yet been put into effect.

ONGOING BATTLES

Russia and South Africa are, of course, not the only countries where the larger
society has a profound impact on Deaf communities. Changes, however, are most

visible in countries where massive changes, for good or bad, are taking place. Deaf people often suffer disproportionately during crises. In the United States, for example, deaf people are far more likely to be infected with AIDS as the population at large.[4] Information about AIDS that has been available since the mid-1980s did not reach deaf people until much later. One of the first systematic programs was begun in 1990 when Deaf Marylander Harry Woosley, Jr., was diagnosed as being HIV positive and founded the Deaf AIDS Project (Family Service Foundation 1998–2000).[5] The situation is even worse in the Deaf communities of nations with higher rates of HIV infection. Countries including Zimbabwe, however, are beginning systematic outreach efforts.

General turmoil also takes its toll on Deaf communities, with deaf people falling victim to the same violence that afflicts their fellow hearing citizens. An unknown number of the 3,000 to 4,000 members of Rwanda's Deaf community died in the 1994 genocide. The community now is just beginning to rebuild with the help of the Ugandan Association of the Deaf (Mutabazi 1998).

A number of specifically Deaf issues also are important internationally. Despite the new Deaf activism and the now extensive body of research on sign language and Deaf culture (see Joachim and Prillwitz 1993 for an extensive bibliography), oralism and medical models of deafness are still powerful. As Dotter and Okorn point out (chapter 3), today's oralists hold up cochlear implants as the new "cure" for deafness without informing parents of the dangers and limitations, leading to unrealistic expectations. Cochlear implants may improve hearing but may not improve it enough to allow children access to normal spoken language acquisition. The resulting delay in exposing children to sign language at a young age can retard the whole process of language acquisition and mental development.

These medical models are not similar across the board and are cultural models themselves (Senghas and Monaghan 2002). Not all supporters of cochlear implants are anti-Deaf community. Children with cochlear implants in Scandinavia are seen as part of the Deaf community and are sent to signing schools. Lakshmi Fjord (1999–2000, 2001) argues that this integration is supported because of the high value placed on childhood peer groups in Scandinavia. She also documents, however, the ongoing battle that Scandinavian supporters of cochlear implants have with implant supporters from Britain and other countries who argue that implants "cure" deafness.

One of the few commonalities among Deaf communities around the world is that most are in periods of rapid change, often for the better. Local political reforms and the international spread of ideas about sign language and Deaf culture offer hope for the greater recognition of rights and greater access to services for deaf people everywhere. New technologies such as e-mail and the Internet allow Deaf people to connect in ways never before possible. New dictionaries are being published around the world, and deaf people are gaining access to higher education and a range of other services, including trained interpreters. Deaf communities are solidifying their organizations. There are even countries such as Sweden and Thailand where signed languages are recognized as national languages.

Final Words

Each of the chapters in this book examines some aspect of Deaf community life, including the history of schooling and community building, forms of language

used, how local events shape particular cultures and the influence of growing
Deaf political movements. Despite the great differences between communities,
certain patterns do emerge.

1. There is no one beginning to Deaf communities. Communities have sprung
   up again and again wherever deaf people have been in contact with each
   other.
2. Schools bring deaf children together. A corollary of this is that a majority of
   the adult communities have sprung up around these educational institutions.
3. Schools, however, are not the only places where communities start. Villages
   with a high degree of indigenous deafness like Martha's Vineyard, Massachusetts, or Bhan Khor, Thailand, can have strong signing populations (Groce
   1985; chapter 15). Urban areas like 18th-century Paris and modern Kano in
   northern Nigeria are other places where deaf people can come together in
   sufficient numbers for language and community to be created (Lane 1984;
   chapter 16).
4. In large modern Deaf communities, all three of these factors—education, hereditary deafness, and urban density—may be present. The balance among
   the influences, however, will vary according to historical accident and the
   etiology of people's deafness.
5. Sign language is a vital part of Deaf and deaf communities. Even if specifically
   banned, sign languages will develop when deaf people, particularly children,
   try to communicate with one another. Even in deaf communities where
   speech is common, such as those that have developed around oral schools for
   the deaf or enclaves of mainstreamed school graduates, members may use a
   version of spoken speech, but even the spoken language will be adjusted to
   make sure all participants see what is happening (Monaghan 1996).
6. The form any sign language takes is intertwined with the nature of the community that uses it. Woodward (chapter 15) lays out four different kinds of
   sign languages—indigenous, original, modern, and link—which were the inspiration for the discussion of how communities start in points 2–4 above.
   The indigenous sign language he describes, Bhan Khor Sign Language, is connected to an isolated rural village with a high degree of deafness; the original
   sign languages with the pre-Western contact languages of urban areas like
   Chiangmai and Bangkok; and modern sign language with the American Sign
   Language influenced form that developed after the opening of schools for the
   deaf in Thailand. His final type, link language, has vocabulary from both original and modern sources.
7. The nature of deaf or Deaf identity in a given community depends on the
   forms of community and language discussed above. A deaf person in a small
   farming village such as Bhan Khor will have a very different concept of deafness than a graduate of Gallaudet University in Washington, D.C. Deaf ethnicity, for example, is a model used in the United States while Boyes et al. use a
   language minority model in their chapter on Switzerland (chapter 6; chapter
   5).
8. Any community of deaf people will be influenced not only by its members'
   deafness but also by the larger sociopolitical and economic realities surrounding it. As many deaf people do not have access to the same resources that

their fellow hearing citizens do, they can be at particular risk from the ravages of poverty.

9. Although many policies that affect deaf people are society-wide policies, others specifically target deaf people. However, even these policies come out of general principles within a society.

10. Particular policies might affect rich and poor differently. While there is often huge pressure for children of the wealthy (we return again to the Velasco brothers' example) or comfortably middle-class to conform to their parents' values, this pressure is less of an issue for the children of the already disenfranchised. It is children in the developed nations of Europe, North America, and Australasia that are expected to use (or be subject to) the latest medical technology and, in many cases, are the most pressured to learn to speak in oralist programs. Poor children, however, be they from the slums of 18th-century Paris or modern-day Cape Town, are often brought together in large institutions where they educate each other in their own sign languages and developing cultures (Lane 1984; chapter 10).

11. The rise of nations has fostered the growth of schools for both rich and poor. Deaf schools in Europe rose with the growing nationalist sentiments of the 19th century, and deaf schools continue to be founded in the relatively new nations of Africa and elsewhere. With these schools come new Deaf communities. The political power of the local deaf communities that develop out of these institutions, however, is often connected to a growing recognition of the rights of deaf people everywhere. Nationalism, therefore, may lead to the founding of deaf communities, but internationalism plays a large role in the empowering of communities.

No one chapter in this book deals with every aspect of community that I have discussed here, but together, they show how people gather in sufficient numbers to create ongoing communities and share traits with both the surrounding hearing cultures and other Deaf communities worldwide. The chapters also show the resilience of these communities under sometimes life-threatening situations and give hope for the future. May the chapters in this book serve as both models for research and models for the ways other communities can build from their strengths.

Acknowledgments

Many thanks to Matthew Levinger and Jennifer Monaghan for helpful discussion of 18th- and 19th-century history, to John Vickrey Van Cleve for his very useful comments on Deaf history, to Dana Fleming for her annotated bibliography, and to Adam Benjamin, Benno Caramore, Donald Grushkin, and Richard Senghas for insightful comments on the text. Thanks also to Charles and Jennifer Monaghan for their careful proofreading and comments as well as to Sharon Kornelly, Mark Wolverton, Robert Coontz, and Constanze Schmaling for proofreading and for their help on the references. Any mistakes, however, are my own.

NOTES

1.   In chapter 8, Barbara LeMaster argues that the Christian Brothers' refusal to use the Dominican methods is one of the keys to understanding the separate sign languages that developed at the boys' and girls' schools in Ireland. Each order went to Paris to learn from the National Institute and brought back separate versions of its teachings. The Irish Deaf community benefited, however, from the fact that both schools were run under vows of silence.

2.   Although Galton's emphasis on heredity was questioned even in his own day by critics including Alphonse de Candolle, a Swiss botanist, Galton had many claims to the mantle of science. He allied himself with the widely respected work of Charles Darwin and used careful statistical methods that were widely accepted as the height of 19th-century scientific procedures (Fancher 1979).

3.   Harry Clay Sharp, an Indiana prison doctor, started carrying out vasectomies in 1899, leading Indiana to pass a law allowing sterilization in 1907. German physician Alfred Plötz invented the concept of *Rassenhygiene* or "racial hygiene" in 1895. The idea of sterilization spread with O. Juliusburger's description of Sharp's work and the Indiana law in a German medical journal. No German was sterilized because of deafness, however, until after the passage of the 1933 Nazi Law for the Prevention of Offspring with Hereditary Diseases (Biesold 1999).

4.   A letter to the *Archives of Otolaryngology* notes that in one study .8% (30/3646) HIV patients were deaf or had hearing loss. This is far higher than the general rate of deafness and hearing loss in the general population (McNaghten, Wan, and Dworkin 2001).

5.   The list of deceased community members is available on the Web at http://www-.deafaids.net/remember/index.html. Information on the topic of HIV/AIDS can be found at the following Web sites: http://www.deafvision.net/dap/; dww.deafworldweb.org/pub/a/aids.html; and http://www.thebody.com/whatis/deaf.html. Additional information is available by calling the U.S. Public Health Service TTY hotline: (800) AIDS-TTY.

REFERENCES

Allen, A. B. 1980. *They hear with the eye: A centennial history of the Sumner School for Deaf Children*. Wellington, New Zealand: School Publications Branch, Department of Education.

Aspden, Peter, John Devere, John Hunt, Leila Monaghan, and Lynette Pivac. 1992. *Celebrating 50 years of deaf schools in Auckland*. Auckland, New Zealand: Kelston Deaf Education Centre.

Baynton, Douglas. 1996. *Forbidden signs: American culture and the campaign against sign language*. Chicago: University of Chicago Press.

Biesold, Horst. 1999. *Crying hands: Eugenics and deaf people in Nazi Germany*. Introduction by H. Friedlander. Translated by W. Sayers. Washington, D.C.: Gallaudet University Press.

Blommaert, Jan, and Jef Verschueren. 1992. The role of language in European nationalist ideologies. *Pragmatics* 3 (2):355–75.

Carlson, Elof. 2000. Scientific origins. In *Image archive on the American Eugenics Movement*. Available on the Internet: <http://vector.cshl.org/eugenics> (accessed in October 2002).

Chao, Chien-Min, Hsi-Hsiung Chu, and Chao-Chung Liu. 1988. *Taiwan Ziran Shou Yu* (Taiwan Natural Sign Language). Taipei, Taiwan: Deaf Sign Language Research Association.

Conrad, Ruben, and Barbara Weiskrantz. 1984. Deafness in the seventeenth century: Into empiricism. *Sign Language Studies* 45:291–399.

Erting, Carol J., Robert C. Johnson, Dorothy L. Smith, and Bruce D. Snider, eds. 1994. *The Deaf Way: Perspectives from the International Conference on Deaf Culture*. Washington, D.C.: Gallaudet University Press.

Family Service Foundation. 1998–2000. Deaf AIDS Project: History. Available on the Internet: <http://www.deafvislon.net/dap/history.htm> (accessed October 2002).

Fancher, Raymond E. 1979. *Pioneers of psychology*. New York: Norton.

Fischer, Renate. 1993. Abbé de l'Epée and the living dictionary. In *Deaf history unveiled*, ed. John V. Van Cleve, 13–26. Washington, D.C.: Gallaudet University Press.

Fjord, Lakshmi. 1999–2000. Voices offstage: How vision has become a symbol to resist in an audiology lab in the U.S. *Visual Anthropology Review* 15(2):121–38.

———. 2001. Contested signs: Discursive disputes in the geography of pediatric cochlear implants, language, kinship, and embodiment. Ph.D. diss., University of Virginia.

Galton, Francis. 1883. *Inquiries into human faculty and its development*. New York: Macmillan.

Garretson, Mervin. 1976. Total Communication. *Volta Review* 78:88–95.

Groce, Nora Ellen. 1985. *Everyone here spoke sign language: Hereditary deafness on Martha's Vineyard*. Cambridge, Mass.: Harvard University Press.

Hepp, Ignaz, and F. Nager, 1926. *Die Taubstummheit im Kanton Zurich*. Zurich: n.p.

Holder, William. 1669. *Elements of speech*. London: Royal Society.

Jankowski, Katherine A. 1997. *Deaf empowerment: Emergence, struggle, and rhetoric*. Washington, D.C.: Gallaudet University Press.

Joachim, Guido, and Siegmund Prillwitz. 1993. *International bibliography of sign language*. Hamburg: Signum. Available on the Internet at <http://www.sign-lang.uni-hamburg.de/BibWeb/>.

Johnson, Robert, and Carol Erting.1989. Ethnicity and socialization in a classroom for deaf children. In *The sociolinguistics of American Sign Language*, ed. Ceil Lucas, 41–84. New York: Academic Press.

Lane, Harlan. 1984. *When the mind hears: A history of the deaf*. New York: Random House.

Lane, Harlan, Robert J. Hoffmeister, and Ben Bahan. 1996. *A journey into the deaf world*. San Diego: DawnSign Press.

Leakey, Tricia. 1993. Vocational education in the deaf American and African-American communities. In *Deaf history unveiled: Interpretations from the new scholarship*, ed. John V. Van Cleve, 74–91. Washington, D.C.: Gallaudet University Press.

Long, Joseph Schuyler. 1909. The sign language: A manual of signs. *American Annals of the Deaf* 54:23–37; 140–60.

Maynes, Mary Jo. 1985. *Schooling in western Europe: A social history*. Albany: State University of New York Press.

McNaghten, A. D., Pei-Chun T. Wan, and Mark S. Dworkin. 2001. Prevalence of hearing loss in a cohort of HIV-infected patients. *Archives of Otolaryngology—Head & Neck Surgery*. 127 (12):1516–518.

Miller, William J., David S. Kopf, Edward J. Lazzerini, and J. Norman Parmer. 1995. *The world of Asia*. Wheeling, Ill.: Harlan Davidson.

Monaghan, Leila. 1993. Contexts of luck: Issues involved with entering the New Zealand Deaf community. *Anthropology UCLA* 20:43–62.

———. 1996. *Signing, oralism and the development of the New Zealand deaf community: An ethnography and history of language ideologies*. Ph.D. diss., University of California, Los Angeles.

Mottez, Bernard. 1993. The deaf-mutes banquets and the birth of the deaf movement. In *Deaf history unveiled: Interpretations from the new scholarship*, ed. John V. Van Cleve, 27–39. Washington, D.C.: Gallaudet University Press.

Mutabazi, Pascal. 1998. After the genocide—Rebuilding the deaf community. *Disability Awareness in Action* (November):3. Available on the Internet: <http://dww.deafworldweb.org/pub/g/genocide.rwanda.html> (accessed October 2002).

Nakamura, Karen. 2001. Deaf identities, sign languages, and minority social movement politics in modern Japan (1868–2000). Ph.D. diss., Yale University.

Ojile, Emmanuel. 1994. Education of the deaf in Nigeria: An historical perspective. In *The Deaf Way: Perspectives from the International Conference on Deaf Culture*, ed. C. J. Erting, R. C. Johnson, D. L. Smith, and B. D. Snider, 268–74. Washington, D.C.: Gallaudet University Press.

Padden, Carol. 1989. The deaf community and the culture of deaf people. In *American deaf culture: An anthology*, ed. Sherman Wilcox, 1–16. Burtonsville, Md.: Linstok Press.

Pearson, Raymond. 1994. *The Longman companion to European nationalism, 1789–1920.* London: Longman.

Penn, Claire, ed. 1992–1994. *Dictionary of Southern African signs for communicating with the deaf.* 5 Vols. Pretoria: Human Sciences Research Council.

Piroux, J. 1842–1843. Notice sur Pierre-Aron Berg. *L'ami des Sourds-Muets* 5:72.

Plann, Susan. 1997. *A silent minority: Deaf education in Spain, 1550–1835.* Berkeley: University of California Press.

Radutsky, Elena. 1993. The education of deaf people in Italy and the use of Italian Sign Language. In *Deaf history unveiled: Interpretations from the new scholarship*, ed. John V. Van Cleve, 237–51. Washington, D.C.: Gallaudet University Press.

Ramsey, Claire. 1989. Language planning in deaf education. In *Sociolinguistics of the deaf community*, ed. Ceil Lucas, 123–46. San Diego: Academic Press.

Sacks, Oliver. 1989. *Seeing voices.* Berkeley: University of California Press.

Schiffman, Harold. 1996. *Linguistic culture and language policy.* London: Routledge.

Senghas, Richard J., and Leila Monaghan. 2002. Signs of their times: Deaf communities and the culture of language. *Annual Review of Anthropology* 31:69–97.

Silber, Käte. 1965. *Pestalozzi: The man and his work.* 2d ed. London: Routledge & Kegan Paul.

Smith, Wayne. 1999. A history of the development of education of the deaf in the Republic of China. Typescript.

Stewart, David Alan. 1991. *Deaf sport: The impact of sports within the deaf community.* Washington, D.C.: Gallaudet University Press.

Stokoe, William C. 1960. *Sign language structure: An outline of the visual communication system of the American deaf.* Buffalo, N.Y.: University of Buffalo.

Stokoe, William C., Dorothy C. Casterline, and Carl G. Croneberg. 1976. *A dictionary of American Sign Language on linguistic principles.* Silver Spring, Md.: Linstok Press.

Van Cleve, John V., and Barry A. Crouch. 1989. *A place of their own: Creating the deaf community in America.* Washington, D.C.: Gallaudet University Press.

Williams, Howard G. 1993. Founders of deaf education in Russia. In *Deaf history unveiled: Interpretations from the new scholarship*, ed. John V. Van Cleve, 224–36. Washington, D.C.: Gallaudet University Press.

Winefield, Richard. 1987. *Never the Twain shall meet: Bell, Gallaudet, and the communication debate.* Washington, D.C.: Gallaudet University Press.

Winzer, Margaret. 1993. Education, urbanization, and the deaf community: A case study of Toronto, 1870–1900. In *Deaf history unveiled: Interpretations from the new scholarship*, ed. John V. Van Cleve, 127–45. Washington, D.C.: Gallaudet University Press.

Witkowski, Jan. 2000. Traits studied by eugenicists. In *Image archive on the American Eugenics Movement.* Available on the Internet: <http://vector.cshl.org/eugenics> (accessed in October 2002).

Wolf, Eric R. 1997. *Europe and the people without history.* 2d ed. Berkeley: University of California Press.

Woodward, James. 2000. Sign languages and sign language families in Thailand and Viet Nam. In *The signs of language revisited: An anthology in honor of Ursula Bellugi and Edward Klima*, ed. Karen Emmorey and Harlan Lane, 23–47. Mahwah, N.J.: Erlbaum.

Wrigley, Owen. 1996. *The politics of deafness.* Washington, D.C.: Gallaudet University Press.

2 British Manual Alphabets in the Education of Deaf People Since the 17th Century

Rachel Sutton-Spence

The British manual alphabet is a set of 26 hand arrangements that allow the manual representation of English orthography through fingerspelling. This ancient system has changed considerably in form and function throughout history. Originally, hearing people used it, but later, it became a tool to teach spoken and written English to deaf people. This use as a teaching tool led to its becoming a medium of language for deaf people and, ultimately, a part of the natural sign language of the British Deaf community.[1] It has been used by educators as a pedagogical tool for the teaching of English to deaf people for more than 400 years. The changes in the manual alphabet and its role in British education are considered here, together with relevant events in Europe and America that have influenced its use in British schools.

FINGERSPELLING IN THE BRITISH DEAF COMMUNITY TODAY

Today, approximately 8.7 million people in Britain have a noticeable hearing loss (Royal National Institute for Deaf People 2001). Most of these people have lived their lives as hearing people, receiving a standard education and acquiring their hearing loss only in later years. However, approximately 1 in every 1,000 people has grown up profoundly, prevocationally deaf and has received special education. Many of these deaf people are part of Britain's Deaf community, with its own culture and language, British Sign Language (BSL).

BSL is a visual gestural language, completely independent of the English language (Brennan 1992; Sutton-Spence and Woll 1999). The grammar and vocabulary of BSL bear no relation to English. "Signed English," in which the signs of BSL follow English grammar with additional markers to represent English morphology (McCracken and Sutherland 1992), is not the natural language of the

Deaf community but has been a tool of educators of the deaf to teach English to deaf children. Although BSL is independent of English and is not a creation of hearing people, the manual alphabet today is used by signers to reproduce English words as part of BSL. Manual alphabets are used in many countries in communication among members of the Deaf community and between deaf and hearing people (Carmel 1981).

The two-handed British manual alphabet consists of 26 basic hand arrangements that correspond to the 26 letters of the English alphabet. Each hand arrangement is a manual letter. Another manual alphabet also is used by some members of the British Deaf community, the one-handed Irish manual alphabet, used by some Roman Catholic signers, especially in Glasgow, London, and northwest England. That manual alphabet will not be considered further here. Fingerspelling is produced when the manual alphabet is used to reproduce the spelling of English words. The British manual alphabet is shown in figure 2.1.

All British signers are bilingual to some extent. A signer may use English through any combination of speech and lipreading, reading and writing, or the production and reception of fingerspelling. Throughout history, many deaf people have learned English through formal education, especially in schools (see Evans 1978). Fingerspelling has played an important but varying role in the education of Britain's Deaf community. The use of the manual alphabet in deaf education also has influenced BSL because fingerspelled words have become a part of

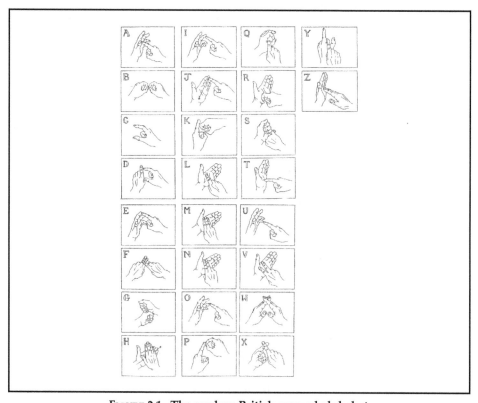

FIGURE 2.1. The modern British manual alphabet

BSL vocabulary in addition to being used for representing English (Sutton-Spence 1994). Today, fingerspelling is used in BSL for a wide variety of reasons and frequently is altered to better fit the phonological and morphological requirements of BSL. Fingerspelling occurs in BSL to represent English proper nouns (the English names of people and place names) and words for concepts that are new to the Deaf community and that have no widespread BSL sign synonym. Fingerspelling is also used for many core vocabulary items, including the signs for many family members as well as units of measurement and time. It is possible for the full English word to be fingerspelled, but more established loans become altered and are frequently abbreviated to the initial letter or a selection of two or three letters (maximally, four). Sometimes, the initial letter will be altered in some way so it receives some additional meaning. For example, the sign for Friday is made using the manual letter F but with a rubbing movement (Sutton-Spence 1994).

The use of the manual alphabet in Britain has changed considerably through history, particularly over the last 400 years. Originally, it was intended for those who could hear and speak but, for some reason (especially for secrecy or religious vows), chose not to. Not until the 16th century was its use formally advocated for those who could neither speak nor hear. Its first recorded use as an educational tool for deaf people was by the Spaniard Pedro Ponce de León in the mid-1500s (DeChaves and Soler 1980). We should be aware, however, that deaf people (probably deafened postlingually) were using fingerspelling before educators picked up the idea (Wilkins 1641).

The history of the British manual alphabet is independent of the alphabets that developed in the rest of Europe and are used in much of the world today. The one-handed, international manual alphabet and many of those used in parts of Europe and America today can be traced back to a common root in Spain (Rossellius 1579). Note, however, that two-handed manual alphabets are also used in many parts of Europe, even if they are not formally recognized by the educational establishments of those countries (Sutton-Spence 1994). Little is known about these "alternative" two-handed systems, and their relationship to the British two-handed alphabet is unclear. In a conversation in 1992, Odd-Inge Schroeder has suggested that the two-handed Norwegian manual alphabet was brought to Norway by British sailors. However, other countries, including Germany, the former Yugoslavia, and the Czech Republic, also use two-handed systems, and some evidence can be found of influence in France and Italy. This whole area needs further research.

The work here will consider only the British manual alphabet as used in Britain. Closely related sign languages such as Australian Sign Language and New Zealand Sign Language have a shared heritage as a result of British colonial policies. However, each sign language has been influenced by the educational policies of the specific country, and attitudes in each country toward fingerspelling and its use by deaf children should not be assumed to be the same.

PHILOSOPHIES OF DEAF EDUCATION

To understand the changing role that fingerspelling has played in the language of deaf people and in deaf education, one must consider the context of educational philosophies during earlier centuries. The philosophies of education of deaf children that were pursued until recently have been polarized into "manual" and "oral." However, such a simple dichotomy is often unhelpful and misleading, and clarification of the terms is necessary here.

ORALISM

"Pure" oralism involves communication entirely by means of speech and lipreading; in cases of complete breakdown in communication, reading and writing are used. Signing and fingerspelling are never used, and pantomimic gesturing is minimal. In 1778, Samuel Heinicke established a school for deaf children in Leipzig who were poor. Throughout the 19th century, the German method in the Leipzig school claimed to be totally oral, at least, in its ultimate intent. Heinicke used various teaching methods, and Lane (1984) reports that Heinicke was inspired by the Dutch cleric Amman, who was known to be a strong believer in oralism. Whether or not Heinicke used a small amount of fingerspelling in his teaching (and there is evidence that he did), Harvey Peet in 1851 mentioned "the modern German teachers who reject the use of the manual alphabet altogether." Behind the oralist philosophy is the belief that deaf children should know and use their community's spoken and written language to minimize the effect of deafness. This philosophy maintains that the use of an identifiably separate language by deaf people alienates them from the rest of society. Knowledge and use of the spoken language is considered necessary for the deaf person to integrate into the "hearing world" (Lane, Hoffmeister, and Bahan 1996).

Within the concept of oralism, however, we find some variation. Oralism may be either an entire philosophy of language and education for the socialization of a deaf person or simply a way to communicate. An oralist may be someone whose ultimate goal is to teach speech and whose approach will use any combination of lipreading, signing, and fingerspelling to accomplish this goal. Alternatively, an oralist could be someone who educates a child entirely through speech and lipreading. Consequently, teachers who teach speech using signs, fingerspelling, or both may be categorized with those who use only lipreading and lip-speaking. Some teachers have tried to teach articulation to deaf pupils but have not expected them to rely on lipreading. Others have expected their pupils to read speech but have not expected articulation and have, instead, relied on fingerspelling or even signing for language production. All these educators may be termed "oralists" by some definitions.

MANUALISM

Manualists have been seen as the polar opposites of oralists. They advocate the use of manual language for communication in schools. The meaning of manualism, however, has changed over the years. The term is also very broad and does not necessarily distinguish the use of signs from fingerspelling nor natural sign languages from either signed systems representing the grammar of spoken language of the surrounding hearing community (Signed English or Signed French) or artificial signed languages using specially created vocabularies.

This lack of distinction is important: Manualists using signed systems related to spoken languages can still claim to be teaching a form of language that allows a deaf person access to hearing society. In contrast, a manualist who advocates the use of the natural language of the national Deaf community is promoting the use of a separate, distinct language. Both groups of manualists are rejecting the sole use of the national language's spoken form, but the former still advocate the use of the national language whereas the latter make a claim for a separate language, culture, and community for deaf people.

Before the widespread use of hearing aids (before the Second World War), full English fingerspelling was the goal of some educators in Britain, especially in Scotland. The intent here was to provide English for deaf people and, hence, to maximize integration into the "hearing world" without relying on the spoken word. Other manualists attempted to achieve perfect representation of the spoken language through the signed version of that language at the expense of the deaf population's natural sign language. Paget-Gorman Signed Speech is one of these systems. The sign language of the Deaf community was not commonly used for the education of deaf children in the past. In many cases, "sign language" was a signed form of the spoken language and was simply a tool to be dropped when the deaf child had learned English.

BILINGUALISM

Since 1945, technological advances have enabled teachers to teach articulation more successfully, allowing those who believe that deaf people should use spoken English to work toward completely integrating deaf people into the speaking world. Despite these advances, this complete integration is still the exception rather than the rule, and a broader approach is now used in many cases. Because national sign languages are now recognized as full, real languages, the possibility exists to argue for genuine bilingualism. Many people (especially parents and teachers) still have a strong desire to integrate deaf people into hearing society as much as possible while recognizing that deaf people will also need to use their own sign language within their national Deaf community. To this extent, although emphasis is still on the spoken language, signed languages may be tolerated or even encouraged. Some schools (such as in Sweden and Norway) educate children in all subjects by means of the community's sign language, teaching the spoken language mainly through reading and writing. This policy of bilingual education in deaf schools is gaining increasing acceptance in Britain, although the primary importance of learning English is still retained. Thus, the present-day debates in deaf education deliberate less about manualism and oralism and more about the use of BSL (i.e., the sign language of the adult Deaf community) and various forms of English.

The key point of this necessarily brief description of deaf educational philosophies is that most educators have tended to see fingerspelling as an acceptable medium of communication, irrespective of their teaching methods. Many oralists, including extreme oralists such as Heinicke and the American Alexander Graham Bell, accepted fingerspelling as being some form of the spoken language (Heinicke, quoted in Arnold 1886; Bell 1883). Manualists (or those advocating the combined method) have accepted it because it is a manual way to provide complete information about an utterance from the spoken language.

Today, the terms *manualist* and *oralist* are less important than they have been in the past, particularly since the emergence of bilingual education of deaf children. However, until about 20 years ago, the debate was firmly polarized, and the history of the use of the manual alphabet and fingerspelling in education is usefully seen in the light of these two philosophies.

Fingerspelling in Manualist and Oralist Philosophies

Joseph Gordon summed up the attitude of many educators in the 19th century:

> Fingerspelling is to the deaf a borrowed art. It was originated neither by them nor by their teachers, nor is it essential to their education, yet its value can hardly be overestimated. To the deaf-born the mastery of common language is an extremely difficult task. Intelligible speech in certain cases is well-nigh impossible. Writing is slow, wearisome, lifeless and often impracticable. Fingerspelling which may have the rapidity of deliberate speech and three times that of writing, permits dramatic action, emphasis, accuracy and easy repetition, thus keeping the senses alert and vivid by impressing the forms of words and sentences upon the mind. It compels practice in our language, and encourages and stimulates the child in his efforts to master it. (Gordon, quoted in Buxton 1886, 83)

Gordon's observation identifies the main arguments of those who rejected the use of speech for the education of deaf children and highlights some of the advantages of fingerspelling over speechreading and speech. Gordon, however, does not question that deaf people need to master "common language," and his goal is clearly to teach English in some form.

Francis Green sent his deaf son to Thomas Braidwood's academy (founded in 1760) in Scotland and described some of the Braidwood family's methods of teaching (Green 1783). Green visited the school and saw boys using writing, lipreading, speaking, and signing. His son signed and spoke simultaneously as well as signed to his school friends. The use of simultaneous speech and sign implies that the signing was something akin to methodical signs, which would follow the order of English. Green also referred to Arnot's *History of Edinburgh* in which the boys of Braidwood's academy were reported to be using the manual alphabet. Clearly, the members of the Braidwood family were not the total oralists they had sometimes been made out to be.

The British educators in particular have been widely considered to be oralists. This view must have been inferred, in part, because the British originally claimed to use pure oral techniques for reasons of prestige, although in reality, they relied considerably on manual and visual media. The American belief that the British were oralists may stem from the fact that Thomas Braidwood refused to give American Thomas Gallaudet his teaching methods without payment. In fact, Braidwood learned much of his method from the French, and Joseph Watson (Braidwood's grandson and headmaster of a school using these oralist methods) revealed in 1809 that he used gestures, signs, pictures, the written word, and lipreading in his broadly based curriculum, which included articulation. That approach was not far from what the manualist Americans learned from Sicard and were using ten years later.

Before we continue to consider the use of the manual alphabet in oralist and manualist philosophies within the schools for deaf children, we must trace the source of the British manual alphabet and the early functions of fingerspelling. In the review that follows, note that (with the possible exception of the author of *Digiti Lingua* [1698] about whom little is known) all the authors of manual alphabets and tracts concerning them were hearing.

THE EARLIEST FINGERSPELLING

The manual alphabets used in Britain have been of two basic types. Before 1698, most manual alphabets were based on methods of allocating letters to joints of the fingers or areas of the hands and pointing these out in succession. In these "arthrological" systems of the 17th century, the shapes of the hands did not change; letters were distinguished by pointing to locations on the hands. For a few letters in some manual alphabets, this system was not used. Instead, a letter was represented by a given hand arrangement. In the later "dactylological" systems of the 18th century onward, the letters were distinguished by different hand-shapes, often reflecting the shapes of the written letters. The most substantial shift from arthrology to dactylology occurred in 1698 with the publication of *Digiti Lingua*, an anonymous tract, describing several forms of manual alphabets.

One popular belief has been that the sign languages of deaf people evolved from monastic sign languages; however, no firm evidence appears to verify this belief, at least in Britain. Undoubtedly, not all monastic sign languages made use of the manual alphabet because descriptions of the old monastic sign languages make no mention of it. For example, the descriptions of the Benedictine sign language by Banham (1991) and Martins (1958) detail signs clearly but mention no manual alphabets. Barakat (1987), however, does describe a Cistercian manual alphabet. This Cistercian system is no doubt strongly visually motivated and unlike any arthrological British alphabet.

Despite this lack of evidence, the possibility still exists that the early British arthrological systems used by deaf people were used originally in some monasteries. Indirect evidence for this idea comes from a manual alphabet very similar to those used in Britain in the 17th century that has been in existence in Britain and Ireland since as early as the sixth century B.C.

THE OGHAM MANUAL ALPHABET

A Goidelic alphabet called Ogham was used during the Celtic period during the sixth century B.C. and was still being used at the time of the Roman occupation of Britain. This alphabet included both written and manual forms and was used by Druids, especially in Ireland, but also in parts of Britain. Robert Graves (1952) claims that the alphabet was designed to be used manually and in writing. The manual form of this alphabet allocated letters to different areas of the left hand. The forefinger of the right hand pointed out the letters.

WILKINS'S ARTHROLOGICAL MANUAL ALPHABET

The same basic arthrological system as the Ogham manual alphabet is described in the first known reference to a manual alphabet used in England, John Wilkins's

1641 publication of *Mercury, the Swift and Silent Messenger*. The book is a work on cryptography, and fingerspelling was referred to as one method of "secret discoursing, by signes and gestures." Although Wilkins did not provide an illustration of the manual alphabet, a reconstruction can be made that is based on his written description.

Wilkins (1641) referred to deaf people's use of signs and gestures, including fingerspelling (or "arthrology," as he called it). He mentioned that arthrology was of "especial note for [its] use and antiquity." Clearly, Wilkins knew that the manual alphabet he described was used among deaf people and by hearing people (see figure 2.2). He made no suggestion that the manual alphabet was of his design.

The letters are arranged very differently in the two arthrological systems described by Graves and Wilkins, but we can reasonably assume that the later system developed out of its earlier counterpart. We know that the Ogham manual alphabet was being used in Celtic monasteries in the early centuries of the Christian era, so the literati of the time would have been aware of it and could easily have adapted the system to accommodate the Latin alphabet.

The development of the alphabets used in Europe was different from that in Britain. In Britain, the modern manual alphabet was not published and standardized until the 18th century, although, clearly, fingerspelling systems were in use

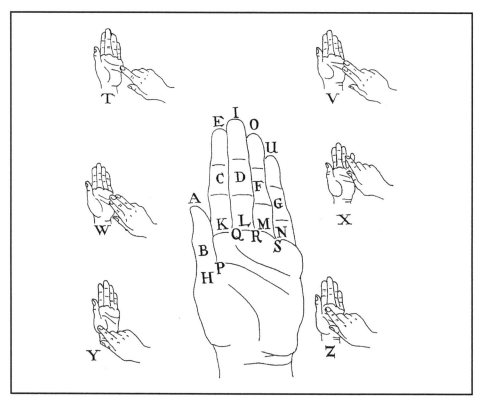

FIGURE 2.2 Wilkins's manual alphabet, reconstructed from his description in
Mercury, the Secret and Swift Messenger (1641)

by hearing and deaf people well before the 17th century for reasons of secrecy, religion, and even for the simple pleasure of language games. On the European continent, one system was steadily handed down through generations of monks, educators, and deaf people and can be dated back at least to St. Bonaventure's system of the 13th century.

OTHER 17TH-CENTURY MANUAL ALPHABETS

Three years after Wilkins's *Mercury* was published, Bulwer's 1644 *Chirologia* arranged various international signs and gestures so they could be used to represent letters of the alphabet and "serve for privy cyphers for any secret intimation" (Bulwer 1644, 150). However, the emphasis was on the use of gestures as a complement to speech rather than as an alternative and was not used by deaf people. The manual alphabet that Bulwer knew to be used by deaf people is mentioned in *Philocophus, or the Deafe and Dumbe Man's Friende* (Bulwer 1648). Here, Bulwer referred to a deafened man, Master Babington of Burntwood, who communicated with his wife using "arthrologie," by pointing to areas of the hand and the finger joints. Although Bulwer did not give any examples of this arthrology, one could reasonably assume that the system was similar to the one described by Wilkins.

The first evidence of this arthrological system being used for the education of prelingually deaf people comes from the writings of William Holder, one of the two earliest British educators of deaf people in England. He wrote in 1669, "Teach him [the deaf child] an alphabet upon his fingers or several parts of his hands, by placing the letters there, which you may devise at pleasure" (Holder 1669, 151). He proceeded to describe an alphabet that involved pointing to joints and areas of one hand with the other. Despite Holder's suggestion that placing the letters on the hand could be devised "at pleasure," the system is remarkably similar to that of Wilkins (see figure 2.3). No doubt, Holder would have been aware of Wilkins's *Mercury*, but Holder also could have simply been using the manual alphabet that was commonly used.

John Wallis, a contemporary of Holder, was also a teacher of deaf people. Wallis seemed to have a similar attitude to the arbitrary nature of the forms of the

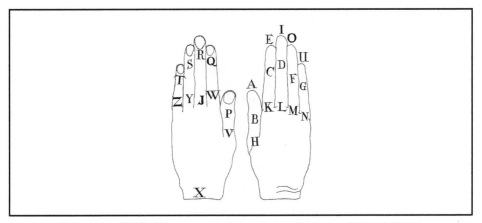

FIGURE 2.3 Holder's manual alphabet from *Elements of Speech* (1669)

manual letters. In his letter to Thomas Beverly in 1693, quoted in Green (1783), he recommended signifying letters by

> the position and motion of the finger, hand, or any part of the body which may be in stead of written letters. For example, that the vowels may be noted by the ends of the five fingers; the other letters b, c, d, &c by other positions and motion, as may seem convenient, and as may be agreed. (Green 1783, 40)

However, despite his claims that any position would be acceptable, the example he gave was not arbitrary (such as his use of the five fingertips for the five vowels). He was clearly referring to the same manual alphabet that was being used throughout the 17th century. Wallis and Wilkins were also well acquainted through the Royal Society, so Wallis would have known Wilkins's form of manual alphabet.

A short time after Wallis and Holder were teaching and writing, George Dalgarno published *Didascolocophus* (1680) in which he provided the first engraving of the manual alphabet in use at that time. Dalgarno was the first British writer to propose that fingerspelling and writing rather than speech could be the main means of communication for deaf people. He did not claim to have invented the manual alphabet presented in his document but only that he had improved on the existing one. He wrote: "After much search and many changes, I have at last fixt upon a finger or hand-alphabet according to my mind, for I think it cannot be considerably mended" (Dalgarno 1680, 73; see figure 2.4).

Dalgarno's system also attempted to provide a means of representing consonant clusters such as *st* or *lt*. This idea was not adopted by later authors and is not used today. For Dalgarno, however, the idea was central to his view of the function of fingerspelling. He saw fingerspelling as being a representation of speech and, thus, felt it necessary to produce a system that reflected speech more clearly. This attitude was seen in other 17th- and 18th-century educationalists. The manual alphabet today is seen as representing writing and not speech.

Although unusual for writers at this time, Dalgarno gave practical advice on

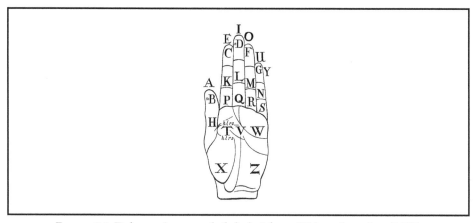

FIGURE 2.4 Dalgarno's manual alphabet from *Didascalocophus* (1680)

the alphabet's best use. For example, he recommended practicing combinations of consonants until they were easy to produce (a technique recommended by many even today). He also suggested "multiple touching" of letters so a whole monosyllabic word could be made simultaneously. (This unusual attempt to move away from production of fingerspelled words as a stream of concatenated letters and toward whole, meaningful units was not picked up by others.) He also suggested using the initial letter of an English word to represent an object or concept. This use of initialization was used by the creators of methodical signs in the 18th century (I. Peet 1868) and has subsequently become an important role of fingerspelling in British Sign Language (Sutton-Spence 1994).

Arthrological systems remained popular even when dactylological systems were in common use. In 1883, Alexander Graham Bell attempted to reintroduce a modification of Dalgarno's manual alphabet (Bell 1883). This version was produced entirely on the surface of one hand, but it read systematically, from left to right, down the hand, making no exception for the vowels (unlike all the early English manual alphabets, which always placed the vowels on the tips of the fingers).

In all these arthrological systems, the manual alphabet was intended for the representation of English as the only language to be considered. Bulwer and Dalgarno both implied that the deaf person would be a fluent user of English. Wallis and Holder, in contrast, saw fingerspelling as a teaching tool but made no suggestion that any language other than English is considered. Indeed, it would appear from the sources available that most fluent fingerspellers were deafened people who were already literate in English.

Digiti Lingua: The First Known Dactylological Manual Alphabet

Digiti Lingua, published anonymously in 1698, presented the first known truly dactylological manual alphabet with most letters represented by distinctive hand arrangements. The vowels, however, remained at the tips of the fingers as in previous arthrological alphabets (see figure 2.5). The roots of the modern British two-handed alphabet clearly lie in this publication.

The author of *Digiti Lingua* claimed not to have spoken for many years and suggested that his alphabet might be used on occasions when silence and secrecy were needed or purely for entertainment. He made no explicit reference to deaf people and it is not known whether he was deaf himself.

Adoption of Fingerspelling by the Deaf Community

The modern British manual alphabet was printed for the first time in a plate published in 1720 in Defoe's *The Life and Adventures of Duncan Campbell*, a semibiographical account describing the life of a deaf fortune-teller who was said to possess second sight. According to Jussen (1973), the plate in the 1720 edition shows a manual alphabet that is very similar to the modern alphabet (although *J* is missing) with only four other letters different from those used today. Jussen provides a copy of that plate. The 1732 edition of the same book contains a different but basically similar illustration of the manual alphabet, which is shown in figure 2.6.

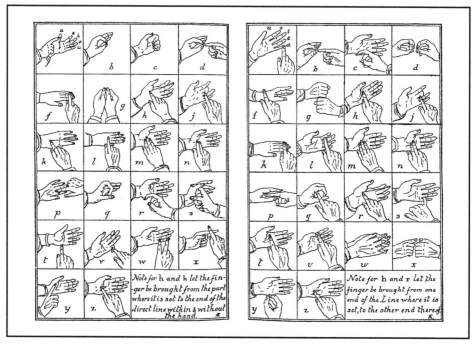

FIGURE 2.5 The first known dactylological manual alphabet, published in *Digiti Lingua* (Anonymous 1698)

Up until this time in England, manual alphabets were not expected to be widely intelligible. Wilkins (1641) had said that the letters might be performed in any way as long as all parties agreed on them. Bulwer (1648) offered several completely different types of alphabets, with no suggestion that they should have anything in common with one another (those in his first book were for rhetoric use, and the one mentioned in his second book was for use by deaf people). Wallis (1674) described his version clearly but added that any choice of alphabet could be used if it were convenient and if all parties agreed. Defoe (1732) described his version, adding "or otherwise it shall be agreed upon" (24).

Throughout the 17th and first part of the 18th century, the expressed goal of manual alphabets was to permit people (deaf or not) to communicate with their immediate friends, coconspirators, or family and between tutors and their deaf pupils. In this last circumstance, if speech were the ultimate goal of the education, then a manual alphabet may have been seen only as a makeshift stopgap. For this reason, perhaps, authors describing these alphabets often left the option open for the readers to devise manual alphabets of their own. Only with the growth of more widespread education for deaf people and the development of a British Deaf community did it become necessary for one standard form of the manual alphabet to be used. Somewhere between 1698 and 1720, the manual alphabet used in Britain became fixed in its form.

Unadopted Manual Alphabets

Where Britain's fixed-form manual alphabet came from is not at all clear. It may have been devised in Britain, or it may have come from an alphabet being used in

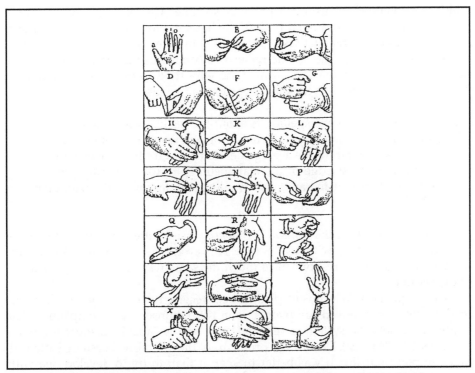

FIGURE 2.6 The manual alphabet that appeared in the 1732 edition of Defoe's
The Life and Adventures of Duncan Campbell

the rest of Europe. Nevertheless, the British manual alphabet also had to face competition from new inventions by hearing people. Lucas (1812) designed a system for *The Art of Reading, Spelling and Ciphering by the Fingers*. This system placed all the letters on the surface of one hand, in the tradition of Wilkins and Dalgarno, but did not place vowels on the fingertips.

Notably, Lucas (1812) also proposed using the initial letter of certain words to stand for those words. He recommended that the signer should point to *l* to mean pounds, to *s* for shillings, to *p* for pence, and to *q* for farthings (a farthing was worth a quarter of an old penny). He also gave a list of words from *a* to *z*, which could be represented by a single manual letter: and, but, can, do, every, for, have, if, judge, king, last, may, nor, own, perhaps, philosopher, question, or, soon, shall, truly, that, you, very, with, which, except, yet, and zeal.

Lucas (1812) also claimed that when only some of the letters of a word will identify a word, it need not be fully spelled, saying "all that is necessary is, to make the word or sentence to be well understood; there being no more need of true spelling in Chyrology, than in Stenography." This approach did not reflect the attitude of the 19th-century teachers who believed that every letter had to be fingerspelled, but Lucas's method is more like the way that fingerspelling is often used in modern BSL. There is no evidence that Lucas's ideas were adopted by any of the English educational establishments.

In another case, E. Abraham, a reviewer writing in the *British Deaf Monthly* in 1897, criticized the *Unique Practical Deaf-Mute Manual Alphabet* by Henry Woolen, which was intended for use with phonetic spelling. The technique was to point to various parts of the front and back of the hand to indicate letters representing speech sounds rather than letters (/sh/, /ch/, /th/) and to indicate commas, full stops, colons, and semicolons. The reviewer's comments on this new system reflect a common complaint leveled at those who tried to introduce a system to "help" deaf people but had no knowledge of their needs:

> Mr. Woollen's phonetic spelling is about the terriblest to look at that we can recall . . . though the phoneticism of Mr. Woollen does not go very deep, it goes too far for the average deaf-mute . . . if Mr. Woollen had any real practical knowledge of manual spelling, he would hardly put forward a system that in rapid use would be almost illegible. (Abraham 1897, 83)

Much of the contents of the *British Deaf Monthly* was written by—and often for—hearing people working with deaf people. However, "the average deaf-mute" undoubtedly would have responded in much the same way, given the opportunity of expression.

Although the newly invented alphabets received cool responses, those already in use also received complaints. John Kitto, himself deaf, complained that "upon the whole the system is very defective and is capable of great improvement" (Kitto 1845, 107). Despite the problems of the established system, Kitto was quick to point out that it was better to keep it than to try to develop one with fewer defects. He observed that too many people already knew the existing alphabet and any changes could discourage others from learning it, which would limit the number of people with whom he could converse. Kitto had been deafened in his early teens and was clearly a highly literate man. He relied on fingerspelling for his conversation with others, especially his family.

One-Handed Manual Alphabets in Britain

Many authors in the past have suggested that deaf people should know both one-handed (the one descended from the original Spanish system, and widely used in America) and two-handed alphabets. John Pauncefoot Arrowsmith reprinted both alphabets with the following advice: "Make the child learn to talk with both hands and with one, agreeable to the manual alphabets subjoined; they are the same as those in general use at home and abroad" (Arrowsmith 1819, 42). This last comment might be another hint that a two-handed manual alphabet was being used outside Britain, alongside the "standard" one-handed systems. Kitto (1845), too, gave both forms. Late 19th-century British pamphlets give the two-handed and one-handed alphabets, designating the one-handed version as Irish (although actually very different from the one currently used in Ireland).

The 1853 report on the Conferences of British Instructors of the Deaf and Dumb (by an unnamed contributor to the *American Annals of the Deaf and Dumb*), states that Mr. Hopper of the Birmingham Institution claimed that the one-handed manual alphabet was very much superior to the two-handed. The conference unanimously agreed that it would be best if the pupils became used to both manual alphabets. The editor commented: "The two-handed alphabet, we will also venture to prophesy, has received its death-blow from Mr. Hopper" (Conferences of British Instructors 1853, 253). This prophecy was not to be. In 1875, Buxton observed the preference of many English teachers for the one-handed alphabet but noted the following:

> The arguments in its [the one-handed alphabet's] favor, like those for the decimal currency, may probably be admitted; it would be better if we had it. But the rival system has got possession and is in familiar use, and persons are apt to think that the inconveniences of making the change would outweigh the advantages to be expected from it. (Buxton 1875, 114)

A more recent attempt to establish the American one-handed alphabet at the Northern Counties School for the Deaf (Evans 1978) was also unsuccessful. Evans claims in many places that the American system is superior to the British one. This judgment was based on the fact that the American, one-handed system can be produced nearer the mouth, hence aiding lipreading, and allows the easier creation of initialized signs. However, British signers tend to focus on the mouth when conversing and perceive fingerspelling through peripheral vision, so the location of fingerspelling relative to the mouth is not an important issue. Further, initialized signs are not necessary for a sign language (and indeed, anecdotally, they are disliked by many deaf people), and BSL uses many other methods of sign formation. From the evidence available, therefore, it seems that a system with its roots in secrecy and confusion is finally evolving through its use by deaf people to become simpler and clearer and more amenable to the sign-formation processes of BSL.

Having followed the course of development of the British manual alphabet, the reader will find the following review of the education methods known since the 16th century a useful way to understand how fingerspelling fit in with the methods and sign language. This historical context explains much of the present status and role of the manual alphabet and fingerspelling in modern BSL.

THE ROLE OF FINGERSPELLING IN DEAF EDUCATION

The history of the use of fingerspelling and sign language is closely bound with the development of deaf education and the growth of schools for the deaf. There is no doubt, however, that sign language was flourishing before schools for the deaf were started.

EARLY DEAF EDUCATION IN BRITAIN

The goal of the first teachers in England was to prove to a skeptical scientific community that prelingually deaf people could be taught to speak. In the pursuit of this goal, all forms of communication were used: signs, pantomime, lipreading, and fingerspelling. Earlier discussion in this chapter has shown that the idea of a manual alphabet was familiar and used by hearing people, especially in cryptography, and that it was a natural tool for the academics to use with deaf people.

John Wallis taught his deaf pupil, William Whalley, to speak English using a grammar of the language he had originally written for speakers of other European languages. Although his goal was to teach his pupil to speak, he taught written language first, using pantomime, pointing, and natural signs, and he also taught fingerspelling. His methods involved teaching the child long vocabulary lists in various categories, short phrases, and then grammatical rules. Only after these steps did he teach articulation and spoken words, which he did through the manual alphabet as well as through reading and writing.

Wallis, in contrast, was adamant that fingerspelling should precede speech. "The position of the finger," he wrote, "may be in stead of written letters. . . . Afterward he is to be taught speech" (Wallis 1693, in Green 1783, 40).

Accepted convention in the 17th century acknowledged that letters were the basic units of speech sound, and hence, writing and fingerspelling were seen as two ways to represent speech. Wallis was particularly concerned that his pupils should not learn to articulate without knowing the meaning of the words. He declared that deaf people who spoke without comprehending were no better than parrots, and he had no time for that form of education. This assertion was probably a barb directed at his contemporary, William Holder.

Holder also taught his pupils the manual alphabet, together with the written alphabet, but only after he had attempted to teach articulation. Holder's results were less successful than Wallis's (although it is possible that his pupil, Alexander Popham, not only was deaf but also had other learning difficulties). For Holder, fingerspelling was a way to increase language skills but not to help speech. He used the letters as a way to link speech sounds with writing. For this reason, he says that the sounds written as *th*, *sh*, and *ng* must be taught "with that faulty way of writing" (Holder 1669). A teacher who was concerned only with teaching written language would not have been concerned that some speech sounds in English are not written with one letter.

Wallis and Holder argued over which of them had been the first to teach a deaf person to speak. Holder published his work in "An appendix concerning the deaf and dumb" in *Elements of Speech* in 1669. According to Conrad and Weiskrantz (1984), Wallis added his preface concerning deafness to the fourth edition of *De Loquela* in 1674, so Holder was definitely the first to publish. Wallis, however, claimed that he had done the teaching first and had been more successful than Holder. Wallis also published a letter to Boyle that antedated the 1669 *Elements* of Holder in an attempt to prove he had been first. Holder retaliated that Whalley had been deaf only since the age of five and, thus, did not count as a prelingual deaf person.

Amid all the bickering, a few things stand out. First, the two men knew each other well and must have known about each other's methods. At different stages in their teaching, Wallis and Holder both used fingerspelling, which was also the same method of fingerspelling and was probably similar to the one that John Wilkins (also a fellow of the Royal Society) described in 1641. Wallis knew Kenelm Digby, the courtier of Charles II, who in 1644 had published an account of Bonet's work (1620), and historians have little doubt that Wallis knew about Bonet's methods. However, Wallis claimed that he did not know Bonet's work. Certainly, he did not use the Spanish manual alphabet. Instead, as has been explained above, he used the one commonplace in England at the time.

Henry Baker (1698–1775) was the first professional teacher of the deaf in England. Although Baker did not leave any published record of his methods, his unpublished manuscripts show that he used writing, drawing, and lipreading in his methods. Evidence also indicates that he was familiar with methods used by Wallis. Baker was married to the daughter of the novelist Daniel Defoe, who, in *The Life and Adventures of Duncan Campbell* (1732), described the education of the deaf Duncan Campbell by methods recommended by Wallis (DeChaves and Soler 1980). Because Baker knew both Defoe's and Wallis's work, he likely used fingerspelling of some type and probably used the manual alphabet in the picture published by Defoe.

The 17th-century scholars who taught deaf people to speak did so to demonstrate that deafness and lack of speech were not inextricably linked. Their primary goal was to demonstrate a deaf person's ability to speak; the deaf person's ability to learn a language that he or she could use for everyday life was of secondary concern. To these educators, fingerspelling was merely a tool to enable them to reach the goal of speech. In the 18th century, the general education of deaf people and, in particular, their education about Christianity became a greater priority. In this and many other respects, Britain was part of a number of international trends in the education of deaf people. In particular, teaching on the continent of Europe and in the United States had influence on and was influenced by events in Britain.

THE USE OF FINGERSPELLING IN BRITISH DEAF EDUCATION SINCE THE 18TH CENTURY

In Britain, although the goal of 18th- and 19th-century educators had been to teach deaf children English, both signing and fingerspelling were used. Educators soon recognized that lipreading and articulation were of limited use for communication but the feeling was strong in some quarters that use of sign language would cut off deaf people from hearing people, so fingerspelling was offered as a solution. It is important to note that this solution to deaf-hearing communication problems required some effort from hearing people. Speech and lipreading usually demand great effort from deaf people but little from hearing people. Use of the manual alphabet still uses the language of hearing people, but in a form that requires some change, so both deaf and hearing people need to work to reach common ground for communication.

Fingerspelling in "Manualist" Schools

The first Thomas Braidwood had claimed to rely on oral techniques, although evidence from Francis Green and Joseph Watson suggests that this claim was based more on a desire for prestige than on truth. When the second Thomas Braidwood (grandson of the first) died in 1825, the French method and methodical signs started to play a more important role in British education again. De Puget, who had studied under Sicard in Paris, succeeded Braidwood at the Birmingham school. The Doncaster school (opened in 1829) proposed to use first natural signs, then methodical signs, followed by fingerspelling and, finally, writing. De Puget had trained Charles Baker, the institute's headmaster. William Neill trained under Baker and, when he became headmaster of the Northern Counties School, he relied on fingerspelling and methodical signs. His successor Andrew Wright claimed in 1892 that the goals of the school were to teach written language through the manual alphabet and natural signs and to teach articulation and lip-reading to those with aptitude or who could benefit. By 1897, the emphasis had shifted toward speech, but he still offered advice to parents on lipreading, signing, fingerspelling, reading, writing, and speech. At the Northern Counties School at the beginning of the 20th century, both the one-handed and the two-handed alphabets were in use, perhaps because of the French influence on the teaching, but by the 1930s, only the two-handed system was used (Savage, Evans, and Savage 1981).

Fingerspelling for Communication between Deaf and Hearing People

The *Eighth Edinburgh Encyclopaedia* in 1813 (cited in Seigel 1969) criticized the French methods used by de l'Epée (1784), claiming that using "artificial" signs was a waste of time and effort when there was an adequate manual alphabet. The basis of the argument was that, when the children left school, they would be unable to communicate with anyone else. Because fingerspelling could be learned rapidly by any literate person, it was proposed as a more sensible alternative for deaf and hearing people to learn. This proposal ignored the fact that fingerspelling is a form of English and a foreign language to deaf people using sign language as their first language. However, the proposal did show willingness on the part of hearing people to use a form of English that was not speech. During Victorian times, deaf organizations proposed that pictures of the manual alphabet be on the walls of classrooms so all hearing pupils could learn it and communicate with deaf people.

This idea that hearing people should learn something new to enable them to talk to deaf people was an important change in attitude. Previously, the emphasis had been on deaf people making the effort to communicate with hearing people and not on hearing people changing their methods of communication to accommodate deaf people. The very large number of published versions of the manual alphabet that we have from this period are evidence of the prevailing interest of hearing people in the manual alphabet. In almost all of these, reference is made to the fact that learning the manual alphabet will enable the hearing person to communicate with deaf people (examples include R. R. 1809; Watson 1809; Arrowsmith 1819; Hippisley Tuckfield 1839; Kitto 1845; Smith 1864; Ash 1889; Roe 1893; Abraham 1895; Dictionary of D & D Signs 1895; Rhind n.d., but definitely 19th century; Manual Alphabets 1903; and many others that may be seen in the collection of Hay and Lee 1994). Although more and more hearing people were using the manual alphabet without any knowledge of sign language, the general acceptance of fingerspelling in deaf education must also have affected the use of fingerspelling within the sign language used.

Fingerspelling in "Oralist" Schools

The Milan International Congress on the Education of the Deaf in 1880 is usually seen as the great turning point in deaf education. At this congress, oralism was recommended as the ideal teaching method. Oralism was advocated for only some children and the "combined method" (signing and lipreading with speech), for others. This approach could have been a positive step and might have provided different educational methods for deaf children with different hearing losses and educational needs. Unfortunately, however, the argument between the oralists and the manualists became a debate of bipolar extremes and the common ground was lost. In fact, in Britain, little was changed immediately by the decision of the Milan Congress. (In 1889, a Royal Commission in England recommended that all deaf children should have the opportunity to be educated orally. This proposal was seen as the official seal of approval for oralism in English schools, but even then, the combined method continued to flourish in many schools.)

Despite the decisions made at the Milan Congress, a survey of British schools in 1881 showed a great variation in the methods of teaching used. In Ireland, both Belfast and Dublin used manual methods. In Scotland, Aberdeen was manual, basically using fingerspelling but using signing with younger children. In Edinburgh, the Henderson Row school used manual and oral methods, and Donaldson's school used signs. In Glasgow, educators also used combined oral and manual media. In Wales, Llandaff used only writing and did not use either signing or speech. In Swansea, educators used manual media and used both one-handed and two-handed alphabets. In England, Bristol and Bath both used manual methods. Doncaster used oral and manual media, but for different children. Edgbaston used signs or signs with speech (this school had a large staff who were deaf). Hull was manual and relied mainly on the manual alphabet. Manchester and the Northern Counties School in Newcastle were both manual. But in London, oralism had the main hold. All six schools in the city used oral methods and only Margate (a branch of the Old Kent Road Asylum for children unable to benefit from oral methods) used the combined method (Fay 1881). This oralist enclave in London was set to spread.

David Buxton, a committed British oralist of the late 19th century took issue with Joseph Gordon from America, who claimed that practice in fingerspelling was tantamount to practice in English and so should be encouraged. Buxton (1886) retorted that this view might indeed be the case but "it is not practice in speech and lipreading, and that is what the pupil wants and what we want." To Buxton's mind, fingerspelling hindered speech and "lipreading," and it should be banned. He wrote in italics for emphasis: "*it* [fingerspelling] *must on no account be admitted into the school*" (Buxton 1886, 83). He did concede that deaf adults who had successfully acquired speech and could speechread might fingerspell if it would help strangers to understand their speech because, by that stage, fingerspelling would not harm the acquisition of "language."

Thomas Arnold had become concerned that the English system of deaf education provided deaf people with only vocational training and not social training. For social success, he believed that oral skills were vital and, in 1888, claimed to be the first English teacher to use the pure oral method.

Eventually, the orally based teacher-training college at Ealing was transferred to Manchester University when the Department of Audiology and Education was opened in 1919. This development provided the only chair of Education of the Deaf in Britain and also provided the teacher training for almost all teachers of the deaf in England and the Empire (and later the Commonwealth). As a result, the oral method of teaching took over in England and large areas of the English-speaking world, and fingerspelling was used considerably less. The notable exceptions to this situation were the Scottish schools. These continued to use fin-gerspelling as a major teaching tool until the 1950s.

The practices in the Scottish schools had important influences on the signing that we still see in older British deaf signers today, especially those from Scotland, Northern England, and Wales. Many of them fingerspell extensively in their sign-ing—in some cases, fingerspelling entire sentences although, more frequently, mixing fingerspelling with signs. When the policy of fingerspelling in these schools was stopped, subsequent education policies left the younger generations unable to fingerspell fluently and incapable of communicating clearly with many members of the older generation. This development has important cultural and practical implications, not least, that elderly deaf people in residential care may be cared for by staff members who have received "sign language training," but only in BSL and not in use of fingerspelling (Pullen and Kyle 1997).

In 1964, the Department of Education and Science (DES) within the British government set up a committee chaired by Professor M. M. Lewis to investigate the possible place of fingerspelling and signing in British schools for the deaf. At the time, most schools in Britain were officially oral, but the resulting report found that some form of manual communication was used on an informal basis in al-most all schools (Lewis 1968).

The report concluded that the linguistic status of fingerspelling is no different from that of written language and could be used by educated deaf adults. In addition, the report admitted that, among signing deaf adults, fingerspelling would be useful for new or technical terms or for parts of speech that are not signed. It also concluded that fingerspelling could be a useful teaching aid when combined with speech. However, the report recognized the problem of speaking and fingerspelling simultaneously: If the speech keeps pace with the slower fin-gerspelling, it becomes unnaturally slow and loses its rhythm; if normal speech is maintained, then the fingerspelling falls behind and the purpose of using the manual mode to support the oral mode is lost. The committee also noted that, in the Soviet Union, teachers fingerspelled immediately under the chin while speak-ing to get the children to associate the fingerspelled word with the lip patterns. The Russian children were required to articulate while fingerspelling and, later, were expected to learn to speechread without fingerspelling. The committee pro-posed that the same system could possibly be used in Britain. However, the over-all conclusion of the report was that, because British schools should be attempting to teach English to deaf children, fingerspelling could be tolerated, provided it was used for this purpose.

In the wake of this report, the Special Education branch of the DES commis-sioned a further report that confirmed that manual communication was widely used in British schools. Because it was informally used and often used against school policy, the teachers had received no training in the field. Their skills were often picked up casually from the children they taught. Moves were then made to try to provide training in manual communication for teachers of the deaf.

Although the schools followed stated policies of oralism during the past cen-tury, sign language flourished within the Deaf community, particularly among families with many deaf members. This sign language, however, would have been influenced by the education received by the adults who joined the Deaf commu-nity on leaving school.

The 1970s were a period of upheaval in the thinking with respect to deaf education. In 1965, Stokoe, Casterline, and Croneberg had published the results of linguistic research, which showed that the sign language used by the American Deaf community was not a mere collection of pantomime and gesture but a real language. Pressure from deaf organizations led to the introduction of signing into schools, and this development was followed by similar demands in Britain.

The current situation in Britain is by no means uniform. No official policy has been adopted by British schools, especially because 85% of British deaf children are now increasingly educated outside deaf schools, a figure that was determined after a survey conducted by the British Association of Teachers of the Deaf in 1994. However, changes are occurring rapidly within the British education system. As Adam Walker, a prominent spokesman for DEX, the society of Deaf ex-mainstreamers, pointed out in a conversation in February 1999, more recently, figures as high as 93% and 97% have been quoted by the National Deaf Children's Society with respect to those deaf children being educated outside of deaf schools. No longer do any schools rely exclusively on fingerspelling for communication. Some schools (in three areas, Leeds, Derby, and Birmingham) have recently introduced bilingualism, attempting to teach English through BSL, but this approach will have problems of its own, not least, the shortage of qualified teachers of the deaf with adequate BSL skills and fingerspelling skills (Llwellyn-Jones 1991). Fingerspelling now has a different part to play in the language of the Deaf community now that BSL is being accepted as a language in its own right.

CONCLUSION

Hearing educators have frequently considered the manual alphabet to be an important pedagogical tool for deaf children because of its link with English. Both manualists and oralists have used the manual alphabet to certain extents, each believing it to be a part of their philosophy. The form of the British manual alphabet has changed throughout the last 400 years from a system used primarily by hearing people to one adopted by the British deaf education system. Acceptance of the manual alphabet in the education system meant that it rapidly became stabilized across the country. From its early use with deaf people to teach spoken and written English, fingerspelling has formed a continuous thread throughout the history of British deaf education. Now that policies of language use with deaf children have been overtaken by integrationist policies that set children in mainstream schools, overt discussion of the use and importance of fingerspelling are rare. However, fingerspelling as a tool for allowing signers to manually represent English-based forms still has a place in the signing of Britain's modern Deaf community.

ACKNOWLEDGMENTS

Much of the research for this paper was funded by the Economic and Social Research Council (ESRC), grant number R00429024933. I would like to thank Bencie Woll, now at City University in London, for ideas and suggestions in this work and also Mary Plackett of the RNID library (a cooperative venture between the Royal National Institute for Deaf People and University College London Library) for her help with the older texts cited here. Bridget Peace drew the illustration in figure 2.1.

Notes

1. An uppercase *D* is used in the word *Deaf* to refer to those who are members of a Deaf culture and community (after Woodward 1978). A lowercase *d* in the word *deaf* refers to those with hearing loss. Where deaf identity cannot be identified, the lowercase *d* will be used.

References

Many of the older references cited here can be found in the Royal National Institute for Deaf People (RNID) Library in London.

Abraham, E. 1895. How to popularise the manual alphabet. *British Deaf Monthly* 5:299.

———. 1897. Yet another alphabet. *British Deaf Monthly* 7:83.

Arnold, Thomas. 1886. Prevention of signs among junior pupils. *Quarterly Review of Deaf-Mute Education* 1:69–76.

———. 1888. *Education of deaf-mutes.* London: Wertheimer, Lea and Co.

Arrowsmith, John Pauncefoot. 1819. *The art of instructing the infant deaf and dumb.* London: Taylor and Hessey.

Ash, Henry. 1889. *Guide to chirology.* Britain: n.p.

Banham, Deborah. 1991. *Monasteriales indicia: The Anglo-Saxon monastic sign language.* Pinner, Middlesex: Anglo-Saxon Books.

Barakat, Robert. 1987. Cistercian sign language. In *Monastic sign languages,* ed. Jean Umiker-Sebeok and Thomas A. Sebeok, 67–322. Berlin: Mouton de Gruyter.

Bell, Alexander Graham. 1883. Upon a method of teaching language to a very young congenitally deaf child. *American Annals of the Deaf and Dumb* 28:133.

Bonet, Juan. 1620. *Reduccion de las letras y arte para ensenar a ablar los mudos.* Madrid: Abarca de Angulo.

Brennan, Mary. 1992. The visual world of BSL. In *The dictionary of British Sign Language/English,* ed. David Brien, 1–133. London: Faber.

Bulwer, John. 1644. *Chirologia: Or the natural language of the hand.* London: R. Whitaker.

———. 1648. *Philocophus: Or the deafe and dumbe man's friende.* London: Humphrey Moseley.

Buxton, David. 1875. Notices of publications. *American Annals of the Deaf and Dumb* 20:114.

———. 1886. The manual alphabet. *Quarterly Review of Deaf-Mute Education* 1:83–89.

Carmel, Simon. 1981. *International hand alphabet charts.* 2d ed. Rockville: Carmel.

Conferences of British Instructors of the Deaf and Dumb. 1853. *American Annals of the Deaf and Dumb* 5:253.

Conrad, Ruben, and Barbara Weiskrantz. 1984. Deafness in the seventeenth century: Into empiricism. *Sign Language Studies* 45:291–399.

Dalgarno, George. 1680. *Didascalocophus, or the deaf and dumb man's tutor.* London: J. Hayes.

DeChaves, Teresa L., and Jorge L. Soler. 1980. Pedro Ponce de León, first teacher of the Deaf. *Sign Language Studies* 5:48–63.

Defoe, Daniel. 1732. *The life and adventures of Duncan Campbell.* London: E. Curll.

De l'Epée, Charles Michel. 1784. *La véritable manière d'instruire les sourds et muets, confirmée par une longue expérience.* Paris: Nyon.

Dictionary of D & D Signs. 1895. *Our Monthly Church Messenger to the Deaf* 2:2, 77, 131.

Digby, Kenelm. 1644. *Treatise on the nature of bodies.* Paris: n.p.

Digiti lingua. 1698. London: P. Buck.

Evans, Lionel. 1978. Visual communication in the deaf: Lipreading, fingerspelling and sign-ing. Ph.D. diss., University of Newcastle Upon Tyne.

Fay, E. 1881. The methods of the British schools. *American Annals of the Deaf and Dumb* 26:187–92.

Graves, Robert. 1952. *The white goddess: A historical grammar of poetic myth*. London: Faber.

Green, Francis. 1783. *Vox occulis subjecta*. London: Benjamin White.

Guide to the silent language of the deaf. [1890?]. Belfast: Francis Maginn.

Hay, John, and Raymond Lee. 1994. *A pictorial history of the evolution of the British manual alphabet*. Middlesex: British Deaf History Society Publications.

Hippisley Tuckfield, Mrs. 1839. *Education for the people*. London: Taylor and Walton.

Holder, William. 1669. *Elements of speech*. London: Royal Society.

Jussen, Heribert. 1973. *Das graphembestimmte Manualsystem als Sprachlernhilfe bei Gehörlosen*. Cologne: Jussen.

Kitto, John. 1845. *The lost senses*. Edinburgh: Oliphant, Anderson and Ferrier.

Lane, Harlan, ed. 1984. *The deaf experience*. Cambridge, Mass.: Harvard University Press.

Lane, Harlan, Robert Hoffmeister, and Ben Bahan. 1996. *A journey into the deaf world*. San Diego: DawnSign Press.

Lewis, M. 1968. *The education of deaf children: The possible place of fingerspelling and signing*. London: Her Majesty's Stationery Office.

Llwellyn-Jones, Miranda. 1991. Bilingualism and the education of deaf children. In *Con-structing deafness*, ed. Susan Gregory and Gillian Hartley, 137–42. London: Pinter.

Lucas, T. M. 1812. *Chyrology, or the art of reading, spelling and ciphering by the fingers*. London: Lucas.

Manual Alphabets . . . . 1903. *The British Deaf Times* 1:2.

Martins, Mário. 1958. Livros de sinais. *Boletim de Filologia* 17:293–357.

McCracken, Wendy, and Hilary Sutherland. 1992. *Deaf-ability, not disability*. Clevedon: Mul-tilingual Matters.

Peet, Harvey. 1851. Analysis of Bonet's treatise on the art of teaching the dumb to speak. *American Annals of the Deaf and Dumb* 3:200–211.

Peet, Isaac. 1868. Initial signs. *American Annals of the Deaf and Dumb* 13:171–84.

Pullen, Gloria, and Jim Kyle. 1997. Deaf elderly people. Report to the Deaf Studies Trust. University of Bristol.

Rhind, Charles. n.d. *Illustrated lessons for the deaf and dumb*. Britain: n.p.

Roe, W. 1893. Illustration of the manual alphabet. *Our Deaf and Dumb* 1:64.

Rossellius. 1579. *Thesaurus artificosae memoriae*. Venice.

Royal National Institute for Deaf People. 2001. Statistics on deafness. Retrieved on Decem-ber 10, 2001, from the World Wide Web: http://www.rnid.org.uk/html/info_factsheets_general_statistics_on_deafness.htm

R. R. 1809. *The invited alphabet; or address of A to B*. London: R. Tabart and Co.

Savage, Robert D., Lionel Evans, and J. F. Savage. 1981. *Psychology and communication in deaf children*. Sydney: Grune and Stratton.

Seigel, Jules Paul. 1969. The enlightenment and the evolution of a language of signs in France and England. *Journal of the History of Ideas* 30:96–115.

Smith, Samuel. 1864. *The deaf and dumb*. London: William Mackintosh.

Stokoe, William C., Dorothy C. Casterline, and Carl G. Croneberg. 1965. *A dictionary of American Sign Language on linguistic principles*. Washington, D.C.: Gallaudet College Press.

Sutton-Spence, Rachel. 1994. The role of the manual alphabet and fingerspelling in British Sign Language. Ph.D. diss., University of Bristol.

Sutton-Spence, Rachel, and Bencie Woll. 1999. *The linguistics of British Sign Language: An introduction*. Cambridge: Cambridge University Press.

Watson, Joseph. 1809. *Instruction of the deaf and dumb*. London: Darton and Harvey.

Wilkins, J. 1641. *Mercury: Or the secret and swift messenger*. London: John Maynard and Timothy Wilkins.

Woodward, James. 1978. Historical bases of American Sign Language. In *Understanding language through sign language research*, ed. Patricia Siple, 333–48. New York: Academic Press.

3 Austria's Hidden Conflict: Hearing Culture Versus Deaf Culture

Franz Dotter and Ingeborg Okorn

The goal of this chapter is to examine the situation of deaf people from an Austrian perspective and to compare this situation to general patterns of social behavior. A key characteristic of the situation is the conflict between hearing and deaf culture, rarely perceived by the larger Austrian society. We see only its result: the suffering of the people in a weaker position—deaf people themselves, many times hearing parents of deaf children, and sometimes interpreters and teachers. The effects of this conflict include inadequate access to the benefits of hearing society, ostracization, illness, and frustration. This conflict has deep-seated, partially tabooed, multifaceted causes. In many hearing and deaf people—possibly also in ourselves, one hearing and one deaf researcher—there are at least residues of thought patterns and behaviors that promote these problems instead of solve them. Before we discuss how this conflict manifests itself today, however, we will look at its origins by considering the history of deaf people in Austria.

EARLY DEAF HISTORY

The first Austrian school for the deaf (Taubstummeninstitut) was established in Vienna in 1779 after a visit by Emperor Joseph II to Abbé de l'Epée's school in Paris. This facility was the third government-sponsored school in Europe, following Paris (1769) and Leipzig (1778). Daughter institutions of the Viennese Institute were founded all over the Austro-Hungarian empire, including schools in Prague and Milan.[1] Confronted by competing methods—the manualist "French method" and the oralist "German method"—the Viennese institution developed a mixed method, using written language, signs, and a manual alphabet as a base for learning spoken language. These teaching methods were supposedly invented by Joseph May and Michöl Venus (Bundes-Taubstummeninstitut Wien 1979; Schott 1995).[2] From 1827 on, courses were provided for teachers of deaf students. Through these courses, the Viennese school of deaf education influenced teaching throughout Europe, including institutes in Germany, Copenhagen, St. Petersburg, Vilnius, and Warsaw. In 1867, the mixed method was discontinued in Austria in favor of the German method, which was also subsequently endorsed by the Milan Congress of 1880.

Deaf Associations

The Viennese institute has always operated as a charitable organization, with major donations from the rich parents of some pupils and from the emperor's family. In 1865, because of the social problems experienced by many former pupils (no social security system existed), a relief association was founded with help from the school. In 1875, this association was renamed Wiener Taubstummen-Unterstützungsverein (WTU); it was dissolved in 1938 after being outdistanced by the rival Wiener Taubstummenfürsorgeverein (WITAF), founded in 1929. The WTU at first accepted only males. Women founded their own association in 1874, though the authorities decided that men should control its budget (Schott 1995, 180–84).[3] Other local deaf associations were founded soon afterwards (Salzburg in 1899, Graz in 1903). Day pupils of the Viennese deaf school founded a sports club in 1901. A journal was also founded at the school (*Taubstummen-Kurier*, later called *Taubstummen-Revue*). In August 1913, at the Eleventh Deaf Meeting (*Taubstummentag*) in Graz, a parent organization of Austrian deaf clubs (or "unions") was founded. It was dissolved during the Nazi period in Austria from 1938 to 1945 but was refounded in 1946.[4]

Under the monarchy in the 19th century, many deaf people came to Vienna, the most important center of Austrian deaf culture. The number of deaf people in Vienna at that time has been estimated at about 1,000, with about ten local clubs. Similar to the hearing culture, certain cafés became meeting places for deaf people. After World War I, in the context of revolutionary movements in Middle and Eastern Europe, the deaf also founded a *Taubstummenrat*, which organized a large assembly in 1919. This assembly demanded a combined method of education, including sign and written language, reminiscent of the former Viennese method. The socialist government of the "Red Vienna" of the 1920s and the director of the deaf school in Döbling organized a working group that helped establish some services for members of the deaf community. These services included some early social science initiatives—compilation of statistics, free legal advice—and some educational activities, including the training of deaf apprentices.

The State of Research on Deaf History in Austria

For a review of Austrian deaf history, we have only Prohazka (1988). Schott (1995) is a useful source for the time from 1779 up to 1918 (though mainly from a hearing perspective). In 1979, a brochure (Bundes-Taubstummeninstitut Wien 1979) was published for the 200th anniversary of the Viennese school. This brochure, however, was totally oriented to oralism, even defending oral methods against other methods.

In Austria, many different deaf clubs operated at various times. Over the years, the records of these clubs have frequently been lost. Additional documents were lost during World Wars I and II as well as other conflicts. The result is a significant lack of written history from a deaf perspective. Prohazka (1988) provides some circumstantial evidence about financial problems and conflicts among various clubs. A signed (or even an oral) history is additionally complicated by memory gaps (or repression), which occur even when deaf people are questioned by deaf interviewers. This lack of information about Austrian deaf history is the reason that our research center mounted an exhibition on deafness in Austria.[5]

THE LINGUISTIC SITUATION OF THE DEAF BEFORE WORLD WAR II

Interpreting the little information we have, the scenario seems to be that deaf education conformed to the general Austrian pedagogical orientation of the period. It was authoritarian, whether or not it followed the Viennese mixed or German oral methods. The decision to change to the German method worsened the situation for deaf people, because signing was forbidden not only in class but also during free time. But—at least from what we know from deaf narratives—there was a sort of schizophrenia during the whole period. Most of the teachers "knew" (though many would not have confessed it officially) that they needed signs or signing in emergency cases, when spoken or written language did not suffice, to convey minimal information. And though signing varied from school to school and from time to time, it was somehow tolerated during leisure time. Additionally, because most deaf children attended boarding school, they had a lot of time to communicate with one another and, thus, acquired sign language and a deaf identity. On a wider scale, however, the moderate demand of the Austrian Deaf Association to use sign language systematically as an aid in education was never realized.

DEAF PEOPLE UNDER NAZISM

For Germany, there is a comprehensive history of the deaf community for the time period (Biesold 1988 [in German], 1999 [in English]; for another English source on all disabled children, see Rogow 1998; for deaf people, see Soudakoff 1999). In short, under the auspices of the German *Rassenhygiene* (race hygiene or eugenics), deaf people fell under the Gesetz zur Verhütung erbkranken Nachwuchses (Law for the Prevention of Offspring with Hereditary Diseases) of July 14, 1933 (Grassl 1990). Under that law, an estimated 15,000 hereditarily deaf people were sterilized. It is not clear, however, how many deaf people were among the estimated 75,000 victims of the euthanasia program for those who were disabled (Vienna's Spiegelgrund, a notorious psychiatric clinic, was a major site for killings of this kind). Jewish members were expelled from Germany's deaf clubs starting in 1933; the same thing occurred in Austria after the *Anschluss* (the occupation of Austria by Germany) in 1938. Jewish deaf institutions were closed by law on June 30, 1942 (Biesold 1996). In spite of the sterilization program and the neglect of deaf schools financially and in personnel matters, deaf youth participated in a Hitlerjugend (Hitler Youth) deaf organization with its own periodical (*Die Quelle, The Fountain*).

Although almost no published material has been found on the subject, we can assume that the situation in Austria after the *Anschluss* in 1938 was similar to that in Germany. Some indirect evidence such as that contained in the short histories of the Austrian regional deaf associations in *75 Jahre . . . Österreichischer Gehörlosen-*

bund 1913–1988 (Österreichischer Gehörlosenbund 1988) seems to confirm this theory.[6] In addition a Jewish deaf institution had operated in Vienna (cf. Schott 1999). At the same time, the Österreichischer Gehörlosenbund (Austrian Deaf Association) merged as Reichsverband Ostmark (The Austrian Empire's Union) into the Reichsverband der Gehörlosen Deutschlands (Reich Union of the Deaf of Germany), which had placed itself under the command of the German National Socialist Party in 1937. (Photos of Austrian deaf people wearing Nazi uniforms have been found.)

In 1938, immediately after the *Anschluss*, representatives of the Lower Austrian deaf founded a club in collaboration with the Reichsverband Ostmark. Similar local clubs (*Ortsbünde*, or local clubs, in Nazi party terminology) have also been attested to in the town of Zell am See and in the Lungau region, both in the province of Salzburg. One of the younger founders of the deaf association during the monarchy, Karl J. Brunner, seems to have been the chairman of the Reichsverband Ostmark.

The Viennese Jewish deaf people were sharply divided between the hereditary deaf and the "accidentally" deaf people. Apparently, an understandable strategy of "everyone for himself" seems to have existed. Many deaf people hoped that joining the Nazi party would save them. This lack of unity and concern for individual survival seems to be the main reason why the time between 1938 and 1945 is not really dealt with in our few sources (especially in Österreichischer Gehörlosenbund 1988).

Following the tendency to ignore this era, many people accept the general rule that "the world begins" only after 1945 (such as the founding of the club in Wiener Neustadt). Any evidence indicating that structures established before 1945 continued after the war is vague or indirect. For example, although the club of St. Veit, Carinthia, had the same chairperson from 1937 to 1948 and although the Deaf Club of Tirol got a new chairman from 1938 to 1944, was closed down in 1944–1945 and was refounded in 1946, we find no evidence showing how the chairpersons of these clubs acted, either for or against the Nazis, or whether they acted politically at all.[7]

POST–WORLD WAR II SCHOOLS, DEAF INSTITUTIONS, AND LANGUAGE

After World War II, an umbrella organization was created, which brought together all Austrian deaf clubs, including those in the provinces. In 1963, Heinrich Prohazka, one of the founders of the Austrian Deaf Association after the war, deplored the low efficiency of the Austrian deaf organization compared with those in other countries. He identified two reasons: the lack of self-identification by the deaf and the lack of support from authorities (Prohazka 1988). The lack of self-identification in particular is very different from the actively involved deaf school graduates before World War I.

THE CONTINUATION OF PRE-WAR EDUCATION

The use of authoritarian methods in (deaf and hearing) education lasted until the 1960s when authoritarianism gradually weakened. This fact partially explains why the relevant history of the 1933–1945 period and the following period into the 1960s has not been examined (see Möckel 1988, 226–32 for a review). The authoritarian system, however, remained in place much longer in deaf education. The following quotation from 1982 and requoted in 1987 could be labeled "isolation and pressure as an educational principle":

> We can assume that a deaf person will acquire the system of the spoken language only if he or she is exclusively trained in spoken language. The investigation results mentioned above point to a longer acquisition period for deaf children in comparison to hearing children. If they are trained in more than one linguistic system, they seem to choose the easier forms . . . and not speech. (Affolter and Bischofberger 1982, 615; in Uden 1987, 171)

This authoritarianism led to split results. Those pupils who could deal with the authoritarian oral method got partially good spoken-language knowledge. The others, suffering from the effects of the method, stopped at a developmental level of language that is almost incredible. For example, the only Austrian hospital department for deaf people (including ambulant patients) is in a Linz hospital run by the Brothers of St. John of God; it has patients who know fewer than 1,000 terms in signed or spoken-written language, and some know fewer than 300.

THE ORALIST VIEW

All following quoted texts with the exception of Köble (1969) were written in the 1980s and later. Most examples are from German authors who are specialists in scientific pedagogy, psychology, or applied psychology (for further examples, see Dotter 1991; for the United States and other countries, see Lane 1993). Substitute *black* for *deaf* in these texts and one understands immediately why these opinions are no longer tolerable. The oralist view asserts the superiority of the hearing population and the inferiority of the deaf. Hearing people are "fully developed" human beings to whom deaf people "should feel attracted" because

> [a]n intimate conversation with a comprehensible, culturally elevated hearing person gives pleasure to a deaf person. Whether a deaf child or adult gets the opportunity to have a relaxed conversation with a hearing person depends on whether the deaf person can speak well, whether he is far enough along in his development (including his spoken vocabulary), and most of all whether he is sincere with others and not too self-centered. (Uden 1987, 241–42)

We can find similar ideas (sometimes put differently) in the attitude toward "underdeveloped ethnic communities" or "humans of a lower level," the same thinking that culminated in imperialist ideologies. This kind of viewpoint almost forces its adherents to see it as their duty to bring their culture to the uncivilized, to undertake the ethical task of forming "the perfect human":

> We are of the opinion that deaf people can be won over to our society and its world view. We are striving to enable hearing-impaired (as well as deaf) children to use the spoken language. We believe that they are

human beings like you and me and are worth the effort. Those in favor of Sign Language firmly believe that deaf people are different from hearing people. Therefore the choice between spoken and sign language is also an ethical decision. (Breiner n.d., 15)

The determined rejection of sign language reveals remnants of attitudes that may be classified as paternalistic and authoritarian, even colonialist and racist, with respect to deaf people. For a long time, the fact that signed languages are languages was denied, and many residues of this opinion are still ingrained in individuals, including government and school officials as well as teachers. They defend their opinion by pointing out the presumed lack of efficiency of signed languages. Note that the following quote is from a linguist who is the son of a proponent of German "content-related grammar" (*inhaltsbezogener Grammatik*), whose advocates were sometimes in close contact with fascism; Helmut Gipper is one of very few linguists who put forth an opinion normally found only among nonlinguists (such as Schulte 1989):[8]

Sign Language can transfer only a small part of the semantic features characterizing linguistic content to the visual mode. In theory, it might be possible to express visually all of the semantically relevant elements. However, this would lead to an uncontrollable torrent of signs and would take too much time to be efficient. (Gipper 1987, 15)

Herbert Breiner (n.d.) provides another example of a psychologically oriented and far-reaching rejection of sign language, this time rationalizing it with aesthetics. He is director of the Pfalzinstitut in Germany, which advocates oral education of the deaf with the help of vibrational stimuli and is one of the most extreme opponents of sign language.

The movements of a sign are big, clumsy, and attract the attention of the addressee. They are dominant, covering the articulatory movements of the mouth, even aggressively pushing them aside. Signs completely differ in form and distribution of energy (in speed, rhythm and realization) from the articulatory movements of the mouth. Thus the structures of spoken language cannot be firmly established. Effective oral instruction is no longer possible. The time needed for the production of signs and spoken language is different. Signing influences the child's temporal perception of linguistic events, making it less subtle. (Breiner n.d., 12)

As modern educational theory opened the way for a more liberal and democratic education, oralists adopted a strategy of misusing modern educational terms to mask their unchanged practice. For example, *integration* when used by oralists camouflages their unchanged goal of deaf assimilation into spoken-language society, thus creating a new way to veil the underlying structural violence. This intention is also clear from oralists' ongoing denigration of deaf associations.

But there was worse to come. Antonius van Uden (1987), director of the famous deaf school of Sint Michielsgestel in the Netherlands and a militant oralist, advocated denying deaf people the right to marry other deaf people and promoted their marriage to hearing people, an interesting reversal of the racial principles of the Third Reich. Uden also maintained that, in addition, these mixed marriages ought to stay childless.

We first thought that the attitudes we have discussed here were typical only of German-speaking countries. Certainly, the fascist era could have reinforced these feelings, but think of all the scientific precursors of fascist theories from 1900 on, for example, Robert von Erdberg, Jean A. Gobineau, or Charles S. Chamberlain, who come from Germany, France, and Great Britain respectively.[9] Although the European Union is relatively progressive in deaf matters, our experience with it (particularly with some officials and representatives from southern Europe) raises doubts about whether these problems are confined to German-speaking areas. The present situation in Germany, Austria, and comparable European countries is that deaf people are the last group to have their human rights recognized. Some scientists, for example, continue to argue against acknowledging autochthonous sign languages.

We also should not forget the professional interests involved in the situation. In the contemporary Austrian educational system, teachers of the deaf are asked to take a certain number of hours of sign language instruction but do not need to pass an exam. Hearing professionals, therefore, do have legitimate though rarely confirmed fears:

> Have we not got various possibilities to render the lessons more intensive and illustrative without automatically pushing aside the hearing teacher? The frequently expressed fear that hearing-impaired education might focus on hearing-impaired teachers need not become reality in a sensible model of scholastic education. (Hintermair 1995, 58)

See Migsch (1987) for an insightful description of the official and psychological situation of the teachers in the Austrian school system before integration.

ILLNESS AND REPAIR METAPHORS

In our opinion, authoritarian ideologies merge with metaphors of illness and repair and are applied more widely than to deaf people alone. These metaphors have been deeply internalized by many professionals working with disabled people. They even affect the professionals' picture of the relationship between a mother and her deaf child. This relationship is seen as "expectedly abnormal." Mothers (and, in other contexts, teachers) are held responsible for incomplete communicative, linguistic, and cognitive development of children.

> The special perceptive situation of deaf people necessitates a therapeutically supervised acquisition period. This is much more difficult than is normally the case, for both the children and their social environment. There is some sort of teacher-pupil contact between the mother and her child if she is at all able and willing to interact adequately with a handicapped person. (Hogger 1990, 120)

As a consequence of this thinking, we find general statements such as Köble's: "There can never exist a deaf child who is psychically healthy" (1969, 156). These metaphors allow many professionals to continue a practice that they themselves recognize as insufficient. Despite the fact that these educational efforts often do not lead to success, it is better, they argue, to try to "repair" children according to some prescribed image of what deaf children should be than to compensate by using strategies such as teaching in sign language.

The last, most absurd step in this pattern of thinking is promoted by Weber (1995), who states that the relationship between mothers and deaf children must be "ill" in psychoanalytic terms, and therefore, deafness must come from a deep conflict between mother and child. This statement is blatantly incorrect but nevertheless accepted by one program in Zurich and published by a distinguished press in the field of deafness (Groos in Heidelberg).[10] Hearing people are not the only ones to use these metaphors. Among deaf people, they surface in the form of feelings of inferiority.

THE STRUGGLE: WEAPONS USED IN THE DEBATE

Limited Acceptance of Signing

In the last few years, some orally oriented educators, psychologists, and politicians have become more open to signing. This development does not mean that sign language is used systematically, and this new acceptance is far from being a bilingual model of education (Dotter and Holzinger 1995). The people who advocate this more open attitude would never think of blaming their predecessors for their failures (see Jussen 1994a). Instead, they draw a picture of deaf education as evolving in an undisturbed, well-designed fashion. This approach is one key strategy, we have learned, to overcome the past without coping with the past. This strategy allows the creation of new niches instead of abolishing "disturbances":

> As a next step we ought to discuss the introduction of a subject like *Gehörlosenkunde* (Deaf science) or *Gehörlosenkultur* (Deaf culture) [into the curriculum for deaf pupils]. . . . There one would have the opportunity of practicing, teaching and cultivating Sign Language. In addition, this would provide us with the chance to deal with Deaf culture: everything deaf people created on the basis of their different perceptions—their own norms, habits, institutions, and works of art. I for one do not see any disturbing effects on the orally-oriented phases of the instruction, but rather think that the variety of opportunities produces additional motivation for spoken-language activities and discussions. (Hintermair 1995, 55)

Pfaffhausen (1995) is in favor of sign language use, but only when it is limited to the training of children with multiple handicaps. This position can be interpreted as another strategy to deal with the demand for sign language: "Use it only with children where normal oral pedagogy is at its end" (see also Tings, Rink, and Pasligh 1995).

Misuse of the Cochlear Implant

Cochlear implants (CIs) have become an increasingly important oralist tool. CIs do improve hearing ability. Completely or nearly completely deaf can improve their acoustic hearing range to that of a person with an average-to-high hearing impairment. Nevertheless, this improvement carries no guarantee that it will be sufficient for the acquisition of spoken language. Much assistance is still necessary. However, especially in German-speaking countries, the CI is not seen as merely a useful technological aid. The oralists view it as an additional important reason to do without sign language.

The extensive use of CIs is seen as drastically reducing the number of "real" deaf people. Thus, it is argued, one has no need to consider other communicative means between the diagnosis and the surgery. We will not go further into this issue here, but other factors in this debate include the clear differences in behavior between hearing and deaf parents of deaf children.[11] A telling indication of the larger oralist orientation of the Austrian government, however, is that CIs are financed by state institutions whereas no supplemental financing of deaf children without implants is provided.[12]

Ignorance, Indifference, and Oralism

Nearly all the officials responsible for deaf education in Austria are either oralists themselves or are uninformed about the question. Therefore, they listen to mostly oralist-oriented experts. At the same time, contradictory information is withheld from political decision makers. A few oralists exercise power by controlling not only networks in the leading deaf educational institutions (such as childhood audiological information centers) but also key government offices and medical institutions. Thus, they are easily able to counter other educational theories. Consequently, many hearing people or institutions controlled by hearing people either do not understand the needs of deaf people or deliberately ignore them. The true source of deaf people's alleged "language handicap" is the lack of access to sign language even as simply one alternative in a bilingual effort. Too many doctors, psychologists, educators, and educational institutions continue to advise against allowing children and adults this vital access (Dotter 1993; for an account on the situation of deaf women, see Kölblinger 1993).

Reactions of the Deaf Community

The Austrian deaf community has had and continues to have almost no reaction to these oralist views except, perhaps, general rejection and resignation. One reason is that many deaf people cannot easily read the texts in which these views are purported, so they simply do not know them and their contents. Because members of deaf culture are often illiterate, they are almost entirely excluded from the discussions about education methods. Jarmer's work (1997) is the first university thesis on the linguistic and pedagogical situation of the deaf community written by a deaf person. The situation could be improved by the passage of the Austrian Antidiscrimination Paragraph, a 1997 amendment to the constitution. So far, however, this paragraph has been used only to analyze other laws and not to combat more general discrimination.

THE PRESENT SITUATION IN AUSTRIA

The previous description is valid not only for Austria but also for parts of other German-speaking countries. Let us now focus specifically on Austria. Awareness of deafness-related issues is still very low. If one mentions these issues, one gets interested but stereotypical questions (Why are they not allowed to use their sign language everywhere? Does sign language fulfill the same tasks as spoken language? Wouldn't sign language be useful for worldwide communication?).

With officials in higher positions and politicians, another pattern is evident. Many may advocate deaf interests at some point; they start wavering on the issue, however, when pressured by the other side. In other words, when pressured, they start arguing that the systematic use of sign language, a rethinking of deaf education, or even acknowledging sign language at all would not be necessary.[13] Moreover, when these hearing officials learn that these issues involve numerous controversies, not only among hearing educators and in the scientific literature but also among deaf people, they stop advocating deaf interests.

EDUCATION SINCE THE 1970s

Sign language has become more important over the last three decades. By law, since the 1970s, a few hours each week must be dedicated to *Gebärdenpflege* (cultivating signs—not sign language) in deaf schools. In addition, the use of visual means of communication (including not only Austrian Sign Language but also Signed German) has grown noticeably since the beginning of the 1990s. Despite this opening, the situation in preschools, elementary and secondary schools, and adult education still has far to go, and there is practically no research evidence to support sign language education in Austria. In addition, no materials for systematic teaching have been developed. Currently, individual deaf people work as assistants with hearing teachers, but—as far as we know—only one deaf teacher is employed (in the Viennese Deaf School).

The law does not yet acknowledge the need for either a systematic bilingual education or a policy permitting a wide range of possibilities for communication. There were and are only a few people (mainly officials) who have the opportunity to influence the Austrian government's policy on deaf people, and none is convinced that a bilingual model or a liberal range of diverse options would improve the situation for the deaf community.[14] We are not arguing that any of these people are enemies of either bilingualism or a diverse range of options, rather, that they remain unconvinced that these methods offer solutions. One of the main arguments they make is that statements from experts are contradictory (cf. Gruber and Ledl 1992: 154).[15]

Beginning in 1993, a number of major reforms in the Austrian school system were made. The New School Organization Law has meant a change from educating disabled children in separate kindergartens or schools to creating the possibility of mainstreaming them in "normal" classes or schools (*gemeinsamer Unterricht*, or joint classes). Given Austria's long history of segregationist and authoritarian school policies, this action is a very positive measure. Our criticism of the alternatives available for deaf students should not be seen as a criticism of this measure. Under this law, within the limits of schools' regional and financial situations, the parents of a child with special needs can opt freely for mainstreaming or for a special school. The option for special schooling was one of the main reasons for the law's political acceptance. We therefore get different regional "solutions." For example, the deaf school in Carinthia closed in summer 1998 and all the children were mainstreamed whereas the special school for the deaf in Vienna has enough pupils to remain open.

Mainstreaming has changed or will change completely deaf children's situations for those regions where the decision for integration is unanimous: Deaf children can stay at schools near home, attending classes where they meet the children from next door. There are several systems of integration that we do not refer to here (see Gruber and Ledl 1992). One of the main characteristics of these systems is a support teacher (*Stützlehrer*) for the integrated disabled children. Because very different special needs are represented in a local classroom, there is little chance that two or more children with the same special needs would be in one place. We, therefore, cannot expect every teacher to be able to sign. The "language problem" of the mainstreamed deaf pupils has not yet been addressed.

SIGN LANGUAGE RESEARCH

Sign language research in Austria is rather new as is research dealing with bilingual education (e.g., see Grbic 1994; Rainer 1996) and began accidentally. The Klagenfurt case is typical in some respects. Magret Pinter and Monika Pöllabauer, two teachers of deaf children, noticed the backwardness of deaf education in Austria and, at their own expense, studied international developments. Although the Ministry of Education refused to grant them funding, the ministry had only shortly before allowed a project on bilingual education in the Klagenfurt Deaf School (compare Pinter 1992). An older student, Julia Gruber, encouraged Pinter and Pöllabauer to contact the local university at Klagenfurt. The first scientific project began in July 1990, and the work is ongoing (see Dotter 1999; and the home page of the Research Center for Sign Language and Deaf Communication <http://www.uni-klu.ac.at/fzgs>).

The Department for Interpreting at the University of Graz opened in 1990, a reaction to information about sign language interpreting on television broadcasts from nearby Slovenia. They modeled their Austrian Sign Language interpreting program after a German Sign Language program in Hamburg. In 1995, Daniel Holzinger became the first clinical linguist at the Department for Deaf Patients in Linz. Since 1997, all three institutions, together with the Austrian Deaf Association, have coordinated sign language activities in Austria. They are also involved in international research. This area is now well established in Austria, and the work is done in close contact with the Austrian Deaf community.

The first issue of a descriptive grammar of Austrian Sign Language was published by the Klagenfurt Research Center in July 2002. A contract with the Ministry of Education, Science, and the Arts provided funding for further work on the lexicon (including a database). The program for interpreters of Austrian Sign Language in Graz was made permanent in the summer of 2002.

RECOGNITION OF SIGN LANGUAGE IN AUSTRIA, GERMAN-SPEAKING COUNTRIES, AND THE EUROPEAN UNION

Some of the Austrian politicians understand the needs of deaf people and try to promote them. As a result, in 1993, the Austrian parliament asked the government to report on the situation in Austria of the deaf, the hard of hearing, and those suffering from tinnitus. A committee with members from several relevant ministries was organized and worked for some time. From our perspective, the result was embarrassing. The report confirmed almost exclusively oralist positions (Dotter 1992, 1993). Deaf people, who were at least sometimes invited to state their case, were represented only by integrating their texts (which were in bad German) into the report. As the protocols show, these deaf people were not given appropriate communication support, which put them at a severe disadvantage, and statements made during the meetings were manipulated and deliberately misinterpreted.

Despite the federal government's hesitation, three provinces have given Austrian Sign Language better status. One province, Upper Austria, even finances some activities for the deaf community. The Austrian parliament has passed some limited measures to improve the situation (e.g., the right to demand a sign language interpreter in court and in official procedures). During the "Big Coalition" between Social Democrats and Conservatives that lasted until 1999, the government refused to recognize Austrian Sign Language, arguing the high costs of such measures, while the opposition parties voted for sign language recognition. In 1999, the government changed, and one of the former opposition parties, the Freiheitliche Partei (Freedom Party), became a coalition partner. But this party did not keep its promise to work for the recognition of Austrian Sign Language. Our contacts in government tell us that achieving recognition will not be an easy task. (However, in Germany, a law on recognition of German Sign Language passed the parliament in May 2002.)

Officially, the situation in the European Community is somewhat better (see Krausneker 1998; Centre for Deaf Studies 1998). In November 1998, the European Parliament renewed its original commitment to improving deaf lives in all member states (originally stated ten years before in 1988). Although deafness-related projects can get funded in some EC venues (the integration of people with special needs being one major goal of the EC), funding through programs that deal with languages or linguistic minorities has been blocked. No funding is available, for example, to develop material for Austrian Sign Language and a bilingual-multilingual education approach.

WHAT ARE THE NEXT STEPS?

We must not close our eyes to the problems of interaction and communication between deaf and hearing people. We need to realize, for example, that hearing people are in some danger of adopting a pattern of treating deaf adults like juveniles (a high official in Carinthia who is actively involved in social issues called deaf people "my children") or of developing a "helper syndrome." One result of this pattern is that when the "children" do not behave as expected, frustration sets in and contact is broken. Deaf people must get the opportunity to form their own scientific research groups and must become informed about the tactics of hearing opponents and the rules of hearing negotiation. One step toward this end would be for deaf groups to plan to mount exhibits at all important international and national conferences of psychologists, sociologists, medical practitioners, and other researchers, highlighting the importance of the responsible research and practices in the field of deafness.[16]

We must also continue to struggle against false "scientific standards" in the Austrian research community. This will not be easy.[17] Scientists who work against the human rights of deaf people must understand their responsibility in this matter. Instead of weighing arguments and results, these oralist researchers use manipulative strategies and misrepresent situations. This approach is especially true of the more militant representatives like Breiner, Diller (cf. 1995), Gipper, Jussen (1994b), Löwe, Schulte, and the late Kröhnert (Jussen and Kröhnert 1998) and Uden. They should not be redressed with emotional accusations, however. Rather, they must be shown that they are not meeting the standards of scientific work. The need for an intensive and comprehensive *Vergangenheitsbewältigung* (societal coping with the past) concerning deaf policy and education is clearly important not only now but also for the Nazi period.[18]

WHAT WILL HAPPEN?

The fact that a proposal for studying how deaf people can become sign language assistants in educational settings (written in 1997 by the Klagenfurt University and the Klagenfurt Institute for the Education of Teachers of Compulsory Schools, *Pädagogische Akademie*) has not gotten any response from the Ministry of Education is not surprising. Another unfunded project is a video with information for parents of deaf children.

Similarly, cases like that of "Anja," a Tyrolean deaf girl, are sadly common. At first, Anja was allowed to attend the specialized vocational school. After one year, however, permission to attend was withdrawn. Supposedly, Anja did not meet the standards for the second school year. But she had no tutoring throughout the first year, even though a former teacher had offered this service. Despite the fact that the ineffectual education given to her was the reason for this situation, Anja was blamed. Authorities said she was unfit for this vocational education, and they recommended that she go to an orally oriented deaf school in Germany instead.

However, in a more positive light, an increasing number of teachers are arguing for more liberal practices (see Fraundorfer 1991), and some institutions have begun to introduce more flexible education programs. More and more teachers of deaf pupils are also learning Austrian Sign Language, voluntarily exceeding required course work. In addition, requests are increasing for help in serving deaf patients in hospitals and emergency situations. The Austrian government has even sent signals (similar to earlier ones from the political opposition in parliament) that Austrian Sign Language could be acknowledged under certain conditions. The next few years may bring not only the recognition of sign language but also its use in educational settings. Unfortunately, rear-guard actions for oralism also continue. We hope, though, that we are witnessing the beginning of a new age in deaf education and politics.

ACKNOWLEDGMENTS

This article is based on work at the Research Center for Sign Language and Communication of the Hearing Impaired of Klagenfurt University—Head: Franz Dotter (hearing); collaborators: Elisabeth Bergmeister (deaf), Marlene Hilzensauer (hearing), Klaudia Krammer (hearing), Andrea Skant (hearing), Ingeborg Okorn (deaf), and Manuela Hobel (deaf). It was funded by Fonds zur Förderung der wissenschaftlichen Forschung, Arbeitsmarktservice Körnten and the European Social Fund. For translation of the quoted texts into English and for extensive help with the text of the article, we thank Marlene Hilzensauer and Andrea Skant. Last but not least, we thank Leila and Charles Monaghan for their careful editing.

NOTES

1.   These institutions include Prague, in 1786; Waitzen (now Vác in Hungary), in 1802 (McCagg 1993); Milan, in 1805; Linz, in 1812; Brixen (Italy) and Lemberg (now Lwiw in Ukrainia), in 1830; Salzburg, in 1831; Graz and Brünn (now Brno in the Czech Republic), in 1832; Pressburg (now Bratislava, Slovakia), in 1833; Goerz (now Gorica/Gorizia, a twin town in Slovenia/Italy), in 1840; Trient (now Trento in Italy), in 1842; St. Poelten, in 1846; and Klagenfurt, in 1847.

2.   Joseph May was a teacher of German who learned Epée's method at the Paris school together with Johann Friedrich Stork. Stork became the first director of the Vienna institute where he and May were the founding staff. May followed Stork as director from 1792 to 1819. Michöl Venus was the third director (1820–1850).

3.   Female teachers for the deaf were first allowed in 1887 by the Prussian government.

4.   Earlier, at the International Deaf Congress in Paris in 1912, the Austrian representatives proposed the foundation of a world association of the deaf. This idea was refused on the grounds that national associations should be founded first (Prohazka 1988, 72).

5.   We found some partners (a museum and a university department on contemporary history) and scheduled the exhibition for 2002.

6.   Although evidence clearly shows that many deaf people were sterilized (if not worse) under the Nazis, no Austrian deaf person has been willing to come forward and apply for compensation, which is now possible.

7.   For Germany, Stepf (1997) gives a short illustration of all (expectable) forms of behavior at this time.

8.   What we have here is a typical situation of an overwhelming majority and a minority whose image is relatively low. The attitudes of the majority about the so-called inefficiency of sign language and its "nonlinguistic" (i.e., not like spoken language) state reflect typical stereotypes. Of course, these evaluations contain some truth when we look at several deaf individuals (and we must not suppress this information). But we have to keep in mind the causes for this situation, which occurs when a speech community may not work at its language, improving it, using it in all (including modern) contexts; when a language is not adequately translated; when its respective culture is not completely understood or acknowledged; when almost all facts are interpreted and analyzed by hearing people (lexicon and grammar of sign languages can be shown as examples for this bias); and when there are inadequate and restrictive educational measures.

9.   In our eyes, fascist "theories" expressed only what was at least latent in important social strata. The fascists, in turn, made these ideas "fit for society" and officially usable. And "predecessor" does not mean that these people advocated fascism directly

(although some of them later publicly supported the Nazis); rather, they represented some schools of thought that made fascism possible. For the German-speaking area this includes the philosophers Nietzsche and Heidegger, the pedagogue Eduard Spranger, and historians such as Othmar Spann and Heinrich von Srbik.

10.   Of course, we must mention the many valuable publications and initiatives of the Hamburg Institute of German Sign Language and Communication of the Deaf as well as the publisher Signum.

11.   Publications such as Kammerer (1997) that look at more than one side of the argument are few. Most publications are in favor of CIs and do not reflect what actually happens to children with them (compare the studies quoted in http://www.liga-fuer-hoergeschödigte.de/ or journals like *ciimpulse*).

12.   We found only a few cases of deaf-community-friendly approaches to cochlear implants. One is from the Innsbruck deaf community where young deaf people meet with those using CIs. In this situation, people with CIs can move in both the deaf and the hearing culture, although most people with cochlear implants do not feel that they totally belong to the hearing community. In another case, the parents decided that their daughter should get a CI but also learn sign language as early as possible to give her the opportunity of deciding for herself later.

13.   Because all school laws must pass parliament with a two-thirds majority, negotiations sometimes continue for a long time before proposals are accepted by both sides.

14.   Because this article is the first publication to deal with the Austrian situation, these supporters should be named: Heinz Gruber (chief official for children with special needs in the Ministry of Education for many years), who pushed for integration after the failure of a first attempt that was formulated by Günther Hartmann when the parents' organizations began to demand it; Ulrich Koskarty (retired director of the Vienna Deaf School); and Karl Rieder (linguist and director of the Vienna School for the Hard of Hearing).

15.   We can illustrate the situation with anecdotal snapshots of deaf children and their parents:

- Deaf parents had to help their deaf daughter to read written texts by explaining them to her in sign language. The daughter told us that, in school, she understood nothing and had to learn everything at home afterwards. In the meantime, she has successfully finished her education.

- A daughter of hearing parents got a cochlear implant and never learned to sign. She went through hearing schools and academic studies successfully. Now she regrets that she has never had the opportunity to sign and to come into contact with deaf culture.

- The deaf son of hearing parents got a cochlear implant and received intensive help from both teachers and parents. He now is put forward as an example for the achievements of CIs. His parents go to many events where they argue against any use of sign language.

16.   Consider, however, when Franz Dotter tried to introduce the deaf theme to the 1996 German Congress on Sociology, the response was "We could not decide in favor of this theme!" When he then asked the presidency of the German Union of Sociologists how to handle the material in the long term, he got no answer at all.

17.   We have not been able to find any deaf people (or their parents) who have sued the government or a school management for deliberately reducing their (or their children's) opportunities by not allowing alternative educational methods.

18.   What we have learned from recent history is that, until the last representatives

of a political system are dead, a full analysis of the past does not seem possible. Residues of "fascist common sense" were strong through the 1960s and 1970s and are not extinct yet.

REFERENCES

Affolter, Félicie, and Walter Bischofberger. 1982. Psychologische Aspekte der Gehörlosig-keit. In *Pädagogik der Gehörlosen und Schwerhörigen*, ed. Heribert Jussen and Otto Kröhn-ert, 605–30. Berlin: Marhold.

Biesold, Horst. 1988. *Klagende Hände*. Solms-Oberbiel: Jarick Oberbiel.

———. 1996. Jüdische Taubstummenerziehung in Deutschland—dargestellt an der Gesch-ichte der "Israelitischen Taubstummenanstalt für Deutschland zu Berlin-Weißensee." In *Verloren und Un-Vergessen: Jüdische Heilpädagogik in Deutschland*, ed. Sieglind Ellger-Rüttgardt, 239–59. Einheim: Deutscher Studien Verlag.

———. 1999. *Crying hands: Eugenics and deaf people in Nazi Germany*. Introduction by H. Friedlander. Translated by W. Sayers. Washington, D.C.: Gallaudet University Press.

Breiner, Herbert L. n.d. *Information zur Arbeitsgemeinschaft Lautsprache und Integration für Gehörlose und Schwerhörige*. Frankenthal o.J.

Bundes-Taubstummeninstitut Wien, ed. 1979. *Taubstummeninstitut Wien 1779–1979: 200 Jahre Gehörlosenbildung*. Vienna: Bundes-Taubstummeninstitut.

Centre for Deaf Studies, ed. 1998. *Sign on Europe : A study of deaf people and sign language in the European Union*. Bristol: University of Bristol.

Diller, Gottfried. 1995. Hörgerichtetheit und psychische Grundleistungen. *Hörgeschädigtenpä-dagogik* 49:307–18.

Dotter, Franz. 1991. Gebärdensprache in der Gehörlosenbildung: Zu den Argumenten und Einstellungen ihrer Gegner. *Das Zeichen* 17:321–32.

———. 1992. Zur jüngsten Entwicklung bezüglich der Gebärdensprache in Österrreich. *Das Zeichen* 19:22–25.

———. 1993. Stellungnahme zum "Bericht der Bundesregierung betreffend Anerkennung der Gebärdensprache Gehörloser in Österreich aufgrund der Entschließung des Na-tionalrates vom 28. Jänner 1993." Klagenfurt. Mimeographed.

———. 1999. Gebärdensprachforschung in Klagenfurt. *Das Zeichen* 49:356–67.

Dotter, Franz, and Daniel Holzinger. 1995. Vorschlag zur Frühförderung gehörloser und schwer hörbehinderter Kinder in Österreich. *Der Sprachheilpädagoge* 27:1–21.

Fraundorfer, Stefan. 1991. Integration oder Assimilation? *Heilpädagogik* 34:51–57.

Gelter, Irmgard. 1987. Wortschatz und Lesefähigkeit gehörloser Schüler. *Der Sprachheilpäda-goge* 3:37–42.

Gipper, Helmut. 1987. Foreword to *Gebärdensprachen von Gehörlosen und Psycholinguistik*, by Antonius van Uden. Heidelberg: Groos.

Grassl, Markus. 1990. "Erbgesundheit" und nationalsozialistisches Recht. In *Nationalsozia-lismus und Recht*, ed. U. Davy, H. Fuchs, H. Hofmeister, J. Marte, and I. Reiter, 68–96. Vienna: Orac.

Grbic, Nadja. 1994. Das Gebärdensprachdolmetschen als Gegenstand einer angewandten Sprach-und Translationswissenschaft unter besonderer Berücksichtigung der Situa-tion in Österreich. Ph.D. diss., University of Graz.

Gruber, Heinz, and Viktor Ledl. 1992. *Allgemeine Sonderpädagogik: Grundlagen des Unter-richts für Schüler mit Schulschwierigkeiten und Behinderungen: ein Studien-und Arbeits-buch*. Vienna: Schulbuchverlag Jugend und Volk.

Hintermair, Manfred. 1995. Von einer "Psychologie der Gehörlosen" zu einer identitätsstif-tenden Sozialisationsperspektive für gehörlose Kinder und Jugendliche, Teil II. *Hörge-schädigtenpädagogik* 49:3–13.

Hogger, Birgit. 1990. Die Initiierung des Verbalspracherwerbs bei Gehörlosen über die Schrift. *Frühförderung Interdisziplinär* 9:120–25.

Jarmer, Helene. 1997. Bilingualismus und Bikulturalismus: Ihre Bedeutung für Gehörlose. Bachelor's thesis, University of Vienna.

Jussen, Heribert. 1994a. In memoriam Herrn Universitätsprofessor Dr. Otto Kröhnert. *Hörgeschädigtenpädagogik* 48:5–17.

———. 1994b. Zur zweisprachigen Erziehung Gehörloser. *Hörgeschädigtenpädagogik* 48:34–42.

Jussen, Heribert, and Otto Kröhnert, eds. 1982. *Pädagogik der Gehörlosen und Schwerhörigen.* Berlin: Marhold.

Kammerer, Emil. 1997. Gedanken zum Stellenwert des Cochlea-Implantats für die Entwicklung jüngerer, stark hörbehinderter Kinder. In *Gehörlos—nur eine Ohrensache?*, 60–66. Göttingen: Deutsche Arbeitsgemeinschaft für Evangelische Gehörlosenseelsorge e.V.

Köble, J. 1969. Zur Psyche des tauben Kleinkindes. *Neue Blätter für Taubstummenbildung* 3:153–61.

Kölblinger, Maria. 1993. Hörbehinderte Frauen: Die Lebenssituation und die sozialen Beziehungen von schwerhörenden und ertaubten Frauen. Ph.D. diss., University of Linz.

Krausneker, Verena. 1998. Gebärdensprachen in der Minderheitensprachenpolitik der Europäischen Union. Bachelor's thesis, University of Vienna.

Lane, Harlan. 1993. *The mask of benevolence: Disabling the deaf community.* New York: Random House.

McCagg, William O. 1993. Some problems in the history of deaf Hungarians. In *Deaf history unveiled*, ed. John V. Van Cleve, 252–71. Washington, D.C.: Gallaudet University Press.

Migsch, Gertraud. 1987. Die Verstummung des Widerspruchs: Ein qualitativer Beitrag zur beruflichen Sozialisation von Gehörlosenlehrern. Ph.D. diss., University of Salzburg.

Möckel, Andreas. 1988. *Geschichte der Heilpädagogik.* Stuttgart: Klett-Cotta.

Österreichischer Gehörlosenbund, ed. 1988. *75 Jahre Österreichischer Gehörlosenbund 1913–1988.* Vienna: Österreichischer Gehörlosenbund.

Pfaffhausen, Jürgen. 1995. Das mehrfachbehinderte hörgeschädigte Kind in der heutigen Schullandschaft—eine Herausforderung an die Hörgeschädigtenpädagogik. *Hörgeschädigtenpädagogik* 49:201–08.

Pinter, Magret. 1992. Klagenfurter Unterrichtsprojekt: Bilinguale Förderung hörgeschädigter Kinder in der Gehörlosenschule. *Das Zeichen* 20:145–50.

Prohazka, Heinrich. 1988. 1963—ein halbes Jahrhundert Gehörlosen-Organisation in Österreich. In *75 Jahre Österreichischer Gehörlosenbund 1913–1988*, ed. Österreichischer Gehörlosenbund, 71–88. Vienna: Österreichischer Gehörlosenbund.

Rainer, Monika. 1996. Das gehörlose Kind. Bachelor's thesis, University of Klagenfurt.

Rogow, Sally M. 1998. Hitler's unwanted children: Children with disabilities, orphans, juvenile delinquents and non-conformist young people in Nazi Germany. Retrieved in 1998 from the World Wide Web: http://www.nizkor.org/ftp.cgi/people/r/rogow .sally/hitlers-unwanted-children

Schott, Walter. 1995. *Das k.k. Taubstummen-Institut in Wien 1779–1918.* Vienna: Böhlau.

———. 1999. Das Allgemeine Österreichische Israelitische Taubstummen-Institut in Wien. Wien: n.p.

Schulte, Klaus. 1989. Gebärdetes Chinesisch? Zum Problem ein- oder zweisprachiger Bildung Gehörloser. *Hörgeschädigtenpädagogik* 43:251–62.

Soudakoff, Sharon A. 1999. History of deaf Holocaust victims. Retrieved in 1999 from the World Wide Web: http://www.jdcc.org/1999/mar-apr/holocaust.htm

Stepf, Hans Jürgen. 1997. Gehörlose im 3. Reich. In *Gehörlos—nur eine Ohrensache?* 21–26. Göttingen: Deutsche Arbeitsgemeinschaft für Evangelische Gehörlosenseelsorge e.V.

Tings, Franz, Claudia Rink, and Berte Pasligh. 1995. Anregungen zum Gebärdensprachgebrauch in der Praxis. *Hörgeschädigtenpädagogik* 49:291–306.

Uden, Antonius van. 1987. *Gebärdensprachen von Gehörlosen und Psycholinguistik.* Heidelberg: Groos.

Weber, Hans-Ulrich. 1995. *Gehörlosigkeit—die gemachte Behinderung.* Heidelberg: Groos.

4

Pedagogical Issues in Swedish Deaf Education

Sangeeta Bagga-Gupta and Lars-Åke Domfors

This chapter brings together two aspects of the Swedish Deaf community. First, we explore how different historical discourses have shaped present ideologies in Swedish Deaf education, including teacher education. Second, we look at what role Swedish bilingual ideology has played in supporting the development of contradictory meanings of Deafness in Sweden, especially in the aftermath of the national curriculum for compulsory schools, which was put into effect in the early 1980s (Lgr 80 1980).[1] The Swedish situation is unique in the sense that a relatively uniform bilingual educational system is made available to all Deaf children in the country.

PROJECT BACKGROUNDS

The first project that we discuss in this chapter reflects the second author's recently concluded doctoral research (Domfors 2000a). This research focuses (a) on a historical analysis of the education of teachers of the Deaf (ToDs) from the inception of this education in 1874 and (b) on a study of present-day understandings of ToD competencies and professionalism at the high school level. The historical analysis included the study of archival documents like syllabi, examination assignments, annual lecturing journals, bills, biographies, and the personal accounts and letters of teachers and school principals. The second part of the study was based on an analysis of classroom observations and in-depth interviews of ToDs at the national high schools of the Deaf and hard of hearing (henceforth called RGD/RGH schools) during the mid-1990s.[2]

Two of the three RGD schools have found that significant numbers of their Deaf students have serious difficulties with reading and writing.[3] In one of these schools, almost two-thirds of Deaf and hard of hearing students were seen as having reading and writing difficulties.[4] The first author of this chapter has studied during two school years the dynamics of classroom interaction at four different high school programs at RGD in what is known as the RGD project: the

Vehicle Engineering, the Construction, the Bakery (Food), and the Media programs (see Bagga-Gupta 2000, 2001b, 2001c, 2002a).[5]

The second project discussed in this chapter, which was led by Bagga-Gupta,
focuses on language spheres in educational settings. ToDs from each of the six
schools for the Deaf (the five regional schools in Örebro, Vänersborg, Stockholm,
Lund, and Härnösand as well as the local school in Gothenburg) and three schools
for the hard of hearing (local schools in Hässleholm, Piteå, and Stockholm) participated in this writing and reading project (SOL project).

And finally, Bagga-Gupta, together with members of KKOM-DS (Communication, Culture, and Diversity-Deaf Studies) research group, conducted ethno-
graphically oriented research (Special Schools or SS project), which studied the
everyday communication, learning, and achievement at the five state regional special schools for Deaf and hard of hearing students (Bagga-Gupta 2002b).

1981 AND THE BEGINNING OF A TRANSITION

> Compulsory schooling for Deaf children in Sweden has been enforced
> since 1889. . . . A great deal has happened since then both in terms of the
> States and the general society's attitudes towards handicapped children
> and within the field of special education and needs-related teaching. . . .
> [These] schools have, through different decisions and changes in the law,
> adapted to the needs which society today considers appropriate for teach-
> ing of children who because of . . . deafness [and] hearing impairment . . .
> or other reasons cannot attend [normal] compulsory schools.[6] (National
> Agency for Education 1997, 3, 62)

In 1981, Sweden became the first country in the world to officially recognize
a sign language, *teckenspråk* (Swedish Sign Language, or SSL), as the "first language" of its Deaf citizens, including immigrant deaf students. This parliamentary decision was a response to a number of different voices present in Sweden in
the 1970s. During the 1960s, minority and immigrant students could get instruction about and in their home languages for the first time. The "home language
reform" (*hemspråksreform*) went into effect on July 1, 1977. This legislation required
school districts to organize home-language teaching and study supervision for
students in their home languages (Hyltenstam and Tuomela 1996).

Research and the Swedish Deaf and parental nongovernmental organizations
(NGOs) were instrumental in getting SSL accepted as an official language. Following the lead of William Stokoe's research on American Sign Language linguistics
starting in 1957 (Baker and Battison 1980), Brita Bergman and Inger Ahlgren researched SSL.[7] Their work and that of Kenneth Eklindh at the National Agency
for Education (SÖ) gave SSL scientific recognition and paved the way for a political shift in language policy. This shift then gradually had an effect in the different
Deaf arenas such as schools for the Deaf, education programs for ToDs, families
of Deaf people, Deaf NGOs, work settings, and service settings.

The official recognition of SSL has had major consequences for the lives of
Deaf and hard of hearing individuals, their relatives, and others in their social
spheres. The 1981 ruling decreed that all Deaf children would receive their compulsory schooling in SSL because this language was officially the "first language"

of all Deaf students regardless of their backgrounds (including children born to hearing Swedes and children of immigrant families). In addition, the 1981 decision created a new, politically accepted social status for Deaf people: Deaf individuals acquired the right to information and services in SSL in various settings such as preschools, after-school centers, youth centers, workplaces, and hospital programs.

Undoubtedly, SSL existed as a language long before researchers started describing it in linguistic terms and long before it was accorded political acceptance. The 1981 decision, however, had an almost immediate political effect because language policies received a new direction in the new national curriculum at the compulsory schools that were attended by Deaf children between the ages of 7 and 17 (National Agency for Education 1983). This change in the curriculum should not be confused with the broader effect that the decision had on the lives of Deaf, hard of hearing, and hearing people in schools, at home, and in other social arenas during the 1980s and, perhaps, even the 1990s. Therefore, 1981 should be pinpointed as the start of a long transitional stage.

Up until the early 1980s, the majority hearing culture and hearing members of Deaf settings, especially hearing parents, siblings, and teachers, were not expected to possess any SSL competency. The importance of SSL education came to the forefront at this time. Language enhancement classes and in-service courses were created for different categories of hearing individuals such as teachers, parents, siblings, grandparents, and interpreters. In light of changes that the 1981 parliamentary decision brought about and despite the report of the "Minority Language Committee" (Minoritetsspråksutredning) (Swedish Government Official Report 1997), we think it is legitimate to discuss issues related to the situation of Deaf people in Sweden in terms of *pre-minority* (pre-1981) and *minority* (post-1981).[8]

LANGUAGE-BASED MEMBERSHIP OF DEAF SPACES

An important by-product of these special structural changes is that increasing numbers of Swedes who are members or potential members of Deaf settings have some competency in SSL. Because 90% to 95% of Deaf children are born into hearing families, estimating the number of hearing and Deaf Swedes who presently use the language on a daily basis is difficult. In addition, the number of competent SSL-proficient professionals such as interpreters and preschool and compulsory school teachers (roughly the equivalent of American elementary and intermediate schools teachers) is growing. In fact, one could say that, if membership were determined by knowledge of SSL, more hearing Swedes are members of Deaf settings than are Deaf and hard of hearing Swedes. In the county of Örebro, where some of the regional and national educational facilities for the Deaf are concentrated, the signing population could be up to 5% of the entire population. Wiklander reports "1,200 individuals (approximately 1% of the region's inhabitants) are dependent on SSL in Örebro" (1998, 1).

SSL is one of Sweden's indigenous languages not only because it has been officially recognized as the "first"—and "natural"—language of one of its subcultures but also because an increasing portion of the country's population uses it on an everyday basis. Even though SSL is regarded as the "first language" of a portion of the Swedish population, it still has not attained official status as a minority indigenous language (see endnote 8).

1981 AND EDUCATION PROGRAMS FOR THE TEACHERS OF THE DEAF: SOME HISTORICAL ASPECTS (1809–1997)

The historical backgrounds of the different discourses within education programs for ToDs exemplify the ways in which the 1981 parliamentary decision has shaped important Deaf institutions in Sweden. Close ties and a common ideological direction have always characterized the relationship between Swedish schools for the Deaf and education programs for ToDs. However, a variety of tensions have existed since the 19th century. Different discourses have been dominant during different periods, but even when one discursive practice has been emphasized during a particular phase, others have coexisted as underlying strands.

PRE-MINORITY ERA (1809–1980)

Manillaskolan, Sweden's first school for the Deaf, was established in 1809 in Stockholm, and in 1889, basic school education for the Deaf became compulsory. In 1874, the first college for ToDs was established (also at Manillaskolan). Little research has been done on 19th-century education of the Deaf in Sweden. Anita Pärsson's (1997) doctoral thesis, however, analyzes the period from 1889 on. Domfors's doctoral thesis (2000a) examines how college education for ToDs has been shaped from 1874. The first college for ToDs continued to be located at Manillaskolan until the 1960s. During this entire period (1874–1960s), whoever was responsible as the director of the ToD college was also the principal of the school for the Deaf.

The period after establishment of the college was characterized by a conflict between the French manual method and the German oral method. The Milan Congress, held in 1880, is said to have had a major effect on Swedish Deaf education. The Congress declared that oralism was the only appropriate form of communication suitable for educating Deaf people.

According to Pärsson, the general European development "after the Milan Congress was a transition away from signing methods towards speech methods" (1997, 70). She describes the Swedish situation as follows: "[D]uring the period 1880–90 even ToDs were not in agreement about which teaching methods were to be preferred. . . . However at the end of the 19th century there occurred a transition towards speech-methods" (1997, 71). During the same period, an 1889 law (*Lag angående döfstumundervisningen*) made Deaf school education compulsory and even included statutes for teacher education for ToDs (*Döfstumlärares utbildning* 35–49§§) (Sweden 1889). "Education imparted at the college, which is mainly theoretical includes the following subjects and exercises: . . . manual communication (*åtbördsspråket*), its origins, development and use in education" (39). So although Swedish Deaf school education was seeing a transition toward an oral communication model, statutes for teacher education for ToDs included the manual communication model. In addition to the influence of the Milan Congress, evidence shows that, from the 1870s to the 1940s and 1950s, Manilla College was influenced by developments in Germany through visits, literature, and teaching methods.

The patronage of the Swedish royal family also characterized and shaped the discourse of Deaf education in the 19th century. College directors always highlighted this patronage in their annual reports. In addition, the members of the Deaf school boards were invariably people in power such as barons, vicars, doctors, and deputy assistants (Prawitz 1913). Even today, Sweden's Queen Silvia is the patron of the Child Audiology Congress and an important promotional symbol for SSL.

Although oralism was the dominant theme of education during this period, it was not the only one. Religious education was also vital and emphasized rote memorization of the Lutheran catechism, education for confirmation, and participation in church services. This emphasis was a key part of all Swedish compulsory school education of this period (Englund 1992). During the 1870s, teacher candidates at Manilla College were required to participate in their students' confirmation education. And according to official regulations, the college director was required to spend "four hours every week . . . participating (by signing) in the education of the Holy Communion for deaf-mute children" and was required "to sign at the Service and other ceremonies" (Manillaskolan 1873).

Between World Wars I and II, significant changes occurred in the college programs for ToDs. The new discourse, reflected in lecture titles, course reports, and examination assignments, highlighted a scientific and theoretical basis for teaching different school subjects. For instance, developmental and differential psychology and small-scale research appeared for the first time in the college syllabi for ToDs. In addition, medical subjects became visible and accepted parts of college programs. For example, one examination assignment paper published in 1941 was titled "Survey of the Structure and Function of the Inner Ear" (Stockholms Stadsarkiv).

Initial analysis of a number of different sources indicates that some official acceptance of signing also was present during this period between the wars. Certain school practices were always conducted in SSL. ToD college syllabi continued to have underlying strands related to signing. Significantly, Deaf classes were divided into three categories: A-classes, where the medium of communication was oral language; B-classes, where school education was handled primarily by means of written language; and C-classes in which "C-children were the weakest and 'sign language' (teckenspråk) was considered their language" (Pärsson 1997, 72; see also Eriksson 1993, 1998). A-classes were considered the best.

Aspects of signing were therefore part of the college programs for ToDs. In a recent conversation, Lars Ohlson commented that, as late as the mid-1950s, teacher candidates at Stockholm were required to study signing (åtbördsspråket) as part of their college program and were required to pass an exam at the end of their studies. However, teacher candidates were forbidden to use signing during their practical work at the school for the Deaf. Note, however, that, so far, no evidence has been found that shows signing was officially forbidden before 1981 (Pärsson 1997; Eriksson 1998; Domfors 2000a). Although one kind of discourse was dominant during these years, it must be recognized that another parallel discourse was alive (and repressed).

Transition to a Minority Era (1981 and After)

The 1981 parliamentary decision had a major effect on Deaf education in general and education for ToDs in particular. Swedish schools for the Deaf could not immediately respond to the political acceptance of SSL in 1981. For instance, not until the end of the 1980s did the government make any response realistically possible (by making available grants to Deaf schools) for hearing ToDs to participate in full-time SSL in-service education programs. These courses are time-intensive and usually stretch over 20 weeks at the university level. Even at the end of the 1980s, teachers who were trained before 1981 were communicating in their classrooms by combining the oral and the signing modes (for instance, see Bagga-Gupta 1989; Heiling 1994). Thus, the 1980s and even the early 1990s can be understood in terms of a transition to a minority period.

The 1980s and 1990s are also characterized by the appearance of a new communicative discourse in Swedish Deaf education. Gustavsson (1994) looks at this discourse, which focuses on mutual understanding through the use of a common language that is based on empathy and participation. Before 1981, few Deaf student teachers managed to get admission to education programs for ToDs in Sweden. Today, Deaf student teachers can gain admission to both the general Initial Teacher Education Program and the post-graduate Course of Deaf Education. Qualified Deaf ToDs are in high demand in all five of the regional state special schools for the Deaf (National Agency for Education 1997; SPM 2000).

These changes have meant a professional shift for the ToD. Competencies that are viewed as crucial for ToDs today include the ability to communicate in SSL, knowledge of bilingualism, and the ability to compare the linguistic structures of SSL and Swedish. Teachers who had received their college education in the pre-minority era are required to take SSL courses as part of their in-service training. In contrast, new student teachers in the 1990s and the 2000s are expected to be proficient in SSL even before they join a college education program. According to the former Swedish University Degree Ordinance for ToD, the teacher student was required before graduation to have the "ability to, without difficulties, communicate with Deaf and hard of hearing in SSL" (Sweden 1998). In the latest Swedish University Degree Ordinance (Sweden 2001) SSL proficiency is not mentioned for ToD students because they now study in "regular" teacher education programs. One could wonder whether SSL proficiency is now taken for granted following the directives of the National Curriculum (see National Agency for Education 1996; http://www.skolverket.se/kursplaner/specialskolan/index.html).

The ToD teacher education that qualifies one to work in Deaf education is decentralized and is now the responsibility of local university departments and colleges of education. The schools can organize their ToD teacher education by using SSL screening interviews and optional courses in the regular teacher education programs. The lower-level schools for the Deaf are involved in this process through field studies and practical training, an important part of the ToD teacher education program.

Although SSL-related research in the area of formal linguistics has had a head start in Sweden, a lag exists in knowledge of pedagogical aspects of bilingualism for Deaf students. According to Lennart Teveborg and Ingrid Toll (1991), bilingual-methods (for the Deaf) move on untrodden ground. Neither teacher education, personal in-service education or the SSL-standard in the (bilingual state) schools have reached the levels of the parliamentary intentions mirrored in the Curriculum for the Special Schools. (3)

In other words, Deaf education in general has not found a clear, well structured direction since 1981. The national curriculum of the early 1980s could not be continued in Deaf education because adequate working tools related to Deaf bilingualism were not available for ToDs. And as we will contend below, a critical discussion has not evolved with respect to Deaf students' "first language," "second language," and "bilingualism" during this period.

A new national curriculum was put into effect in 1994 (Lpo 94 1994 for compulsory schools; National Agency for Education 1996 for special schools, including revisions in 2001; and Lpf 94 1994 for high schools) and is currently followed by both hearing and Deaf schools.[9] Now, the curriculum has more precise requirements, for instance, in achievement goals for both teachers and students in different subjects. These new precise targets are significant because educational practices begin to be shaped by the very fact of their introduction.

Guidelines concerning the meaning of bilingualism in Deaf education, however, continue to be vague. A specific syllabus for Swedish as a "second language" of the Deaf at RGD/RGH schools, for example, was only recently officially defined (see http://www3.skolverket.se/ki/SC/0102/sf/12/01/index.html), and little instructional material exists for teaching Swedish as a "second language" to Deaf students. In many high school programs, teachers do not have access to any teaching material that takes into account the fact that written Swedish has been conceptualized as the Deaf students' "second language." This lag in the bilingual (SSL-Swedish) developmental work in the areas of policy and pedagogy has major implications for the education of Deaf students, ToD university and college education programs, and everyday language practices.

The Ideology of Bilingualism and the Organization of Deaf and Hard of Hearing Preschool, Compulsory School, and High School Education in the Minority Era

The two languages of the (Swedish) deaf are Sign Language and the written variant of the national language (Swedish). The element of spoken language in deaf (Swedish) bilingualism is very limited. (Andersson 1994, 93)

All Deaf and many hard of hearing children in Sweden have access to an organized educational structure that is probably unique in the world. First, as has been implied above, SSL's official status makes it necessary for preschools, compulsory schools, and high schools to employ staff members who are competent in SSL and to carry out programs to reeducate the staff. Second, the tradition of compulsory schooling makes this expertise available to all Deaf and many hard of hearing children in the country.

SSL is now a school subject studied in many Swedish schools. It is considered to be the "first" school language for Deaf students and the "second" school language for hard of hearing children who study in hard of hearing classes in Deaf or hearing schools. It also can be studied by hearing children in hearing schools as their "third" language. The bilingual ideology that exists in general Swedish school education (including Deaf education) has, since the mid-1970s, been grounded on the principle that, if minority and immigrant children were to receive early stimulation in their home or "first" language, then they would pick up their "second" language (i.e., Swedish) more easily (see Hyltenstam 1996; Svonni 1996; Viberg 1996; Wingstedt 1998). The carrying out of Deaf bilingual programs is based on this research and these bilingual policies and is not grounded in more recent work in language development among minority and immigrant groups or in research in the literacy or communication studies traditions. This lack of connection to more recent research has a bearing on how education policies for Deaf bilingualism and especially Deaf literacy have been framed.

Once a child is identified as deaf, he or she is usually placed in a preschool where SSL is one of the working languages. The overwhelming majority of Deaf children are born into non-SSL-literate families and, thus, have not had any exposure to SSL during the first 10 to 12 months of their lives. Because their numbers are small, Deaf children are usually gathered at one or two signing preschools in each county.[10] Hearing siblings and other hearing children can also join most, though not all, signing environments.

Each of the five state schools for the Deaf, situated in different parts of the country, functions as its own regional intake center. In 1994, a sixth school for the Deaf and hard of hearing was established in Sweden in the city of Gothenburg (the classes are situated on the campus of a hearing school). More recently, a second school for the Deaf that comes under local government authority has been established in Stockholm. Until June 2000, each of the five regional state special schools for the Deaf had attached to it a Regional Knowledge Center that coordinated, among other things, issues related to Deaf and hard of hearing children's school placement. Following a parliamentary commission directive, all five of these regional state special schools (and a sixth national state school for Deaf children with developmental disabilities) have, since July 2000, been merged under one special school authority (Specialskolemyndigheten [SPM]). This authority has its national office in the city of Örebro, and the hope is that school developmental efforts will be more effectively channeled through this authority.

In comparison to the Deaf, hard of hearing children are in a somewhat different situation. Spoken Swedish is officially considered their "first" and "natural" language, and in certain situations, SSL is considered to be their "second" school language (see below). Children are individually integrated in hearing preschools or they attend signing preschools together with Deaf children. Hard of hearing school-aged children are organized according to three different strategies (see also Bagga-Gupta 1999b).[11] Some are integrated into hearing schools with the support of technical systems such as loops and microphones. A significantly smaller number of hard of hearing children are grouped into a class or a few classes within hearing schools with technical and other support resources. Today, at least three schools in Sweden offer educational services for large groups of hard of hearing children. During the early 1990s, a third strategy has clearly evolved: Hard of hearing classes are being integrated into Deaf school environments.[12] Parents work with a team of professionals to decide which environment will best suit the child's needs.[13]

The five regional state schools for the Deaf and hard of hearing offer a compulsory ten-year education for their students. This plan contrasts with the nine years of schooling that hard of hearing children receive if they are individually integrated into hearing schools. Although the five regional state schools continue to be the responsibility of the central government, children placed in the local schools, including the new Deaf schools in Gothenburg and Stockholm, are the responsibility of local governments. All preschools are managed by local government authorities. The situation changes when children complete their compulsory education and wish to continue at the high school level.[14] The National High Schools for the Deaf (RGD) and the hard of hearing (RGH) were established in Örebro in 1967 and 1984, respectively, to concentrate SSL expertise and resources for Deaf and hard of hearing children who wish to receive more than ten years of compulsory schooling. In contrast to hearing children, whose high school studies extend over three years, bilingual RGD and RGH students are almost always required to spend four years in high school.

Language and Social Policy Practices in the Minority Era: Discourses of Normality and Special Needs

One result of the 1981 parliamentary decision and the direction given in the new national curricula (Lgr 80 1980; Lpf 94 1994; Lpo 94 1994) has been normalization of the Deaf and hard of hearing groups. These groups are now no longer looked on as handicapped but, instead, as a minority language group. The 1981 decision, therefore, had a major bearing on the ideology behind and the organization of institutionalized Deaf settings such as education programs for ToDs, Deaf schools, and preschools.

"First" and "Second" Language Competencies in Institutionalized Deaf Settings: Some Reflections and Implications

> Communicative competence involves knowing not only the language code, but also what to say to whom, and how to say it appropriately in any given situation. . . . The concept of communicative competence is one of the most powerful organizing tools to emerge in the social sciences in recent years. (Saville-Troike 1989, 21)

As mentioned earlier, full-time university-level SSL courses for teachers of the Deaf first became available at the end of the 1980s.[15] The first evaluation study of the five regional state schools for the Deaf and hard of hearing that was carried out in 1997 reveals, however, that not even half of the teaching staff members who are hearing at these schools have had the opportunity to attend these SSL courses (National Agency for Education 1997). In 2000, 138 (of a total of 284) teachers had been given the opportunity to study SSL at the university level (SPM 2000; see also Bagga-Gupta 2002b). Even though Swedish Deaf education emphasizes making opportunities available for the total development of the child (*helhetsperspektiv*), a large proportion of the schools' nonteaching staff members have no possibility to attend in-service SSL courses at the university level. At RGD, many teaching staff members continue to feel less than competent in SSL, their students' "first" language. Some of them rely on interpreters in their own classrooms. In the five regional state schools for Deaf and hard of hearing however, ToDs themselves report that they are competent in SSL. Interpreters are rarely, if ever, used in classrooms in these schools.

A very small minority of Deaf students (about 5%–10%) come from homes where SSL has been a full-fledged functioning language throughout their childhood. The principally hearing caregivers of the overwhelming majority of Deaf children go through a chain of language courses and frequently consider themselves to be incompetent in SSL—a language that is perceived as their "second" language—through their active parenting years.[16] In fact, most of the Deaf children in these situations first come into contact with SSL in the context of an institutionalized Deaf setting. In this respect, language socialization becomes a crucial task for preschools, compulsory schools, and high schools for the Deaf, and there is a need to reconsider what the term "first language" or "native language" means in this context (see also Bagga-Gupta 2001a, 2002a).

Both the national curricula (Lgr 80 1980; Lpo 94 1994) that have been in effect during the minority period at the compulsory school level have recognized Swedish as a text-based second language for Deaf students. However, even at the end of the 1990s, few didactic perspectives exist either in the discussions on the teaching of written Swedish to Deaf students or in how they should be evaluated in this subject.

The 1990s have seen a growing awareness and concern for Deaf children's "poor" performance in their "second" language, written Swedish. In our view, these discussions are often carried out in the absence of a pedagogical and sociocultural analysis of the institutionalized communicative contexts in which teaching and learning are supposed to occur. Until very recently, the official guidelines for Swedish that were followed by the RGD/RGH schools expected Deaf students to be able to "talk, read and write Swedish"(GyVux 1994.2.190 1994). However, our data suggest that language teachers at the RGD schools followed their own local curricula, which were more finely tuned to the 1981 decision. In the absence of a critical discussion of language issues in the post-1981 period, ToD education and the Deaf schools continue to be informed by traditional prescriptive models as to how they should handle the special "second" language situation of their Deaf students. Although ideologies have changed, as long as teachers, students, and staff members at schools for the Deaf are not adequately equipped with the basic language competencies for working in the institutionalized educational Deaf settings in Sweden and as long as there is an absence of a critical analysis of a bilingual ideology informed by empirically driven research that focuses on the teaching of written Swedish for the Deaf (see also Sweden 1999), a special-needs situation lingers on.

Bilingual Deaf students in the minority era are required to follow almost the same curriculum and guidelines that have been established for monolingual hearing children. The main differences are in the area of language learning. For Deaf students, SSL is obligatory, and Swedish and English are required to be studied as written languages. This situation means the same demands are being made on the educational institutions of the Deaf as on schools for hearing children. The

ToDs are hampered by a lack of informed theoretical direction in bilingual issues and by a scarcity of second-language teaching resources. Some ToDs may also lack not only linguistic competency in SSL but also communicative competency in SSL.

These two issues—problems with SSL communicative competencies of ToDs and inadequate pedagogical discussions related to Deaf bilingualism—constitute important aspects of what we would like to call the "paradox of bilingualism" in the Deaf minority era in Sweden. This paradox is often forgotten in discussions that focus on the evaluation demands of the latest national curricula for compulsory schools (Lpo 94 1994) and RGD/RGH schools (Lpf 94 1994). Highlighting broader perspectives instead of "individual reductionism" (Wertsch 1998) can help us understand why Deaf students in the 1990s can be considered handicapped by some measures (see also Grosjean 1996).

FROM EVALUATING READING AND WRITING TO STUDYING LITERACY PRACTICES: SOME SOCIOCULTURAL AND PEDAGOGICAL PERSPECTIVES

No adequate methodology exists to directly compare the Swedish language competencies of hearing students (for whom Swedish is the "first" language both for everyday out-of-school life and in school) and Deaf students (for whom Swedish is a "second" language in the written form and a language that, by and large, gets treated as a school-based language). A general notion exists that, compared to hearing students, Deaf students are "failing" and are unable to master Swedish in the manner that "they are supposed to." This notion is often based on either comparisons of national test results for Deaf and hearing groups of same-age students or content analysis of texts written by Deaf students (for instance, see Heiling 1993, 1994; Persson in National Agency for Education 1997). Although our colleague Ronny Andersson (1994), a Deaf linguist, gives credit to the national curriculum that was put into effect at the beginning of the minority era (National Agency for Education [SÖ] 1983), saying that "a growing number of the deaf students now reaching high school level are educationally and emotionally equipped" to participate in further independent study or the job market, he also points out that "there are, however, still deaf students who read and write their second language poorly" (Andersson 1994, 91; see also Heiling 1993).

Kerstin Heiling's (1993) doctoral thesis showed that Swedish Deaf students who had received early stimulation in SSL fared considerably better in the mastery of written Swedish in school when compared to an earlier, pre-minority Deaf cohort from the late 1960s. Her comparative work "point[s] to the importance of easily accessible communication, i.e. a visual/gestural language mode, to social as well as intellectual development in deaf children" (1993, 222). However, Heiling also says that "although deaf subjects in the eighties have made substantial gains in writing skills compared to their age-mates in the sixties, they are still far from the fluency and flexibility achieved by hearing subjects" (1993, 221). Furthermore, the new goal-oriented 1994 National Curricula (Lpf 94 1994; Lpo 94 1994) in Sweden makes deaf students' achievement levels more visible.

In addition, Heiling's further research (1994) and recent comments in conversation indicate that Deaf student cohorts from the early 1990s are not faring as well as could have been expected from Heiling's initial (1993) findings. Most of these Deaf students

> started school with a general level of knowledge and social competence that were not common in earlier groups of deaf children. . . . General level of knowledge is certainly an important foundation for reading. How come then that the younger pupils have such difficulties learning to read? They are well oriented in lots of matters—information mainly acquired in SL. (Heiling 1994, 10)

Our own developmental project at all nine compulsory-level schools for the Deaf and hard of hearing in Sweden as well as our different empirical projects were in part initiated in the latter half of the 1990s to help us understand why, according to some authorities and teachers, minority-era Deaf cohorts are not faring "as well as could have been expected" (a ToD in the SOL project).

Even if we take into account the effect of Deaf children's general delay in becoming members of Deaf settings, how can we understand their performance in their "second" language? Why does early exposure to SSL not lead to better performance in Deaf students' "second" language? From our perspective, an understanding of these issues goes far beyond tests, performance, and achievement as well as beyond commonly accepted notions of "first" and "second"language acquisition (for instance, see Bagga-Gupta 1999a, 2000, 2002b).

"Problems arise when individual competence is judged in relation to a presumed ideal speech community, or assessed with tests given in a limited subset of situations" (Hymes in Saville-Troike 1989, 25). Since the 1980s, several studies have focused on the acquisition of literacy skills in bilingual and multilingual cultures. These studies show that acquisition of literacy (including literacy in writing systems) exists in different domains and that these domain-specific skills are closely related to specific social practices (Scribner and Cole 1981; Grosjean 1982; Heath 1983; Street 1984; Barton 1994; Bagga-Gupta 1995; Grosjean 1996).

The 1981 Swedish decision created a situation whereby the emphasis in many preschools moved from Swedish language use (i.e., oral Swedish, signed Swedish, and use of Swedish texts) to only SSL use. Ronny Andersson points out that "the deaf do not start really learning the national language (Swedish) until they go to school" (1994, 94). Although no systematic research has been published in this area, anecdotal evidence, including our own experiences in the field, does suggest that the position of written Swedish was downgraded in many signing childcare centers and preschools for the Deaf (for instance, see Heiling 1994). Heiling describes the compulsory school and preschool situation as follows:

> [In the] stricter bilingual setting . . . Swedish and Sign Language have been kept apart. In most of the pre-schools this meant that *written Swedish was almost excluded* as well. Fingerspelling of names was replaced by personal signs and written names on hangers and drawers were replaced by pictures. These very strict conditions have been dissolved but the situation is different from the late seventies and early eighties when reading and writing was more common and also used in a playful way in preschool activities. (1994, 9, italics added)

Even today, preschools for the Deaf are called "signing preschools" (*teckenförskola*) and not "bilingual preschools" (*tvåspråkig förskola*). Paradoxically, one of the suggestions the parliamentary FUNKIS commission put forward in its 1998 final report was to change the term *bilingual schools* (*tvåspråkigskolor*), used for the five regional state schools for the Deaf and hard of hearing, to *signing schools* (*teckenspråksskolor*) (Swedish Government Official Report 1998, 66).[17]

Some evidence indicates that the view of SSL during the latter half of the 1980s and beginning of the 1990s had become so rigid that hearing parents and teachers of Deaf preschools and compulsory schools felt compelled to think more about the structure of what they said to their child rather than to communicate with their child (Heiling 1994, 1997). From her experience as a clinical psychologist over a long period of time at a large regional state school for the Deaf, Heiling raises thought-provoking questions. During this period, she points out, that

> demands for a "real sign language" were growing fast. Tied to these demands were warnings about the negative effects of not supplying the children with a "pure language." As the possibilities to acquire this genuine sign language through education was lacking at least in our part of the country, many teachers and parents began to feel uncomfortable and incompetent. I noticed that much of the joyfulness disappeared and that communication was seen as a permanent test of language achievement for the hearing adults (both parents and teachers). (Heiling 1994, 10)

A 55-year-old hearing ToD at one of our RGD project schools echoes Heiling's concerns when he reflects on the situation from the late-1980s: "Suddenly we had these people coming and telling us that we were not signing genuine SSL. I communicate in SSL with my students don't I, so what is wrong if I don't always use some genuine Deaf expressions?" In other words, in addition to bilingualism being emphasized only at the compulsory and high school level and not being valued in the preschool sphere, a view of language purity became established, and this view, perhaps (paradoxically), had detrimental consequences for communicative practices in various Deaf settings within society where hearing individuals lived and worked during the post-1981 years.[18]

Our RGD and SS projects attempt to illustrate some of these issues connected with institutionalized literacy practices. In a number of the bilingual program settings that have been studied at the high school level, hearing teachers' SSL competencies are often, though not always, inadequate for the purposes of carrying out needed in-depth and theoretical discussions. In high school practice-centered programs such as the Bakery, Vehicle Engineering, and Construction programs, hearing teachers rarely rely on the use of interpreters. One might suppose that the teachers would therefore be forced to rely more on written communication with their Deaf students. This situation does not occur. If anything, the teachers' notions of Deaf students' poor skills in written Swedish almost seem to stop them from even considering this strategy as an option. Instead, teachers often simplify any written texts that they might be forced to use with their Deaf students.

Realistic production criteria (for instance, making baked products for sale in the school shop and repairing cars) mean that production goals almost invariably supersede any direct focus on literacy learning. Because each class is made up of two to ten students and teachers or assistants are always around, students often do not need to read any classroom texts (for instance, recipes, car manuals, or construction designs) to complete their tasks. From the student's perspective, what makes more sense is to point to the oven or the baking ingredient or the part of the car being discussed and to solve problems in SSL by turning to older, more experienced Deaf students and, sometimes, to Deaf assistants than to use written Swedish as a form of natural communication with the hearing professional teacher in the classroom. In both compulsory and high schools for the Deaf, (written) Swedish is an obligatory "theoretical core subject" (*kärnämne*) for all students. Our data from RGD project show that Swedish is studied and experienced by Deaf high school students as both a "school" and "theoretical" (*teori*) subject. Analysis of everyday communication in classrooms at the compulsory level in special schools also shows a focus on studying the formal structures of written Swedish rather than the communicative aspects of the language. Analysis of data from these two projects have so far indicated that more creative and concerted efforts need to be made to integrate the everyday practices of literacy and the formal practice of Swedish at bilingual high schools and compulsory schools for the Deaf.

Our two-year-long collaboration with the teachers at all six of the state and local compulsory schools for the Deaf and hard of hearing as well as the three local schools for the hard of hearing (and our data from the SS project) also indicate a split between everyday literacy practices and the formal teaching of Swedish. Therefore, we are not surprised that the initial findings of Heiling (1993) have not continued but, rather, that Deaf children on average seem to be faring poorly on standardized evaluation tests. Is this situation the result of (rather than the cause of) literacy approaches not being used in areas within Deaf schools where text-related strategies would have been used in hearing schools?

When students fare poorly on standardized tests, educational underachievement also becomes part of the creation and marking of cultural boundaries (see Ogbu 1985, 1993; Jacob and Jordan 1993; Smith 2001). In the Swedish context, Hyltenstam and Tuomela (1996) stress that, although the learning of Swedish, the "second" language, is usually made easier if a (hearing) child already has some fluency in his or her "first" language, we find "situations where the motivation to learn the majority's language get extinguished, namely if the majority (group) display segregative or generally oppressive attitudes towards the minority" (1996, 40).

We wonder whether some Deaf students do not want to be or, in some sense, resist being perceived as smart in their "second" language because they do not want to be identified with the majority non-SSL Swedish culture—not only because Swedish is the language of the majority culture but also because it is a language that is strongly associated with the pre-minority era when SSL was not an officially accepted language. We also wonder how Deaf students in the Swedish

> bilingual schools model and perceive their own linguistic status. Do the Deaf students see themselves as "belonging" to both SSL and Swedish or do they see themselves as "belonging" to SSL? In what way does this

ownership of language impact Deaf students' perceptions of their abilities and aspirations to skills in Swedish? (Bagga-Gupta 2001a)

A few students in our project who are perceived as having poor skills in Swedish by almost all their teachers and who show very little interest in any "literacy event" (Heath 1983) connected to the formal practice of Swedish are nevertheless adept at surfing on the Internet and are regular users of e-mail.

ALLOWANCES

For our third example of the complexities woven into notions of Deafness in the post-1981 period, we look at some aspects of Swedish social policy during this period. Swedish families who have a Deaf child are entitled to a special financial "care-allowance" (vårdbidrag).[19] This money is paid by the social insurance authorities and is seen as a "compensation for the extra care and extra costs" the family experiences because of the presence of the disabled child—in this case, the Deaf child (Swedish Institute 1995, 4). To receive this financial care-allowance, the parents are required to send a written application describing their handicapped child and the family's special circumstances after the child is diagnosed as being deaf. The parents receive this allowance until the child reaches high school age. In a precedent-setting court judgment in the middle of the 1980s, a Deaf high school student was awarded a "sick allowance" (sjukbidrag) until he completed his high school education. After this judgment, all social insurance authorities now pay this allowance to Deaf high school students. Since 1994, the sum paid has decreased, though the label "sick allowance" continues to be used. Another allowance that Deaf individuals receive is called "disability compensation" (handikappersättning). This compensatory allowance is paid for life.

Because of a nationwide rethinking of subsidies, however, social insurance authorities and the counties have started questioning the various allowances that Deaf students receive. Compared to the situation in the 1980s, the awarding of these allowances is now more restricted.

NOTIONS OF NORMALITY AND SPECIAL NEEDS IN THE TRANSITION-TO-MINORITY ERA

Discourses are not composed by randomly choosing words and statements. Instead, rules constitute and regulate language use. . . . Such rules help shape a discursive practice that produces a specific discourse. (Cherryholmes in Östman 1996, 40)

Two decades have passed since a historic parliamentary decision made SSL the cornerstone of Swedish Deaf education. That period has been a time characterized by shrinking resources and attempts to give Deaf educational research a direction. We have, in this chapter, made an attempt to pause and reflect on the tensions that exist between the discourses about minority and normalcy, on the one hand, and the discourses about handicap and special needs, on the other.

The entire system of Deaf education has been restructured to reflect the new ideology of bilingualism and builds on the concepts of minority groups and of a normalizing discourse. Special resources, however, such as appropriately trained teachers and SSL school environments, have had to be concentrated in a few cities in Sweden, a practice based on a concept of special needs for which special resources must be earmarked.

Other aspects of the school system also reflect this notion of special needs. Swedish Deaf children's schooling stretches over two extra years when compared to hearing children's schooling. Explanations related to Deaf children's special bilingual situation are often offered to account for these extra compulsory school years.[20] One begins to question this reasoning, however, after noting that the extra school year was added at the compulsory school level in the 1950s. This action was taken during a period when an oral discourse in Deaf education was dominant, and it was done to compensate for the extra time that deaf children needed to learn a spoken language. Despite the shift in policy and the implications of the new discourse in Deaf bilingualism, the extra school year has been retained at the compulsory school level; moreover, one extra school year was added for deaf and hard of hearing students at the high school level when this school form was instituted in 1967 and 1984 respectively. The extra year in high school is often explained by claiming that it allows Deaf students "to get to know and adjust to Örebro" (an administrator and ToD in the RGD project; for further discussion on this issue, see Bagga-Gupta 2002b).

This discourse that focuses on the needs of Deaf students is so well entrenched in the institutionalized educational Deaf settings of the minority era that other explanatory models (for instance, what we have called the "paradox of bilingualism," which concentrates on, among other things, the needs of the ToDs and the broadening of our research agendas) would probably be difficult to hear. It is not the lack of skills of students and teachers that must be addressed but the nature of opportunities and resources that have been and are now available.

Another aspect of the paradox of bilingualism can be seen in the tension between the organization of the educational system for the Deaf, which rests firmly on a normalizing discourse, and the new national curricula (Lpf 94 1994; Lpo 94 1994) that emphasize evaluations. Without giving appropriate attention to the educational implications of Deaf bilingualism, the 1994 national curricula emphasized evaluations in such a way that Deaf students have unwittingly become labeled as underachieving and handicapped. We find a marked absence of critical discussions about, for example, "first language," "second language," "bilingualism," "language ideologies," and "practices of language" both in Deaf education and, until very recently, even in research on Deaf education.

As we have outlined, the implications of the 1981 parliamentary decision created a situation in which bilingual Deaf children are expected to perform at levels considered normal for monolingual hearing students (or even bilingual hearing students). In our view, this situation needs to be rethought. Although the latest national curricula (Lpf 94 1994; Lpo 94 1994) urge a normalizing discourse with Deaf students, the "normal" treatment of Deaf people predisposes them to being viewed as handicapped because they are compared directly to the hearing population in assessment tests.

Today, Deaf student-teachers can participate in regular teacher education programs (with interpreters) and thereafter get employment at Deaf compulsory and

RGD/RGH schools. Although this practice is part of a normalizing trend, a discourse about the special needs of these students in post-graduate ToD education programs continued until very recently. These programs were, until recently, more often associated with special education programs than with general education programs. More significantly, however, research on Deaf bilingualism has only very recently started focusing on the pedagogical and didactic aspects of the problem (compare with Sweden 1999). Consequently, bilingual studies in teacher education programs focus almost entirely on "a formalistic conception of language," (i.e., grammatical aspects of language comparison and training) at the expense of a "functionalistic conception of language," which here would mean a pedagogically informed notion of communication practices (Linell 1998). In addition, SSL courses at the university level are, for the most part, informed by only research in structural linguistics and not sociolinguistics. We contend that the paradox of bilingualism creates a special needs situation for ToD education programs and, as a result, creates a special needs situation in Deaf education in general.

The structure of Swedish society rests on an emphasis on general welfare policies (Swedish Institute 1995). The responsibilities for achieving the objectives of disability policies are borne by the entire Swedish society. By exploring different phenomena in the institutionalized Deaf settings of the minority Swedish period, we have highlighted the coexisting and often contradictory meanings that go into constituting Deafness since the beginning of the 19th century. These contrasting sets of meanings, which are supported by different discursive practices, become more visible at the end of the 20th and beginning of the 21st century because the general welfare policies that have been the traditional backbone of Sweden have been weakening.

ACKNOWLEDGMENTS

This chapter has grown from a paper that was presented at a panel titled "Ethnically Deaf," which was organized by Karen Nakamura and Leila Monaghan at the 96th annual meeting of the American Anthropological Association, November 1997, in Washington, D.C. We would like to thank the organizers for giving us an opportunity to develop some of these ideas and Nancy Fishberg for critical comments at the AAA meeting. We would also like to thank Leila for her detailed comments and her editorial assistance. This assistance helped us remain focused on relevant issues. Our text has also benefited richly from critical comments by several of our colleagues in Sweden, including Marjanna de Jong, Robbin Battison, and Kerstin Heiling. Each of these people has helped us in different though complementary ways to distance ourselves from the ideological nature of the discourses within the field. By taking a critical stance in relation to Swedish Deaf education we, as researchers with a background in communication and pedagogy, hope to contribute only to furthering present day understandings of these complex issues.

NOTES

1. Lgr 80 is the accepted abbreviation for "National curriculum for compulsory schools." The Swedish schools for the Deaf received their supplementary curriculum to

Lgr 80 in 1983 (National Agency for Education 1983), and this document had a major consequence for bilingual education for the Deaf and hard of hearing. In a nutshell, Swedish bilingual education for the Deaf acknowledges SSL (Swedish Sign Language) as the students' "first" language and the language of instruction. Swedish is recognized as the students' "second" language, which primarily involves the written form of Swedish in education.

2.   The National High School for the Deaf (Riksgymnasium för döva) and National High School for Hard of Hearing (Riksgymnasium for hörselskadade). The three national RGD/RGH schools are housed on three locally governed hearing school campuses in the city of Örebro.

3.   We must point out that, because of a sorting mechanism within the Swedish context, Deaf students who are good at reading and writing are very often channeled into the third national high school, which has a more academic orientation. The principals from the other two schools, who had initiated what is known as the RGD project, had invited participation from the third school. The third school was not interested in participating in the project, which could be interpreted as meaning that these teachers experienced their Deaf students as being good readers and writers. The RGD project was funded for two years by the National Social Services Board (Socialstyrelsen) and by the National Agency for Education (Skolverket) for one year.

4.   The new high school curriculum (Lpf 94 1994) is presently under evaluation. Many students from the hearing population do not appear to be faring well in Swedish, English, and mathematics. However, the numbers who are not faring well in the general population are far below the numbers from the project national high schools for the Deaf.

5.   The new high school curriculum (Lpf 94 1994) allows for specializing in 17 different national programs. In addition to these, students can choose to follow a customized individual program if they have not received passing grades in one or more of Swedish, Mathematics, and English. Together, the three national RGD/RGH schools offer all these different programs. Thus, the Bakery and Media programs are offered in one of the three national RGD/RGH schools while the Vehicle Engineering and Construction programs are offered in another RGD/RGH school.

6.   We have translated the original Swedish quotes into English.

7.   Brita Bergman was installed as the first professor of SSL at the Department of Linguistics, University of Stockholm in 1992.

8.   The committee concluded that Tornedalers, Swedish Finns, Roms, and Jews fulfill the four criteria that identified minority groups and thereby recommended to the government that these four groups be accorded national minority status. Swedish Deaf culture and SSL are not mentioned in this report.

9.   The main exception is that Deaf students study their "second" and "third" languages primarily in their written forms.

10.   Here, Deaf and hearing adults competent in SSL are employed.

11.   Often, this organization occurs with the support of itinerant teachers who have some competency in SSL.

12.   This kind of shift took place for some of the five regional state schools for the Deaf in the early 1990s. In these schools, all hard of hearing and Deaf students are geographically integrated in one school campus, though the two groups attend classes defined by their "first" and "second" languages. In one Deaf school, this integrated situation has existed for several years. In other countries, for instance in the United Kingdom, students with a higher degree of hearing loss are placed in hearing schools, which is rarely the case in Sweden.

13.   Progress evaluations allow children to be shifted among these different organizational forms throughout the school years. In fact, children tend to drop into the third

organizational form described above throughout their school years (see National Agency for Education 1997).

14.   About 95% of all school children, including Deaf and hard of hearing children, continue into high school today.

15.   The category labeled teachers of the Deaf (ToDs) does not include other personnel (child-care personnel, service staff, accommodation staff, etc.) who work at preschools, compulsory schools, and the high schools for the Deaf.

16.   A 1996 parliamentary committee directive (*TUFF-utredning*) suggested improvements in the existing possibilities that parents have in accessing SSL courses (Swedish Government Official Report 1996, 102; Sweden 1997). Parents now have the right to 240 hours of paid SSL courses. A recent national evaluation of TUFF education commissioned by the National Agency for Education and carried out by the second author of this chapter (Domfors 2000b) suggested that the number of hours offered to parents should be increased.

17.   However this suggestion was not endorsed in the ensuing FUNKIS commission report (Sweden 1999).

18.   No national curriculum or guidelines for preschools existed until 1998. The first curriculum for ages 1 to 6 years is currently being carried out, and its effect on Deaf and other bilingual preschool settings needs to be studied.

19.   This system came into force sometime in the middle of the 1970s and covers families where children also have other types of functional disabilities.

20.   In contrast, hearing immigrant children are offered only nine years of (bilingual) compulsory school and three years of high school education in Sweden.

REFERENCES

Andersson, Ronny. 1994. Second language literacy in deaf students. In *Bilingualism in deaf education*, ed. Inger Ahlgren and Kenneth Hyltenstam, 91–101. Hamburg: Signum.

Bagga-Gupta, Sangeeta.1989. The education, integration, and segregation of the deaf and the hard of hearing in Sweden: A focus on social definitions. Department of Communication Studies, Linköping University, Sweden. Typescript.

———. 1995. *Human development and institutional practices: Women, child care and the mobile creches*. Linköping Studies in Arts and Science 130. Ph.D. diss., Linköping University, Sweden.

———. 1999a. Deaf children: Practising literary or participating in literacy practices? Lecture at the first European Days of Deaf Education conference, Sept. 23–26, Örebro, Sweden.

———. 1999b. Tecken i kommunikation och identitet: Specialskolan och vardagsdeltagande (Signs in communication and identity: Special schools and everyday participation). In *Möten: Vänbok till Roger Säljö* (Meetings: In honor of Roger Säljö), ed. Ullabeth Sätterlund Larsson, Kerstin Bergkvist, and Per Linell, 111–39. Linköping, Sweden: Linköping University.

———. 2000. Visual language environments. Exploring everyday life and literacies in Swedish deaf bilingual schools. *Visual Anthropology Review* 15 (2):95–120.

———. 2001a. Discursive-technological practices and belonging to a language: Explorations of diversity and signs of deaf and hearing membership. Paper presented in the panel "Desire, technology and language: The discursive power of technologies in deaf arenas" at the 100th annual meeting of the American Anthropological Association, November–December 2001, Washington, D.C.

———. 2001b. Diskursiva och teknologiska resurser på visuella tvåspråkiga pedagogiska arenor (Discursive and technological resources in visual bilingual pedagogical arenas). *Utbildning och demokrati* (Education and Democracy) 10 (1):55–83.

———. 2001c. Tid, rum och visuell tvåspråkighet (Time, space and visual bilingualism). In *Interaktion i pedagogiska sammanhang* (Interactions in pedagogical contexts), ed. Sverker Lindblad and Fritjof Sahlström, 125–42. Stockholm: Liber.

————. 2002a. Explorations in bilingual instructional interaction: A sociocultural perspective on literacy. *Journal of the European Association for Research on Learning and Instruction* 12(5): 557–87.

————. 2002b. *Vardagskommunikation, lärande och måluppfyllese i tvåspråkiga regionala specialskolor* (Everyday communication, learning and goal achievements in bilingual regional special schools). Stockholm: Skolverket (National Agency for Education).

Baker, Charlotte, and Robbin Battison, eds. 1980. *Sign language and the deaf community: Essays in honor of William C. Stokoe.* Silver Spring, Md.: National Association of the Deaf.

Barton, David. 1994. *Literacy: An introduction to the ecology of written language.* Oxford: Blackwell.

Domfors, Lars-Åke. 2000a. *Döfstumlärare—specialpedagog—lärare för döva och hörselskadade: En lärarutbildnings innehåll och rationalitetsförskjutningar* (Deaf and dumb teacher—special teacher—teacher for deaf and hard of hearing: A teacher education's content and rationality shifts). Örebro Studies in Education 1. Ph.D. diss., Örebro University, Örebro, Sweden.

————. 2000b. Utvärdering av TUFF: Teckenspråksutbildning för föräldrar: Ett Skolverksuppdrag (Evaluation of TUFF: SSL education for parents: A National Agency for Education project). Project report. Örebro, Sweden: National Agency for Education.

Englund, Tomas. 1992. Tidsanda och skolkunskap (The spirit of the times and school knowledge). In *Ett folk börjar skolan* (A people start a school), ed. Gunnar Richardson, 88–111. Stockholm: Allmänna Förlaget.

Eriksson, Per. 1993. *Dövas historia: En faktasamling, Del 1* (The history of the deaf: A collection of facts, Part 1). Örebro, Sweden: National Swedish Agency for Special Education.

————. 1998. *The history of deaf people: A source book.* Örebro, Sweden: Daufr.

Grosjean, François. 1982. *Life with two languages: An introduction to bilingualism.* Cambridge, Mass.: Harvard University Press.

————. 1996. Living with two languages and two cultures. In *Cultural and language diversity and the deaf experience*, ed. Ila Parasnis, 20–37. Cambridge, Mass.: Cambridge University Press.

Gustavsson, Kjell. 1994. *Vad är idrottandets mening? En kunskapssociologisk granskning av idrottens utveckling och läromedel samt en organisationsdidaktisk kompetenssanalys* (What is the meaning of sporting? A sociology of knowledge analysis of sports development, textbook materials and an organizational didactic competence analysis). Acta Universitatis Upsaliensis. Uppsala University, Sweden.

GyVux 1994.2.190. 1994. *Programmaterial för gymnasieskola och gymnasial vuxenutbildning: Byggprogrammet: Programmål, kursplaner, betygskriterier och kommentarer* (Program material for high school and post-compulsory adult education: Building program: Program goals, course plans, grading criteria and comments). Stockholm: National Agency for Education, Fritzes.

Heath, Shirley Brice. 1983. *Ways with words: Language, life and work in communities and classrooms.* Cambridge: Cambridge University Press.

Heiling, Kerstin. 1993. *Döva barns utveckling i ett tidsperspektiv: Kunskapsnivå och sociala processer* (The development of deaf children in a time perspective: Academic achievement levels and social processes). Stockholm: Almqvist and Wiksell.

————. 1994. Reading and writing in deaf children: Comparison between pupils in different ages from oral and bilingual schools. Paper presented at the International Workshop on Bilingualism and Literacy, Oslo, Skådalen Resource Centre, November 10–13.

————. 1996. Deaf children's reading and writing: Comparison between pupils of different ages from oral and bilingual school. In *Bilingualism and literacy concerning deafness and deaf-blindness: Proceedings of an International Workshop, 10–13 Nov. 1994*, ed. Arnfinn

Muruvik Vonen, Knut Arnesen, Regi Theodor Enerstvedt, and Anne Varran Nafstad, 101–14. Oslo: Skådalen Resource Centre.

———. 1997. Döva barns språkliga situation (Deaf children's language situation). In *Från joller till läsning och skrivning* (From babbling to reading and writing), ed. Ragnhild Söderbergh, 199–211. Malmö, Sweden: Gleerups.

Hyltenstam, Kenneth, ed. 1996. *Tvåspråkighet med förhinder? Invandrar- och minoritetsundervisning i Sverige* (Bilingualism with restraint? Immigrant and minority teaching in Sweden). Lund, Sweden: Studentlitteratur.

Hyltenstam, Kenneth, and Veli Tuomela. 1996. Hemspråksundervisningen (Home language teaching). In *Tvåspråkighet med förhinder? Invandrar- och minoritetsundervisning i Sverige* (Bilingualism with restraint? Immigrant and minority teaching in Sweden), ed. Kenneth Hyltenstam, 9–109. Lund, Sweden: Studentlitteratur.

Jacob, Evelyn, and Cathie Jordan, eds. 1993. *Minority education: Anthropological perspectives.* Norwood, N.J.: Ablex.

Lgr 80. 1980. *Läroplan för grundskolan* (National curriculum for compulsory schools). Stockholm: Liber Utbildnings Förlaget.

Linell, Per. 1998. *Approaching dialogue: Talk, interaction and contexts in dialogical perspectives.* Amsterdam: Benjamins.

Lpf 94. 1994. *1994 Års läroplan för de frivilliga skolformerna, särskilda programmål för gymnasieskolans nationella program: Kursplaner i kärnämnen för gymnasieskolan och den gymnasiala vuxenutbildningen* (1994 Curriculum for the noncompulsory school forms, special program goals for the high school national program: Course plans in theory subjects for high school and the postcompulsory adult education). Stockholm: Ministry of Education, Fritzes.

Lpo 94. 1994. *Läroplan för det obligatoriska skolväsendet: Grundskolan, sameskolan, specialskolan och den obligatoriska särskolan* (Curriculum for the compulsory school system: Compulsory school, sameer school, special school and the compulsory-special school). Stockholm: Ministry of Education.

Manillaskolan. 1873. *Reglemente för ett seminarium till bildande af lärare och lärarinnor för döfstummas och blindas uppfostran och undervisning* (College regulations to educate teachers for the upbringing and teaching of deaf-mute and blind). Stockholm City Archives.

National Agency for Education. 1983. *Läroplan för specialskolan: Kompletterande föreskrifter till Lgr 80* (Curriculum for special schools: Complimentary texts for Lgr 80). Special School Supplement. Stockholm: Liber Utbildningsförlaget Skolöverstyrelsen.

———. 1996. *Specialskolan. Kursplaner, timplaner, betygskriterier och kommentarer* (Special schools: Course plans, time plans, grading criteria and comments). Special School Supplement. Stockholm: Statens Skolverk, Fritzes.

———. 1997. *Utvärdering av den statliga specialskolan—organisation och resultat* (Evaluation of the state special schools—organization and results). Dnr: 97:01591. Stockholm.

Ogbu, John U. 1985. Research currents: Cultural-ecological influences on minority school learning. *Language Arts* 62 (8):860–69.

———. 1993. Variability in minority school performance: A problem in search of an explanation. In *Minority education: Anthropological perspectives*, ed. Evelyn Jacob and Cathy Jordan, 83–111. Norwood, N.J.: Ablex.

Östman, Leif. 1996. Discourses, discursive meanings and socialization in chemistry education. *Journal of Curriculum Studies* 28 (1):37–55.

Pärsson, Anita. 1997. Dövas utbildning i Sverige 1889–1971: En skola för ett språk och ett praktiskt yrke (The education of the deaf in Sweden 1889–1971: A school for language and practical trade). Ph.D. diss., Gothenburg University, Sweden.

Prawitz, Johan. 1913. *Manilla Dövstumskola 1812–1912* (Manilla School for the Deaf Mute 1812–1912). Stockholm: Manillaskolan.

Saville-Troike, Muriel. 1989. *The ethnography of communication: An introduction.* 2d ed. Oxford: Basil Blackwell.

Scribner, Sylvia, and Michael Cole. 1981. *The psychology of literacy.* Cambridge, Mass.: Harvard University Press.

Smith, Nathaniel W. 2001. Truth as resistance: Critical pedagogy in the high school classroom. Paper presented in the panel "Life in Schools: Issues of Access, Equity and Critical Pedagogy" at the 100th annual meeting of the American Anthropological Association, November–December 2001, Washington, D.C.

SPM. 2000. *Årsredovisning: Specialskolemyndigheten* (Annual Report: National Agency for Special Schools for the Deaf and Hard of Hearing). Örebro, Sweden.

Street, Brian V. 1984. *Literacy in theory and practice.* Cambridge: Cambridge University Press.

Survey of the structure and function of the inner ear. 1941. Stockholms Stadsarkiv (Stockholm City Archives). Examination papers in journals of education from the deaf-mute college collection.

Svonni, Mikael. 1996. Skolor och språkundervisning för en inhemsk minoritet: Samerna (Schools and language teaching for an indigenous minority: Sameer). In *Tvåspråkighet med förhinder? Invandrar- och minoritetsundervisning i Sverige* (Bilingualism with restraint? Immigrant and minority teaching in Sweden), ed. Kenneth Hyltenstam, 148–86. Lund, Sweden: Studentlitteratur.

Sweden. *Swedish code of statutes.* 1889, no. 27. Lag angående döfstumundervisningen (Law concerning the deaf-mute education). Stockholm: Ministry of Education and Science.

———. *Swedish code of statutes.* 1997, no. 1158. Förordning om statsbidrag för teckenspråksutbildning för vissa föräldrar (Ordinance of state allowances for Swedish Sign Language education of some parents). Stockholm: Ministry of Education and Science.

———. *Swedish code of statutes.* 1998, no. 1003. Appendix 2. Examensordning (The degree ordinance). Stockholm: Ministry of Education and Science.

———. 1999. *Elever med funktionshinder—ansvar för utbildning och stöd* (Students with disabilities—responsibility for education and support). S. Proposition 1998/99: 105. Stockholm: Ministry of Education.

———. *Swedish code of statutes.* 2001, no. 23. Appendix 2. Examensordning (The degree ordinance). Ministry of Education and Science.

Swedish Government Official Report (SOU). 1996. In *TUFF: Teckenspråksutbildning för föräldrar* (TUFF: Swedish Sign Language education for parents), 102. Stockholm: Fritzes.

———. 1997. In *Minoritetsspråksutredning slutbetänkande* (The Minority Language Committee final report), 193. Stockholm: Ministry of Agriculture.

———. 1998. In *FUNKIS: Funktionshindrade elever i skolan* (FUNKIS: Functionally disabled students in school), 66. Stockholm: Fritzes.

Swedish Institute. 1995. *Disability policies in Sweden.* Fact sheets on Sweden. Stockholm: Swedish Institute.

Teveborg, Lennart, and Ingrid Toll. 1991. Preface to *Dövas två språk: Metodbok* (The two languages of the deaf: Methods book). Service Material, National School Agency, S 91 Nr. 7. Stockholm: Skolöverstyrelsen.

Viberg, Åke. 1996. Svenska som andraspråk i skolan (Swedish as a second language in school). In *Tvåspråkighet med förhinder? Invandrar- och minoritetsundervisning i Sverige* (Bilingualism with restraint? Immigrant and minority teaching in Sweden), ed. Kenneth Hyltenstam, 110–47. Lund, Sweden: Studentlitteratur.

Wertsch, James W. 1998. *Mind as action.* Oxford: Oxford University Press.

Wiklander, Lena. 1998. *Utbildningsvägar till yrken där teckenspråk ingår som ett kompetenskrav* (Educational pathways in occupations where sign language is required as competence). Örebro, Sweden: Department of Health and Social Services.

Wingstedt, Maria. 1998. Language ideologies and minority language policies in Sweden: Historical and contemporary perspectives. Ph.D. diss., Centre for Research on Bilingualism, Stockholm University.

5

Romance and Reality:
Sociolinguistic Similarities
and Differences between
Swiss German Sign
Language and Rhaeto-
Romansh

Penny Boyes Braem, Benno Caramore,
Roland Hermann, and
Patricia Shores Hermann

Switzerland is known and generally admired for the several languages spoken by its citizens living in different regions of the country. The well-known Swiss languages are Swiss German, French, Italian, and Rhaeto-Romansh. Not so well-known or recognized is a fifth language used by many deaf Swiss citizens—Swiss German Sign Language (Deutschschweizerische Gebärdensprache, henceforth referred to as DSGS).

The Sociolinguistic Situation of Swiss German Sign Language (DSGS)

DSGS is used by an estimated 7,000 deaf people scattered throughout the 18 German-speaking cantons of Switzerland. Deaf people living in the one predominately Italian-speaking or in the six French-speaking cantons have their own, separate signed languages.

DSGS is composed of five related dialects that have historically developed within and around the five regional public schools for the deaf (in Basel, Bern, Zurich, St. Gallen, and Lucerne). Deaf children who have hearing, nonsigning families have typically learned DSGS from other children in the dormitories and in activities outside the classroom.

The first educational programs for deaf people in both the German and French parts of Switzerland were established between 1811 and 1838. At the beginning, all of these schools were private, having been founded by Catholic priests or Protestant ministers or family and friends of deaf individuals. Although the ultimate goal of all these schools was to teach the deaf pupils how to speak, the first teaching methods, which were directly influenced by Abbé de l'Epée's *signes méthodiques*, included manual signing. Deaf teachers were employed in many of these schools.

Close to 1840, well before the Congress of Milan in 1880, the schools in German Switzerland began to switch to the "German method" of teaching, which allowed no signing at all. This change occurred as more and more school directors were recruited from Germany, there being at that time no training program for teachers of the deaf in Switzerland. These new directors, together with the Swiss teachers, forbade signing in the schools and dismissed all the deaf teachers (Caramore 1988, 1990).

This tradition of teaching deaf children to speak, speechread, read, and write the spoken language while forbidding the use of signing has remained strong in German Switzerland.[1] Only one school for the deaf in German Switzerland (Zurich) has ventured slightly from the traditional oralist method with its introduction in the 1980s of a system of Signed German into the classroom (Maye, Ringli, and Boyes Braem 1987). In the 1990s, most schools for the deaf in German Switzerland began to mainstream as many of their pupils as possible into hearing classrooms of public schools, providing no DSGS interpreters or any other kind of signed language support. Currently, hearing people who are training to become teachers of the deaf are not required to have any competence in DSGS.

Because entrance to all Swiss universities requires a special degree (the *Matura*) from higher secondary schools, people graduating from the schools for the deaf—which are not able to give this degree—have little hope of attaining a university-level education in Switzerland. Over the past ten years, the training program for deaf teachers of DSGS (Gebärdensprachlehrerausbildung, GSLA) has developed into a kind of alternative college for a small group of young deaf adults. During this three-year, part-time educational program, the deaf students take courses in not only teaching DSGS but also higher-level psychology, sociology, pedagogy, and linguistics. All of these courses are taught in DSGS, so the students are able for the first time to have full access to broad areas of information, which were lacking in their orally oriented public education.

Several regional clubs and associations of deaf adults have been established, the most active of which have historically been sports clubs. However, in the mid-1980s, the Swiss National Deaf Association set up the first DSGS courses in German Switzerland and began political advocacy for the public recognition of their language. The group has been helped in this effort by the small, private Association for the Support of Deaf Sign Language (Verein zur Unterstützung der Gebärdensprache der Gehörlosen), which over the past 18 years has published a series of booklets about signed language and Deaf culture.[2]

Professional interpreter training programs and services have been in place for less than 12 years in German Switzerland. There is no signed language used regularly by deaf people or interpreters on any Swiss German television programs, with the exception of a half-hour bimonthly program aimed at deaf and hard of hearing viewers. Unfortunately, in 1998, the Swiss German television, as part of its efforts to save money and despite the loud but fruitless protests of the Deaf community, cancelled this program.

Although a small handbook of illustrations of basic DSGS signs was published (Tissi 1992), a full descriptive dictionary of this language does not yet exist. A five-year computer databank project was begun in 1996 to begin the analysis and collection of DSGS and will serve as a basis for a book, CD, and Internet form of this lexicon.

Currently, no research on DSGS is being carried out in any Swiss university. Most research has been done by one private institute (Center for Sign Language Research in Basel), some of whose projects have been financially supported by the Swiss National Science Foundation (Boyes Braem 1996), and by the Association for the Support of Deaf Sign Language. In addition, the deaf students in the Sign Language Teachers' Training Program have also conducted several valuable studies on DSGS (for example, Tissi 1993; Jauch 1994; Gut 1996; Ribeaud 1998).

WHY COMPARE DSGS AND RHAETO-ROMANSH?

Both the spoken language, Rhaeto-Romansh (RR), and the deaf sign language, DSGS, are languages used by minority groups in Switzerland. Both languages consist of a number of dialects and both face similar problems as a result of not having a standardized form that is used in daily face-to-face communication. Neither of these two minority languages can look for support from a large community in another country that uses the same or a closely related language, unlike the other languages used in Switzerland (Italian, French, and Swiss German). Neither language can claim a city in Switzerland as its primary linguistic-cultural center.

The users of both these languages are minority groups according to several different criteria.

- Both groups are numerically relatively small.

- Neither group, except for a few small RR communities in the canton of Grisons, represents a politically or economically dominant group in its area.

- The group members identify themselves as a minority. Both the RR and the DSGS communities have their own cultures and institutions, including local clubs, sport groups, and theater groups.

- The users of both these languages share the social and economic pressures of having to be bilingual in the language of the majority Swiss German group.

- Both languages enjoy the support of some academics in various fields who have become advocates for the language. "When scientists finally bring themselves to step down from their ivory tower, it's when the fate of a minority language hangs in the balance" (Bauer 1996, 38).

An important difference between the two languages, however, is that the dominant group of hearing Swiss Germans is much more aware of the RR minority than of the DSGS minority. We have two basic reasons for juxtaposing these two languages and their cultures: (a) a comparison of the striking similarities between these two minority groups might encourage the deaf DSGS community to think of itself as not being a totally unique sociolinguistic case; and (b) the discussion of DSGS might make members of the dominant hearing community more aware of a native deaf minority group that has been living within their midst for a long time.

Why the Title "Romance and Reality"?

In our initial research on this question, we repeatedly found areas in which the commonly held view of both these minority Swiss languages contrasts with the reality of their sociolinguistic situations. Furthermore, many of the commonly held opinions could be characterized as "romanticized" views that correspond to other widely held beliefs of the majority culture.

Both languages, for example, tend to be perceived by members of the majority culture as being closer to ancient forms of language and simpler, more natural lifestyles. RR has acquired an aura of the antique from the fact that the language is historically a mixture of "Rhaetian" spoken by the pre-Roman inhabitants of the Rhaetia alpine region and the Vulgar Latin of Roman soldiers, merchants, and officials who invaded the Alps in approximately 15 b.c.[3] The agricultural, mountainous regions of Grisons where this language is spoken also easily evoke a popular, romanticized image of Switzerland in which farming families live a "simple alpine life," "close to nature."

Hearing people often express the belief that signed language is a more direct, honest, emotional form of expression than spoken language. Many hearing non-signers ask, for example, whether it is possible to lie in a signed language. Hearing people often misinterpret the use of specific facial expressions for grammatical functions as particularly vivid and direct nonverbal expressions of the signer's feelings. Another common belief is that signed languages are historically closer to the gestural precursors of spoken language. The following comments in a booklet on sign language, made by a hearing writer 170 years ago, could just as well have been made by hearing people in Switzerland today:

> What new social improvement could be accomplished (through sign language) can now only be imagined, not yet predicted. . . . Sign language is a language which existed earlier than all spoken languages and because of this, is extremely simple, bound to none of the arbitrary forms to which the expression of speech was later subjected. (*Die Zeichensprache der Taubstummen* 1829, 217–19)

For both RR and DSGS, one reality is that the closer the daily interaction with members of the minority culture, the more likely that the romantic view of the language will be shaded with more negative opinions. For example, the largest vote against making RR an official language of Switzerland was from another minority group, the Walser Swiss Germans, whose villages are close geographic neighbors of RR communities in Grisons (Deutsch-Bünden sagt leise ja 1996). Similarly, the greatest opponents of DSGS in this century have traditionally been people who work most closely with sign language users. Teachers and administrators of schools for the deaf have repeatedly characterized signed languages as being either degraded forms of the spoken language or, more derogatorily, as "monkey languages" (Caramore 1988).

Both RR and DSGS have also gone through periods in which they have had to fight against attacks from academics. For example, the status of RR as a separate language in its own right was heavily attacked by researchers of another Romance language, Italian, during World War I (Gross, Cathomas, and Furer 1996). Some spoken-language linguists who have never themselves studied a signed language nevertheless have concluded that these languages do not have a full language status because they are not based on sound and do not display some of the language features such as articles and copula verbs that these linguists would expect in a "real" language. This parallelism breaks down when it comes to the majority culture's views of the users of the two languages. The average Swiss German's view of the RR speaker tends to be that of a "heroic" or "archetypal" Swiss. The deaf signer of DSGS is, however, more often seen simply as a physically handicapped person.

THE LEGAL STATUS OF RR AND DSGS

Among the aspects of language use that are addressed by the Swiss Federal Constitution and current legal doctrine are

- the individual's right to use any language in private ("language rights");
- the "territorial principle" of language use;
- "national languages" used in the different territories; and
- "official languages" that are used for administrative purposes.

THE INDIVIDUAL'S PRIVATE LANGUAGE RIGHTS

The Romanticized View of the Individual's Language Rights

People living in Switzerland have the basic human right to use any language for private purposes. This right stems from the legal interpretation of the Language Article 116 of the Swiss Federal Constitution and from Switzerland's 1992 signing of the Council of Europe's European Charter for Regional or Minority Languages (Gross, Cathomas, and Furer 1996). According to the last census in 1990, other languages that are used privately as first languages by a large number of people living in Switzerland are, in descending order of number of users, Spanish, Slavic, Portuguese, Turkish, English, and Albanian (Franceschini 1996).

The Reality of the Individual's Language Rights

Rhaeto-Romansh

RR speakers are not overtly denied the right to use their language in private. However, RR speakers often find themselves in situations familiar to minority language speakers throughout the world wherein social pressures marshal against the use of their language. There are, for example, situations in which using RR is considered offensive or even overtly political (Viletta 1984). A specific example of this reaction occurred at a recent cantonal music festival in Grisons where Swiss German- and RR-speaking people participated. Everything went along well until the list of winners was read in RR with no translation into German. A speaker of a Swiss German dialect later commented, "It was more than impolite; it was an affront, inexcusable" (Bundi 1996, 69).

DSGS

For DSGS signers, the basic individual human right to use any language for private purposes is more severely violated. Parents, schools, or other authorities often forbid deaf children to use DSGS, even for private conversations. In the cases where DSGS is not strictly forbidden in the private life of deaf children outside the classroom, it still is often actively discouraged.

The use of DSGS in public situations where nonsigning hearing people are present is also considered offensive by many deaf members of the older generation who prefer speaking to signing in public places. Many hearing people who are bilingual in a spoken language and a signed language also do not switch to the signed language if a deaf person joins a conversation. Deaf people in Switzerland, accustomed throughout their whole lives to accommodating to the oral language of the hearing majority, will switch to a contact language form of signing, which uses many spoken-language elements (including vocalization), when a hearing person joins a conversation. This occurs even if the deaf person knows that the hearing people present have some command of DSGS (Lucas and Valli 1989; Boyes Braem 1996).

THE "TERRITORIAL PRINCIPLE" OF LANGUAGE USE

The Romanticized View of the Territorial Principle

There are four main geographical areas, or territories, of Switzerland. In each it is commonly believed that the majority of the population speaks the same language, which is (depending on the territory) either Swiss German, French, Italian, or Rhaeto-Romansh (see figure 5.1).[4] Public road signs and advertisements clearly signal which language is the language of the region, and sometimes, even the crossing of the regional border can be clearly marked. For example, in the train from Basel to Geneva, all train announcements over the loudspeaker are first given in Swiss German and, after the train has passed a territorial boundary, then change to being announced first in French.

RR is used primarily in the large mountainous canton of Grisons in southeastern Switzerland. The Grisons, with Chur as its capital, has the distinction of being the only trilingual (German, Italian, Rhaeto-Romansh) canton in the Swiss Federation. The canton is further subdivided into five territories (Sursilvan, Sutsilvan, Surmeiran, Putèr, and Vallader) in which RR speakers have in the past been the majority language-users.

DSGS is used by deaf people in all of the Swiss German cantons and in Grisons. The regional dialects of the signed language used in German Switzerland

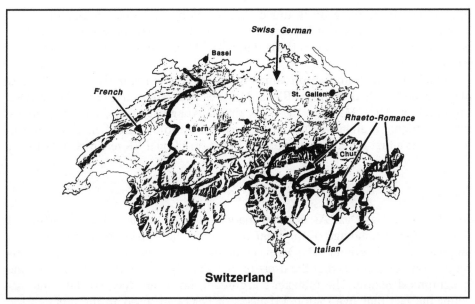

Switzerland

FIGURE 5.1 The regions of Switzerland where the four national languages have traditionally been spoken by a large part of the population. The dialects of DSGS are centered around the schools for the deaf in Basel, Bern, Luzern, St. Gallen, and Zürich.

are those centered around the schools for the deaf in Basel, Bern, Lucerne, St. Gallen, and Zurich (Boyes Braem 1984). There are no official statistics for DSGS users; however, the most cited figure estimates somewhat more than 7,000 deaf users of this language. Moreover, many hearing people also have learned DSGS either from their deaf parents in the home or in signed-language courses.[5]

The Reality of the Territorial Principle

Rhaeto-Romansh

The traditional territory of RR has been shrinking since 1880 when 40% of the population in Grisons stated that it was their "native language." In 1990, only 17% of the Grisons population claimed that RR was the language over which they had the "best command." This desolate figure for "language of best command" is offset by somewhat more positive figures for RR as a language in which one has some competence in speaking (34% of the Grisons population) or understanding (42%) (Gross, Cathomas, and Furer 1996). However, when only 72 of the 213 communities in Grisons have a Romansh-speaking majority, the need to revise the old map of traditional RR territories is clear.

The territory in which the majority of the population uses RR as a first language is becoming increasingly fragmented because of the growth of the Swiss German-speaking population—a phenomenon known as "creeping Germanism." For economic survival, almost every RR speaker must know Swiss German and written German. In addition, more and more native Swiss German speakers either have moved to or spend long vacations in areas that were traditionally part of the RR regions in Grisons. As a consequence of these trends, an ever larger number of children are growing up in this canton speaking Swiss German as their first language. The situation of RR had become so acute that the Swiss population voted in March 1996 to amend the Federal Constitution to protect the endangered RR (Bundeskanzlei 1996, 4).

In all of Switzerland, approximately 70,000 people regularly speak RR, and about 40,000 of them say that RR is their best mastered language (Bieler 1996; Franceschini 1996). Many of these RR first-language speakers, including many who are highly motivated to make a special effort to be sure their children also learn RR as a first language, do not live in the traditional RR territory of Grisons.

DSGS

In 1993, the Swiss Deaf Association made a request to the federal government that the signed language of the Deaf community be considered a fifth national language of Switzerland. The Minister of the Interior wrote back refusing this request on the grounds that the users of this language were not all located in one geographical region. The minister's argument, however, does not take into account the fact that five regional dialects of DSGS are used in the areas of the schools for the deaf. Many of the deaf people who graduate from these schools continue to live in the same cantons. Thus, one could argue that DSGS does indeed fulfill many of the basic territorial principle requirements that the Swiss Minister of the Interior cites as necessary for languages to be officially recognized.

In 1994, both chambers of the Swiss parliament did approve a petition proposed by the Swiss Deaf Association, which "recommends sign language for the integration of the deaf and urges, together with the oral language, its support in the fields of education, training, research and communication" (Parlamentsdienste 1994). This action was an encouraging first step for the signing Deaf community. However, the Minister of the Interior gave the responsibility for carrying out this petition back to the individual cantons where what counts is not the idealistic intent of the postulate but, rather, the comparative political power of different lobbies. The signing Deaf community represents only a very small and unimportant lobby compared with those groups that oppose any recognition of signed languages in Switzerland (many educators of the deaf, doctors, proponents of cochlear implants, hearing aid specialists, and associations of parents of deaf children).

The National Languages of Switzerland

The Romanticized View of National Languages

In the Swiss Constitution, the four languages that have been traditionally associated with specific territories are recognized as being the national languages (*Landessprachen*) of Switzerland. They are German, French, Italian, and Rhaeto-Romansh. For most non-Swiss, the common assumption is that the four national languages of Switzerland represent four different standardized mother tongues used by the Swiss people.

The Reality of National Languages

Rhaeto-Romansh

The reality of the national language situation is different from common beliefs not only for RR but also for spoken Swiss German. Although RR has been one of the four national languages of Switzerland since the constitutional reform of 1938, what is actually being referred to in the constitution is not one standardized language form because the term *Rhaeto-Romansh*, like the term *Swiss German*, refers to a number of language varieties spoken in different geographical regions. Furthermore, unlike the Swiss Germans, who can use a standardized written form of a related language from another country, the Romansh-speakers can look to no other country for a standardized, written form of their language.

Whether or not to use RR as a language of instruction in primary schools is a decision made by the local communities. Bilingual (German and Romansh as well as Italian and German) schools are officially encouraged as a means of maintaining the minority languages. In the upper secondary schools in the canton of Grisons, Romansh is recognized as a native tongue. For entrance exams to the cantonal college, the law specifies that "Candidates whose native tongue is Romansh shall be examined in that language" (Gross, Cathomas, and Furer 1996, 38–39). However, because the canton of Grisons has no university, RR speakers who want a university education are forced into the "German Language Diaspora" (Lämmler 1996, 43).

DSGS

No signed language has been recognized as an official Swiss language. DSGS is also far from being a language of instruction because it is forbidden in the classrooms of all schools for the deaf in German Switzerland with the exception of the Zurich School. The Zurich School does not use DSGS as an official teaching language but has, since 1995, allowed it to be used by a deaf teacher's aide for two hours a week with three classes of deaf pupils (Bachmann 1997).

But even if a signed language were an official language, what would be its form? Would it be the signed language used in the German part of Switzerland or the quite different ones used in the French or Italian regions of the country? Even if this question about which signed language were resolved, the problematic situation (analogous to that of Swiss German and Rhaeto-Romansh) remains because the language consists only of dialects with no standardized form. To make things more complicated, deaf children in German Switzerland, like their hearing counterparts, learn how to read and write in Standard German. Unlike their hearing counterparts, however, deaf children are also taught to speak and speechread Standard German rather than Swiss German, which means they do not use the Swiss German dialect spoken by their hearing relatives and neighbors in everyday life.

THE OFFICIAL LANGUAGES OF SWITZERLAND

The Romanticized View of Official Languages

Using a "national" language in multilingual Switzerland has not meant that one could automatically use that language for all administrative contacts between individuals and federal authorities. Until recently, only German, French, and Italian could be used as an official language for all federal government business and interactions with the Supreme Court. Although RR has been an official language of the canton of Grisons, it was not until the spring of 1996 that the Swiss population voted to accept it also as an official language on the federal level.

The Reality of Official Languages

Rhaeto-Romansh

After the Swiss citizens voted for the official status of RR, it was uncertain which form of RR would be used. A standardized written form of RR, Rumantsch Grischun, was created in 1982 by the linguist Heinrich Schmid of the University of Zurich. There is a small but growing number of publications in this standardized language, including picture dictionaries, children's books, and lexicons on different semantic areas such as professions, technology, biology, and sports. An interregional newspaper in this new language was attempted but given up in 1995, partly because of the competition from existing newspapers published in the regional varieties of RR.

The basic problem seems to be that this newly created written language is not yet widely accepted by the speakers of the various dialects. A 1996 survey among RR speakers has indicated that 66% were in favor of a standardized written form of their language; of these, only 44% favored the new Rumantsch Grischun over a written form of one of the existing dialects (Zur romanischen Sprache 1996, 65). Some RR speakers have particular problems with some of the new Rumantsch Grischun words that have been invented to cover concepts for which no words exist in the older dialects and for which the RR speakers have traditionally borrowed terms from Swiss German.

At least for the Federal Supreme Court, the question about which form of RR should be used was settled by a ruling in June 1996. The only federal judge (of 30 judges) who happened to know RR wrote his decision in Rumantsch Grischun. He then had to translate his deliberations himself into German so his colleagues could read them. The actual use of RR as an official language will take some time and will no doubt face numerous obstacles, including what to do about interpreters.

DSGS

The use of a signed language as an official language for administrative purposes is extremely unrealistic because a widely accepted, standardized form for writing (or documenting) this visual-corporal language does not yet exist. Signed languages can be easily documented by using videotape and film, but at present, the legal system does not recognize audiovisual representation of documents. This attitude might conceivably change in time as the modern multimedia technology that is so advantageous to signed languages continues to evolve and become more generally applied. Unlike the situation with RR, professionally trained interpreters already translate both DSGS and the signed language used in the French part of Switzerland.

PAST AND PRESENT ATTITUDES TOWARD RHAETO-ROMANSH AND DSGS

ROMANTICIZED ATTITUDES

The outsider's picture of either the RR or DSGS minority groups usually tends to be that of a fairly homogeneous subgroup whose members support one another, their language, and their culture. For the Swiss Germans, this assumption is quite likely an extrapolation from their own experience of strong self-identification with their own dialect subgroups. Strong identification with local groups is also reinforced by the federal structure of Switzerland because most of the important legal and administrative aspects of life are handled within the domain of the local communities rather than through the central government in Bern. Indeed, the local community where the citizen lives even issues Swiss passports.

MORE REALISTIC ATTITUDES

Rhaeto-Romansh

Romansh speakers not only are divided by their different dialects but also are geographically separated from one another by the mountains. Some RR speakers have, in fact, characterized their primary loyalty and support of local groups and institutions as having a "mountain mentality," which is one of the reasons why interregional associations for RR (for example, the Lia Rumantscha) do not always enjoy enthusiastic support among local inhabitants. The RR language itself is not held in highest esteem by all its speakers, as one journalist observes:

> [The average RR speaker] . . . seldom values his mother tongue as a spiri-
> tual source of strength but rather finds it a kind of second-rate language,
> just good enough for home, stable, children and the kitchen. Yes, even
> a burden which hinders improvement and makes exams more difficult.
> (Sprecher 1994, 5)

DSGS

The Swiss German Deaf community is also composed of subgroups who often have more loyalty to their regional organizations—local deaf clubs, sports groups, church groups—than to the central Swiss Deaf Association (Schweizerischer Gehörlosenbund) in Zurich. Like the RR's Lia Rumantscha, the Schweizerischer Gehörlosenbund is often faced with a wall of indifference if not outright opposition when it attempts to initiate new interregional projects. Not every deaf person in German Switzerland is an ardent supporter of DSGS. A very small but very vocal association of "spoken-language oriented deaf people" was recently founded in German Switzerland. Sentiments very similar to those attributed above to some RR speakers have been made about signed languages by exclusively orally educated deaf people.

THE REFLECTION OF HISTORICALLY CHANGING SOCIAL CONDITIONS AND ATTITUDES IN THE LANGUAGES

RHAETO-ROMANSH FROM A HISTORICAL PERSPECTIVE

Rhaeto-Romansh has a long tradition of literature written in the different dialects of RR. According to one author (Riatsch 1996), the past 450 years of this literature can be divided into three large historical periods. During the "religious-confessional" phase (1550–1850), translations of the Bible and religious writing were the main texts, although some lyrics, biographies, and translations of philosophical works such as Rousseau's *Contrat Social* were also published.

In the next period (1850–1950), under the influence of the 19th-century ideas of the Romantic Movement and of Nationalism, most of the writings focused on the fight for the official recognition of the RR language and culture. Common themes in the literature of this period were nature and seasons; love and death; emigration, homesickness, and return; and the beauty of and threats to the language as a mother tongue. Many of these themes were handled in the form of fairy tales and legends. In the last phase, which began about 1950 and extends to the present, the themes have been greatly expanded to include those that were previously taboo: drugs, sex, racism, and incest. Along with new themes came new genres such as detective novels as well as experimental prose and poetry. Parody and satire also began to appear, including a biting satirical work about the "save the Romansh movement" itself. Other more recent works have made fun of the myths, the self-importance, and personal infighting related to the local literary scene. Because the authors of the works in this most recent period typically have been bilingual in RR and German or Italian, we find a freer mixing of the languages in the texts.

A great deal of linguistic research has been conducted on RR, especially on the linguistic changes resulting from the different language contact situations over the centuries. The new standardized written language, Rumantsch Grischun, has itself been expanded, with 176,000 newly coined words to meet the needs of its speakers living in a modern society. Although a databank of these newly coined words is available on the Internet home page of the Lia Rumantscha (http://www.spin.ch/liarumantscha/), they are not yet always found in the daily conversation of many RR speakers (Pult 1996).

Swiss German Sign Language and Deaf People in Different Historical Periods

Changing German Words for Deaf People

How deaf people in Switzerland have been viewed and have viewed themselves has gone through several historical changes. Looking at the past 200 years, the influence of the medical-technical perspective of the hearing majority has greatly affected German words describing deaf people, replacing an earlier, more culturally oriented view that the Deaf community had of itself. Beginning in the 1990s, members of the signing Deaf community began to describe themselves with more culturally derived terminology. Table 5.1 summarizes this changing terminology that will be discussed in more detail below.

In the period between 1800 and 1900, deaf people were referred to as "deaf," "deaf and dumb," or "language-fragile" (*taub, taubstumm,* or *sprachgebrechlich*). During this time, deafness was also often associated with idiocy. After 1870, a law was passed that allowed the foundation of private associations, creating a new era for deaf people in Switzerland. Despite strong resistance from hearing circles—above all, teachers of the deaf and many of the directors of deaf schools—

Table 5.1   Changing German Terminology for Deaf People in
German Switzerland over the Past 200 Years

Year	Culturally Determined Terminology	Technologically Determined Terminology
1800	deaf (taub) deaf and dumb (taubstumm) language-fragile (sprachgebrechlich)	
1900		hearingless (gehörlos) hard of hearing (schwerhörig)
1926		mild hearing-impaired (leicht hörbehindert) severely hearing-impaired (stark hörbehindert) hearing-handicapped (hörgeschädigt)
1990	deaf (taub) gelos	

deaf people began to found their own associations. Deaf culture was supported and developed with a variety of activities in which the Deaf community took great pride.

By the early 20th century, however, the development of new technologies such as hearing aids led the hearing authorities to categorize deaf people in new ways, creating a new distinction between "hearingless" and "hard of hearing" people (gehörlos and schwerhörig). Deaf people themselves seemed to be proud, at first, of these new labels that were imposed on them because they implied that deaf people were no longer considered "speechless idiots" but were capable of speaking.

Not only terminology for the deaf but also the lives of Swiss deaf people themselves were greatly affected by another factor in the early 20th century: the growing influence of the theories of eugenics. In 1938, a book appeared, titled *Prevention of Descendants with Hereditary Diseases* (*Verhütung erbkranken Nachwuchses*) and edited by S. Zurukzoglu, professor for Public Health and Bacteriology at the University of Bern. In his foreword, Zurukzoglu writes: "In view of the many victims of congenital sicknesses who must lead sad lives within or outside of institutions, the question arises of whether it would be possible to protect the next generation from such a calamity" (1938, 7).

The background for posing this kind of question involved the delicate social and economic situation at the turn of the century and the emerging science of genetics. The eugenics movement was an offshoot of Social Darwinism. In fact,

Francis Galton (1822–1911), a relative of Darwin, coined the word *eugenics* in 1883, defining it as the science of the improvement of the human race through breeding. Whereas pure Social Darwinism explained and defended current social behaviors as products of an evolutionary biological process of survival of the fittest, the proponents of eugenics did not want to leave this selection process solely to nature but, rather, wanted to plan it with social intervention on a scientific basis.

The basic premise of eugenics was that certain parts of the population, because of hereditary factors, social factors, or both, endangered the survival of a healthy race and, thus, the nation as a whole. For eugenicists, the success and well-being of the nation took precedence over the care of single individuals. Therefore, much discussion took place over how one could eliminate congenital diseases and their carriers while, at the same time, trying to keep the cost of reaching these goals as low as possible.

The teaching of "race hygiene" in the Third Reich in Germany was one of the outcomes of these eugenic ideas. Along with the rise to power of the National Socialists (Nazis), came, on July 14, 1933, the "Law for the Prevention of Descendants with Heredity Diseases" (Das Gesetz zur Verhütung erbkranken Nachwuchses).[6] One of the lesser-known consequences of this law was that, during the Nazi regime in Germany, more than 16,000 deaf were killed, and many others were sterilized or forbidden to marry (Biesold 1988, 1999).

It would be wrong to refer to only the crimes of the Nazis. In many western and eastern European countries, including Switzerland, measures were taken to prevent future generations with hereditary illnesses. In these countries, many different minorities and subcultures were hugely damaged.

In Switzerland, the eugenic measures taken affected the so-called "degenerate" parts of the population (Zurukzoglu 1938, 347). This included the following groups of people: all people with congenital illnesses, the deaf, the blind, the mentally retarded, people with psychological problems (depressives, psychotics, schizophrenics), epileptics, psychopaths, people with querulous or contentious behavior, gypsies, and unmarried mothers.

The Swiss deaf were especially vulnerable to eugenic ideas. While the total Swiss population after the World War I was stagnating, deaf school populations (especially in Zurich and St. Gallen) were dramatically rising (Hepp and Nager 1926, 12).[7] The eugenics movement saw this rise not only as threatening an increase in the number of congenitally deaf in future generations but also as a striking confirmation of its theory that congenitally impaired elements of the population could increase at the cost of nonimpaired members of society.

In this atmosphere then, Ignaz Hepp, director of the "Deaf and Dumb Institute" in Zurich, together with Dr. Nager, director of the Ear-Nose-Throat Clinic of the University Hospital in Zurich, decided in 1926 to make a survey of the deaf population. To collect the medical data for this survey, the hearing authorities needed to make yet further distinctions among degrees of deafness, which resulted in labels for new deaf subgroups: "hearingless," "slightly hearing impaired," and "severely hearing impaired" (*gehörlos, leicht hörbehindert*, and *stark hörbehindert*).

The main purpose of this survey was to establish the number of deaf and hard of hearing people. However, Hepp adds the following comments:

The aim of the caretaking of the deaf and dumb is, and must remain, to make itself superfluous. We should not let ourselves be satisfied with raising our children to be people who strive to be good, capable and able to take care of themselves. We have the duty to help shape the research and to stem the tide of deafness. . . . Precise statistics are one of the best means for recognizing the sources and effects of diseases of the people and for providing a sure basis for maintaining resistance. (Hepp and Nager 1926, 11)

This discussion would be unjust if it ascribed only eugenic intentions to the 1926 survey. That survey also had numerous other purposes. However, the fact remains that the resulting statistics on the number of congenitally deaf people provided the basis for introducing eugenic measures.

The survey's eugenic thrust was certainly recognized by some deaf people and their families. In at least one known case, a mother refused to fill out the questionnaire because she feared the resulting eugenic measures. At the moment, too little is known about how other deaf adults and, especially, the deaf associations reacted to this census. However, in view of how the planned measures would affect deaf people, one would expect that the Deaf community must have resisted to some degree. Nager indicates this resistance was the case in a comment he makes in his discussion of the sterilization laws:

Our many hard of hearing persons, who also need medical care and advice, are afraid to visit their doctor. This makes it even more difficult, if not impossible, to obtain reliable information about family medical histories, as out of exaggerated anxiety, the patient avoids everything that might indicate a suspicion of an hereditary illness. (Zurukzoglu 1938, 187)

During this same period, the Seminar for Special Education was founded in Zurich. The Seminar's new head, alarmed by the statistics of the recent census, made the prevention of more deaf babies one of his priorities (Hanselmann 1935). None of these Swiss medical or pedagogical authorities, however, wanted to adopt the extreme measures being put into practice by the Nazis at the time in Germany. The list of measures used in Switzerland were drawn up by professionals such as Zurukzoglu, Nager, Hepp, and Hanselmann and included the following:

- forbidding the marriage of deaf people;
- marriage counseling with the introduction of a "certificate of fitness for marriage";
- follow-up welfare work;
- obligatory or voluntary sterilization;
- placement in asylums out of "eugenic necessity";
- abortion; and
- measures against incest.

Although the scientists provided the theoretical basis for these measures, it was up to welfare agencies to carry them out. In the case of deaf people, this was above all, the ministers for the deaf who worked together with the teachers of the deaf and the responsible government agencies. In contrast to Germany's practices, involuntary sterilization of deaf women was a measure of last resort in Switzerland. Sterilization without the deaf woman's consent was officially allowed, but only if no other means were available to convince the woman of the surgical procedure's necessity. These other means included encouraging the clergy to dissuade deaf people from marrying one another and placing deaf women in institutions where their likelihood of becoming pregnant was deemed smaller and where the deaf person was under some control.

Members of the older generation of Swiss deaf people today relate many individual stories of how this pressure to prevent deaf babies was exerted. This form of the drive to eliminate deafness continued until at least as late as the 1950s. In 1955, for example, the deaf and hearing members of the Swiss Council for the Deaf and Dumb (Schweizerischer Taubstummenrat) held a meeting at which the following question was discussed, "Do you find it right that deaf people of marrying age receive the advice of genetic researchers?" The answer was concise and unanimous: "Yes, genetic research is today absolutely necessary and possible!" (Pfister 1986, 32).

Until very recently, the reaction of the Deaf community to this historical effort to discourage deaf women from marrying and having children has been one of painful silence. Only within the past decade have deaf women begun, in small groups, to rediscover their identity and past history. A deaf woman in one of these groups has studied deaf women born in the period between 1904 and 1924 (Winteler 1995). In the course of gathering material for this research, elderly single deaf women were encouraged to begin discussing the period in their lives in which they had been approached by social or church workers who persuaded them to lead single lives.

The younger generation of deaf women, between the ages of 20 and 40, are now becoming more insistent on knowing the truth about this period. They do feel, however, that they must conduct their questioning with discretion. Many older women are still afraid to speak openly about the past, knowing that some of the hearing professionals in their stories are still alive. These women experience conflict between feeling grateful toward those who shaped their lives and feeling the desire to criticize these same people.

The evolving differences between the beliefs of the older and younger generations is reflected in current discussions among the younger deaf about how they want to label themselves. With more frequent European meetings and more overseas travel and contacts with non-Swiss deaf communities during the past 20 years, younger Swiss deaf people have evolved a new image of themselves based on cultural rather than technological considerations. The way these younger deaf people now prefer to define themselves is as "normal people who cannot hear." During a workshop on the identity and language, one group of young deaf adults rejected the traditional labels such as *gehörlos* (hearingless) or *hörbehindert* (hearing-impaired), which they felt had been imposed on them by hearing people and connote abnormality as well as deficit. Even the much older term *taub* (deaf) was preferred as being a more neutral term.

Another group of young deaf adults then came up with a new German word for self-identification: *gelos*. This word provides insight into how Swiss deaf people consciously intermingle aspects of their Deaf culture and identity in the coining of new words. *Gelos* is based on a conscious association with two existing German words: *gehörlos* (hearingless) and *gelöst* (resolved, at ease).

By taking the reference to hearing (*hörend*) out of the middle of the word, the deaf group felt a major problem with the word was "resolved" (*gelöst*), and with the result, they felt more "at ease." Formally, what is left are the morphemes *ge* and *los*, components that a hearing German speaker would probably never string together because the resulting word is essentially two affixes without a root morpheme. However, the newly coined word was satisfying to the deaf group, which seemed to be following a metonymic coining technique of DSGS rather than the processes of German word creation. One pleasing aspect of the new German word, they reported, is that its two segments can be produced on the lips in synchrony with the two locations of the hand when accompanying the sign meaning "deaf" (see figure 5.2). In DSGS—wherein the role that is played by fingerspelling in other signed languages is performed by a voiceless mouthing of spoken language-like words or word parts on the lips—this synchronization of manual and mouthing components can be an important phonological consideration (Boyes Braem 2001).

COCHLEAR-IMPLANT: A Sign That Reflects Historical Events and Social Attitudes

Often, not only German words but also DSGS signs reflect aspects of deaf history and culture, both in the coining of new signs and in the playing with old signs found in much Deaf humor. A good example of this reflection is the sign CO-CHLEAR-IMPLANT, the medical procedure to improve hearing in which a device is implanted in the head behind the ear. The scientific evidence so far has not indicated that this medical technological "fix" for deafness will eradicate deafness—and, hence, eradicate the need for signed language—any more completely than did earlier technologies such as hearing aids.[8] However, this technology is cur-

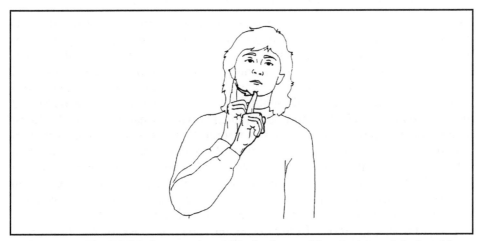

FIGURE 5.2 The DSGS sign DEAF in which the first and last position of the hand is synchronized with the newly coined word *gelos*

rently being used on an ever increasing number of prelingual deaf infants in Switzerland, and professionals are holding out the promise to parents that the resulting ability to hear a doorbell ring or a bird sing will somehow naturally lead to the acquisition of a spoken-aural language.

The Swiss medical and educational proponents of this procedure, which is totally financed by the Federal Insurance for the Handicapped, heavily discourage children who have received an implant from using a signed language and strongly encourage these deaf children to be mainstreamed into hearing classrooms where only the spoken language is used. As a result, a large percentage of the younger generation of deaf people in Switzerland is growing up having no contact with the local Deaf community and its signed language. Because the Association of Parents of Deaf Children is also strongly behind the cochlear-implant and mainstreaming philosophy, the Swiss German Deaf community not only has no contact with this younger generation but also often does not even know who or where they are.

In this sociological context, the Swiss German sign COCHLEAR-IMPLANT is interesting. The form of the Swiss German sign has a different handshape (a bent-V handshape; see figure 5.3a) than those used in either the Swiss French or German Sign Languages for this concept. The Swiss German sign might originally have been a borrowing from a similar form for COCHLEAR-IMPLANT in American Sign Language. Interestingly, this verb form is used by Swiss deaf people to refer to operations only on deaf children, not on adults (see figure 5.3b). The bent-V handshape component of the Swiss German sign is, according to reports of Swiss deaf signers, a conscious association with several other existing signs in DSGS that have the same handshape—SCOLD, ORALISM, and DRACULA—all of which have negative connotations within the local Deaf culture (see figures 5.3c, 5.3d, 5.3e). The Swiss German deaf people who borrowed the DSGS sign COCHLEAR-IMPLANT were thus also incorporating into their sign their opinion of the medical procedure.

A New Sign for a New Deaf Cultural Center in Passugg

The polysemous association of sign subcomponents with different meanings is the source of much Deaf humor. An example of the way that these separate components can consciously reflect aspects of the history as well as the cultural and sociolinguistic concerns of the deaf signer is seen in a new sign that was coined by a deaf group for the name of a new adult education center in the Grisons village of Passugg. The establishment of this new center was an important event for the Swiss German Deaf community, which previously had no national cultural center. The new center also represents an important new spirit in the Deaf community that reflects a renewed awareness of its own culture and a strong determination to foster continuing education with "full access" to information through DSGS. The center, opened in 1996, has been used by a variety of deaf groups from all over German Switzerland for information exchanges, workshops, and courses, most of which have to do with signed language and Deaf culture.

With the inauguration of the new center came the need for an appropriate name sign for the building and what it represented. The village near the center is widely known for its mineral water springs and a brand of bottled mineral water.

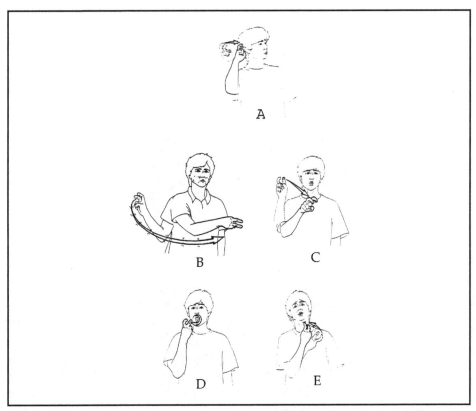

Figure 5.3 DSGS signs (a) cochlear-implant; (b) serially-implant-a-great-many-deaf-children; (c) scold; (d) oralism; (e) dracula

However, the group of young deaf adults who decided during a workshop at the center to coin a new name sign did not feel that simply adopting the existing sign for the town (a gesture associated with drinking and a homonym sign meaning "drunk") was adequate. They came up with a new sign, passugg (see figure 5.4a), which for them consciously evoked metonymic associations with a number of other existing DSGS signs. The different associations discussed by this group were documented by a deaf member of the coining group (Gut 1996).

The deaf coiners associated the initial closed-fist handshape and the initial outward orientation of the palm with their sign stone, making an association with a stable foundation and with the rocky Grisons landscape where the center is located. They found that the path of the movement component was similar to that of an existing sign, upward. The upward orientation of the palm together with the simultaneous opening movement of the closed handshape into an open-5 handshape they associated with other DSGS signs founding, new, and growing (see figure 5.4b and c).

The final handshape of the new sign was associated with the conventionalized hearing gesture for swearing-an-oath, a gesture often seen in folklore and historical paintings of the founders of Switzerland swearing an oath on an alp in central Switzerland (see figure 5.4d). The handshape in passugg, however, is not oriented outward, as in the traditional oath-taking gesture, but inward, toward

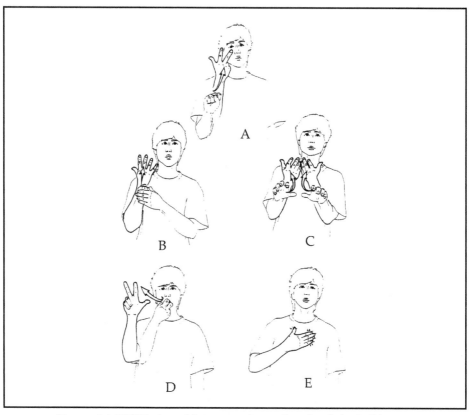

FIGURE 5.4 DSGS signs (a) PASSUGG (a newly coined sign); (b) NEW;
(c) FOUND; (d) SWEAR-AN-OATH; (e) MY

the signer. The deaf coiners made this distinction to associate PASSUGG with the possessive signs MY and OUR (see figure 5.4e). The deaf group also saw this handshape as representing the number 3, which they associated with a variety of other aspects of the canton of Grisons (for example, the three parts of its flag) as well as with specific historical and physical aspects of the new deaf center (the three founding members of the center and physical attributes of the building such as its three floors and three main windows). Not all new signs, of course, are coined with such an elaborate process of conscious associations. However, it is interesting that this associating technique is so deliberately used to create the sign for a center that represents great positive social and cultural importance to the Swiss German Deaf community.

FUTURE PROSPECTS OF THE TWO LANGUAGES

RHAETO-ROMANSH

Since the 1980s, many RR speakers have experienced a new consciousness of their language and culture. This awareness is reflected not only in new kinds of literature discussed earlier but also in a generally innovative cultural scene. Several operas and theater plays have been written in RR, and an annual Literature Days festival and regular (if minimal) TV programming have been established. The RR speaker also benefits from the fact that Swiss society as a whole is becoming more accepting of multilingualism and multiculturalism within individual official language regions (Franceschini 1998).

However, the RR culture is still being threatened with extinction as its traditional territory becomes inhabited by majority language speakers and as more and more RR children learn Swiss German at an early age to prepare for the economic realities of life in German Switzerland. Although efforts by the Lia Rumantscha, the federal government, and other organizations have done much to stem this trend, the fate of RR is still unclear for the coming generations of Swiss who live in an area where Swiss German, German, and English have become the languages necessary for economic survival.

DSGS

Supporters of signed languages share a general belief that this form of language will always have a secure future as long as deaf people are allowed to communicate naturally with one another. The most obvious threats to this presupposition are two possibilities: not allowing deaf people to communicate freely with one another and promoting new attempts to eradicate deafness itself.

Both of these threats loom in the efforts to promote early cochlear implants combined with the mainstreaming of young deaf children into public schools where they have no contact with the local sign language. This combination of cochlear implantation with mainstreaming and no signed language is currently very popular with parents of deaf children. Consequently, the Zurich school, which allows signing in the form of Signed German and a few hours per week of DSGS, had no children scheduled for entry into the first grade in fall 1998. The Lucerne School, although firmly in the "oral education" tradition, has allowed minimal inclusion of DSGS on the school campus by means of deaf adults working in the dormitories. This school has also experienced decreasing enrollments over the past several years.

The school for the deaf in Basel presents a contrasting picture. This school is strongly in favor of cochlear implants for young deaf children and tries to "mainstream" as many of its pupils as possible, with no tutoring or DSGS interpreter support. All adult deaf signers, who in the past taught nonacademic classes like "religion," have been fired, and the school has recently totally shut down its residential program. Thus, one of the traditional routes for the transmission of Deaf culture and DSGS from generation to generation, through signing in the dormitories or in nonacademic classes with deaf adults, has been effectively eliminated in this area of Switzerland. The philosophy and methods of the Basel school have apparently been so appealing to Swiss German parents of young deaf children, that the school had approximately 40 new deaf children registered in fall 1998.

From the Deaf community's point of view, this "lost generation of deaf children" who have no contact with a sign language has made a current Swiss National Science Foundation project for a bilingual, multimedia databank for DSGS even more relevant. In addition to its academic importance, this project will serve as a "bank" for conserving signs until the current generation of cochlear-implanted deaf children reach an age when they can decide for themselves whether they want to learn this language.

Another technological "fix" for deafness, which is waiting on the horizon, is the possibility of parental or prenatal diagnosis of deafness along with gene manipulations made possible by new developments in gene technology. The government is currently drafting a law that would require an individual's agreement before taking a gene-determining test, which would prevent insurance companies from making such tests obligatory (Gentest: Das Gesetz liegt bereit 1998). The spirited public debate about a referendum on whether to allow gene-altering research also indicates that the practical application of any aspect of gene technology to human beings will be preceded by lengthy philosophical and political discussions, at least within Swiss society.[9]

Despite these threats, however, other trends might have a positive influence on the future of signed languages in Switzerland. For example, the fact that the country of Switzerland is becoming more open to being a multilinguistic society is generally positive (Franceschini 1998). The group of people using a signed language is expanding beyond the traditional group of early deafened people as the awareness of the linguistic status and expressive power of signed languages grows among a hearing majority. There is a long waiting list of hearing people wanting to take DSGS courses. Popular commercial films and theater productions,[10] as well as new multimedia technologies (such as CD-ROMs with text and video clips, information on the Internet) will help to make this language more accessible to more people.

Segments of the Deaf community are becoming increasingly active in the research into their own language, history, and culture. Inspired by the founding of a cultural center in Passugg, a group of deaf people in Basel sponsors regular lecture and information evenings as well as the only preschool play group to use signing in German Switzerland. On the national level, the Swiss Deaf Association held a conference in fall 1998 to plan ways and means of ensuring that the 1994 parliamentary statement supportive of signed language is put into effect.

As Grosjean (1992) has commented, there are important differences between those who are bilingual in oral languages and deaf people who are bilingual in signed language and spoken language. Future generations of those who are bilingual in spoken languages have a good chance of becoming monolingual in the language most useful to them. In contrast, future generations of deaf signers will probably remain bilingual because they will continue to have a need in different spheres of their lives for both the economically important spoken language and the perceptually and fully accessible signed language.

One could thus predict that DSGS, although a language still relatively unknown to the hearing majority in Switzerland, will remain a realistically useful language for its deaf users whereas the more well-known and officially more supported RR language perhaps runs a greater risk of become a romantic memory.

ACKNOWLEDGMENTS

All illustrations of DSGS signs are by Katja Tissi. Earlier versions of this study have appeared in German in the information series of the Verein zur Unterstützung der Gebärdensprache, Zurich, as well as in Gogolin, Graap, and List's *Über Mehrsprachigkeit* (Boyes Braem, Caramore, Hermann, and Hermann 1998). The original German portions of the texts have been translated into English by Penny Boyes Braem.

The authors would like to thank the following people for their helpful comments on earlier drafts of this text: Thüring Bräm, Gerald Bennett, Bernard Cathomas, Rita Franceschini, François Grosjean, and Leila Monaghan.

NOTES

1.   The methods and philosophy of oral education have been so pervasive in Switzerland that many deaf parents in the past have been reluctant to use a signed language with their own deaf children. This fact has meant that researchers cannot always rely on the description "deaf child of deaf parents" as ensuring that a signed language informant has a "native" acquisition history. The following categories for informants have been used: "early first-language learners" (deaf children of hearing or deaf parents who learned signed language before the age of 7 years), "later bilingual learners" (deaf people who acquired sign language between the ages of 7 and 13 in the school for the deaf) and "deaf second-language learners" (deaf people who learned signed language after puberty).

2.   VUGS, Oerlikonerstrasse 98, 8057 Zurich, Switzerland.

3.   Little is known about the language of the pre-Romanized Rhaetians. Gross, Cathomas, and Furer (1996, 15) write that the language was neither Etruscan nor Celtic but still somehow related to both.

4.   According to the 1990 census figures, the four languages with their own traditional territories represent the following percentages of the total population of Switzerland: 64% Swiss German, 19% French, 7.6% Italian, and 0.6% Rhaeto-Romansh (see Morgenthaler and Fankhauser 1997, 5).

5.   The most recent census of Switzerland we have access to (1990) did not collect data about the use of a signed language as a first or second language. The estimate of 7,000 deaf signers is based on an internationally used formula: one signing deaf person per thousand of the population. According to this formula, of the approximately 7,000 deaf people in Switzerland, about 5,000 live in the German part, 1,500 in the French part, and 500 in the Italian part. The Swiss Deaf Association in German Switzerland (Schweizerischer Gehörlosenbund, SGB) has taught an average of 500 students yearly for the past ten years, which suggests that at least 5,000 hearing people have some knowledge of DSGS as a second language.

6.   Reichsgesetzblatt I, July 14, 1933, p. 529.

7.   Although heredity or other illnesses were still the primary cause of deafness, data show that fully one-third of this deaf population lost its hearing from a hyperthyroid disorder (Hepp and Nager 1926).

8.   See, for example, Lane (1994; 1995) as well as Lane and Bahan (1998) for critical reviews of the medical literature's claim that cochlear implantation devices will help the acquisition of spoken language as a first language by deaf children.

9.   Viewed on a wider scale, most of these highly technological attempts to wipe out deafness also will be limited to those countries that can afford them and, thus, probably will not affect future generations of deaf people in Third World countries.

10.   In addition to the influential film and foreign language stage productions of the American play, *Children of a Lesser God*, several recent European films have dealt with deaf people and their signed languages, among them, the films *Tanz der Hände* (1997), *Les Enfants du silence*, *Vole mon dragon*, *Hanna*, *Le pays des sourds*, and the Swiss theater hearing and deaf productions *Sprache im Raum—Ungehörte Simme*.

References

Bachmann, Peter. 1997. *Laut-, Schrift- und Gebärdensprachaufbau durch bilinguale Förderung an Gehörlosenschulen mit Beispielen zum kontrastiven Sprachunterricht an der Kantonalen Gehörlosenschule Zürich.* Informationsheft No. 31. Zurich: Verein zur Unterstützung der Gebärdensprache der Gehörlosen.

Bauer, Arthur. 1996. *Allegra genügt nicht! Rätoromanisch als Herausforderung für die Schweiz.* Chur, Switzerland: Verlag Bündner Monatsblatt Desertina AG.

Bieler, Carl. 1996. Mit der Stimme für eine Sprache. *Zurich Tages-Anzeiger,* 29 February, p. 2.

Biesold, Horst. 1988. *Klagende Hände: Betroffenheit und Spätfolgen in Bezug auf das Gesetz zur Verhütung erbkranken Nachwuchses, dargestellt am Beispiel der Taubstummen.* Solms-Oberbiel: Oberbiel.

———. 1999. *Crying hands: Eugenics and deaf people in Nazi Germany.* Introduction by H. Friedlander. Translated by W. Sayers. Washington, D.C.: Gallaudet University Press.

Boyes Braem, Penny. 1984. Studying Swiss German Sign Language dialects. In *Recent research on European sign languages,* ed. Filip Loncke, Penny Boyes Braem, and Yvan Lebrun, 93–103. Lisse: Swets & Zeitlinger.

———. 1996. *Eine Untersuchung über den Einfluß des Erwerbsalters auf die in der deutschsprachigen Schweiz verwendeten Formen von Gebärdensprache.* Informationsheft No. 27. Zurich: Verein zur Unterstützung der Gebärdensprache der Gehörlosen.

———. 2001. Functions of the mouthing component in Swiss German Sign Language. In *Foreign vocabulary in sign languages,* ed. Diane Brentari, 1–47. Mahwah, N.J.: Erlbaum.

Boyes Braem, Penny, Benno Caramore, Roland Hermann, and Patricia Shores Hermann. 1998. Romantik und Wirklichkeit: Soziolinguistische Ähnlichkeiten und Verschiedenheiten zwischen der Deutschschweizerischen Gebärdensprache DSGS und dem Rätoromanischen. In *Über Mehrsprachigkeit: Gudula List zum 60. Geburtstag,* ed. Ingrid Gogolin, Sabine Graap, and Günther List, 157–87. Tübingen, Germany: Stauffenburg.

Bundeskanzlei. 1996. *Volksabstimmung vom 10. März 1996: Erläuterungen des Bundesrates.* Bern: Bundeskanzlei.

Bundi, Hanspeter. 1996. Sie sind anders als wir, heißblütiger und stolz. *Zurich Die Weltwoche,* 18 April, p. 96.

Caramore, Benno. 1988. *Die Gebärdensprache in der Schweizerischen Gehörlosenpädagogik des 19. Jahrhunderts.* Hamburg: Verlag Hörgeschädigte Kinder.

———. 1990. Sign language in the education of the deaf in 19th century Switzerland. In *Current trends in European sign language research,* ed. Siegmund Prillwitz and Tomas Vollhaber, 23–32. Hamburg: Signum.

Deutsch-Bünden sagt leise ja. 1996. *Zurich Tages-Anzeiger,* 11 March, p. 9.

Die Zeichensprache der Taubstummen. 1829. Aarau, Switzerland: Bibliothek der neuesten Weltkunde.

Franceschini, Rita. 1996. Welche Sprachen spricht die Schweiz? Auswertung der Volkszählung 1990. *VPOD Magazin für Schule und Kindergarten* 99:22–30.

———. 1998. Code-switching and the notion of code in linguistics: Proposals for a dual-focus model. In *Code-switching in conversation: Linguistic perspectives on bilingualism,* ed. Peter Auer, 51–75. London: Routledge.

Gentest: Das Gesetz liegt bereit. 1998. *Zurich Beobachter,* 29 May, p. 22.

Grosjean, François. 1992. The bilingual and the bicultural person in the hearing and in the deaf world. *Sign Language Studies* 77:307–20.

Gross, Manfred, Bernard Cathomas, and Jean-Jacques Furer. 1996. *Rhaeto-Romansch: Facts and figures.* Chur, Switzerland: Lia Rumantscha.

Gut, Veronika. 1996. Passugg hat einen neuen Namen. *SGB Nachrichten* 51 (July/August):15–16.

Hanselmann, Heinrich. 1935. Sterilisation und nachgehende Vorsorge. *Heilpädagogik* 4:13–16.

Hepp, Ignaz, and F. Nager. 1926. *Die Taubstummheit im Kanton Zürich.* Zurich: n.p.

Jauch, Claudia. 1994. *Eine Studie der nonverbalen Kommunikation beim Erzählen eines Erlebnisses in Deutschschweizerischer Gebärdensprache.* Informationsheft. No. 25. Zurich: Verein zur Unterstützung der Gebärdensprache.

Lämmler, Rüdi. 1996. Rätoromanen ohne Wirtschaftszentren. *Neue Luzerner Zeitung Wochenende Journal,* 14 September, p. 43.

Lane, Harlan. 1994. The cochlear implant controversy. *World Federation of the Deaf News* 2–3:25–27.

———. 1995. Acquisition of speech perception ability in prelingually deaf children with a multi-channel cochlear implant. *American Journal of Otology* 16:393–99.

Lane, Harlan, and Ben Bahan. 1998. Ethics of cochlear implantation in young children: A review and reply from a Deaf-World perspective. *Otolaryngology—Head and Neck Surgery* 119 (4):297–313.

Lucas, Ceil, and Clayton Valli. 1989. Language contact in the American deaf community. In *The sociolinguistics of the deaf community,* ed. Ceil Lucas, 11–40. New York: Academic Press.

Maye, Claude, Gottfried Ringli, and Penny Boyes Braem. 1987. The use of signs in Switzerland: Projects in the Zurich and Geneva schools. In *Sign and school: Using signs in deaf children's development,* ed. Jim Kyle, 162–70. Clevedon: Multilingual Matters.

Morgenthaler, Bernhard, and Urs Fankhauser. 1997. *Taschenstatistik der Schweiz.* Bern: Bundesamt für Statistik, Sektion Information und Dokumentation.

Parlamentsdienste. 1994. Für die Anerkennung der Gebärdensprache. Press release, May 27. Bern: Parlamentsdienste.

Pfister, Willi. 1986. *Gemeinsam unterwegs.* Muri and Bern: Pfister.

Pult, Chasper. 1996. Zur Befindlichkeit der rätoromanischen Schweiz: pop-rock/engles/um/viv/lom/pop-rock. *Neue Luzerner Zeitung Wochenende Journal,* 14 September, p. 41.

Riatsch, Cia. 1996. Von der Abgrenzung zur Grenzgängerei. *Neue Luzerner Zeitung Wochende Journal,* 14 September, p. 42.

Ribeaud, Marina. 1998. *Wie verstehen gehörlose Kinder eine Videogeschichte in Gebärdensprache?* Informationsheft No. 32. Zurich: Verein zur Unterstützung der Gebärdensprache.

Sprecher, Margrit. 1994. Das Rätoromanische liegt auf der Intensivstation. *Zurich Die Weltwoche,* 27 October, pp. 3–5.

Tissi, Katja. 1992. *Illustration der Grundgebärden der Deutschschweizerischen Gebärdensprache.* Zurich: Schweizerischer Gehörlosenbund.

Tissi, Tanja. 1993. *Namengebärden in der Deutschschweizerischen Gebärdensprache.* Informationsheft No. 23. Zurich: Verein zur Unterstützung der Gebärdensprache.

Viletta, Rudolf. 1984. Die Rätoromanen. Geduldetes Relikt oder gleichberechtigter Teil der Eidgenossenschaft? In *Minderheiten in der Schweiz: Toleranz auf dem Prüfstand,* ed. Alfred Cattani and Alfred Häsler, 95–134. Zurich: Verlag Neue Züricher Zeitung.

Winteler, Gerta. 1995. Ich hätte gerne geheiratet: Aus dem Leben gehörloser Frauen im 20. Jahrhundert. Diploma thesis, Höhere Fachschule für Soziokulturelle Animation, Zurich.

Zur romanischen Sprache. 1996. *Chur (Switzerland) Terra Grischun* 4 February, pp. 64–65.

Zurukzoglu, Stavros. 1938. *Verhütung erbkranken Nachwuchses.* Basel: Benno Schwabe Verlag.

6

The Dilemma of the Hard
of Hearing within the U.S.
Deaf Community

Donald A. Grushkin

Members of the American Deaf culture have long taken what is commonly perceived as a disability to be a "way of life," creating a worldview that maintains a different reality: deafness as the "normal" state of being.[1] To be Deaf has traditionally and primarily been defined as using and valuing American Sign Language (ASL) as well as conforming to a set of culturally defined behavioral and attitudinal norms (Padden and Humphries 1988; Kannapell 1993).

Hard of hearing individuals, being neither fully deaf nor hearing, share characteristics of both yet, at the same time, also share many of the problems and issues faced by Deaf people and have long attempted to tread a fine line between the cultures to which they belong. Despite this effort, hard of hearing individuals frequently report rejections or alienation from both groups, their commonalties notwithstanding. As a result, hard of hearing individuals have often had difficulty developing a secure, complete sense of identity as Deaf, Hearing, or bicultural individuals.

The dilemma of identity has been further compounded for hard of hearing people by a new "Deaf militancy," which asserts that some aspects of being hard of hearing are proof of nonmembership within the Deaf culture. One possible resolution to the hard of hearing person's identity dilemma lies in granting hard of hearing people the means to gain cultural knowledge of, and acceptance by, the minority Deaf culture through education and socialization within enculturating sites such as schools for the deaf, social and recreational activities, and Deaf clubs.

METHODOLOGY

Much of the information presented in this chapter comes directly from my doctoral dissertation (Grushkin 1996) in which I conducted participant observation and interviews (Spradley 1980; Hammersley and Atkinson 1983; Emerson, Fretz, and Shaw 1995) with four hard of hearing high school students at a residential school for the deaf in the United States that used the ASL-English, bilingual-bicultural (bi-bi) philosophy. Students were selected according to criteria for hearing status, length of enrollment within the program, age, and cognitive as well as linguistic ability. Attempts were made to balance selected students for age, gender, and racial composition.

I have a congenital severe-to-profound hearing loss, which with amplification is corrected to a "hard of hearing" level, although I have poor speech discrimination through aural means alone and, therefore, identify myself as Deaf. I was raised orally and in public schools without any contact with other deaf and hard of hearing individuals until I enrolled at the age of 13 at Model Secondary School for the Deaf, a national residential school program for deaf and hard of hearing students connected to Gallaudet University. Since that time, I have been a member of the Deaf community. I attended Gallaudet University and have worked within educational programs for deaf and hard of hearing students for all of my adult life. Some of the information presented in this chapter, including anecdotal commentaries and direct observation, comes from my experience and knowledge as a member of the Deaf community, although the greater portion is, of course, research-based.

BEING HARD OF HEARING: DEFINITIONS

One will quickly learn from reading the literature that determining exactly where the boundaries are that separate being deaf, being hard of hearing, and being hearing is an extremely difficult task. The definitions of these terms vary along audiological, cultural, and ideological lines. In addition, a variety of terms have been developed to describe hearing loss, some of which are considered pejorative or not culturally validating for the Deaf community, for example, *hearing impaired, hearing handicapped, deaf and dumb,* and *deaf-mute* (Levitan 1993).

AUDIOLOGICAL ASSESSMENT AND CATEGORIZATION OF HEARING LOSS

Hearing loss is measured by presenting a series of auditory signals at varying frequencies and degrees of intensity (loudness). The testee's responses (or lack of responses) to these signals are then plotted on a graph called an audiogram. The audiogram's horizontal axis is used to chart the sound frequencies, represented by Hertz (Hz), which refers to the "speed" of the sound waves. Sounds in the lower frequencies (125–250 Hz) are perceived as deeper whereas sounds in the higher frequencies (2,000–4,000 Hz) are higher in pitch. On the vertical axis, the sound intensity, or loudness, (represented by decibel or dB) is graphed. Standard audiological practice is to quote the average of a person's responses (Pure Tone Average or PTA) across several frequencies. People with a greater amount of hearing loss in the higher frequencies are said to have a high frequency loss, and a person with less response to lower frequencies is said to have a low frequency loss.

Rosen (1980) provides a clear, informative explanation of the different degrees of hearing loss and their implications:

- *-10 dB to 25 dB: Normal Range*—Normal breathing is heard at 10 dB; leaves rustle at 25 dB.

- *25 dB to 40 dB: Mild Impairment*—Soft sounds cannot be heard. Repetition may be required to understand what is said. It is hard to understand in noisy places and when more than one person talks. A quiet home at night or whispering occur at around 30 dB.

- *40 dB to 55 dB: Moderate Impairment*—Sounds such as soft speech at 50 dB are not understood without amplification. Normal conversation is barely audible and may sound distorted.

- *55 dB to 75 dB: Moderately Severe Impairment*—Normal conversation level, which is about 60 dB, will be inaudible without amplification, and may sound distorted.

- *75 dB to 95 dB: Severe Impairment*—Only very loud sounds are heard, such as a vacuum cleaner or a shout at a distance of one foot (80 dB). Conversation must be amplified, however, some speech sounds will still be inaudible or distorted.

- *95 dB and up: Profound Impairment*—Even loud noises, such as a power lawn mower (95 dB), a noisy factory (100 dB), music from a rock band (110 dB), or a propeller plane at takeoff (120 dB) may only be sensed as an indistinguishable rumble rather than actually being heard. (2–3)

Difficulty of Using Audiological Definitions

A person might have varying degrees of loss in different frequencies yet maintain an average loss similar to another person with a different frequency range response. Ross (1990) clarifies this point:

> Consider a child with a 40 dB hearing loss at the frequencies of 500, 1,000, and 2,000 Hz. The average hearing loss is 40 dB, and it is this figure that is usually used when describing the degree of the hearing loss. Now consider a child with a zero threshold at 500 Hz, a 40 dB threshold at 1,000 Hz and an 80 dB threshold at 2,000 Hz. The average hearing loss for this child is also 40 dB. The auditory performance and general behavior of these children will, however, differ considerably. The child with a flat hearing loss is consistent in his or her diminished ability to respond to speech and other sounds. The child with the high frequency loss, on the other hand, can respond to low intensity (and low pitched) sounds normally, but because he or she cannot perceive the full spectrum of speech frequencies, the child's responses to meaningful stimuli are inconsistent and inadequate. Furthermore, this child will usually display more severe speech and language problems than the one with a mild-to-moderate flat hearing loss (1990, 8).

Cultural and Attitudinal or Ideological Definitions

Measurable definitions of hearing loss such as those provided above may serve well for bureaucratic purposes, but within the interpersonal realm, they frequently possess little meaning. As an illustration, Witcher (1974) describes her daughter as "hard of hearing," yet she states that her daughter has a severe to moderately severe high frequency loss, which enables her to hear only some sounds such as thunder and car motors. To many observers, this description would be indicative of a deaf, not hard of hearing, person.

Similarly, Ross and Calvert (1967) describe how, by referring to all deaf and hard of hearing children as "deaf," the educational system is creating a self-fulfilling prophecy through which the hard of hearing children indeed become deaf. Although Ross and Calvert's words express some truth, it is clear that both their, as well as Witcher's (1974), comments indicate their desire to avoid placing the stigma (Goffman 1963) of deafness upon the hard of hearing child. That is, both authors appear to imply that being deaf is less desirable than being hard of hearing, just as being hard of hearing is less desirable than being hearing. The avoidance of stigma is what has spurred educators and the general public to use euphemisms such as "hearing impaired," "audiologically handicapped," and so forth to describe hearing loss.[2] In using these labels, the society as a whole is attempting to engage in the process of normalization (Lane 1992) or "hearization" (Nover 1993) of deaf and hard of hearing children and adults. Nover observes:

> [H]earization leads many deaf children into wishing or thinking they will become hearing some day. Others prefer to be called "hearing impaired" or "hard-of-hearing" rather than deaf. Unfortunately, deaf and hard-of-hearing children may learn to view hearing people as superior to those who are deaf. (1993, 16)

Yet, the Deaf community, in a cultural inversion (Levine 1977; Basso 1979; Ogbu 1987) or rejection of Hearing values, has embraced the term *deaf* to apply to themselves. Cultural inversion is common to minorities, especially "involuntary minorities" (Ogbu 1987). Ogbu defines involuntary minorities as those groups who have been placed into a minority status within a nation through means not of their own choosing, for example, the African Americans who were brought to America through slavery or the Mexican Americans living in formerly Mexican portions of this country at the time of American annexation of Mexican territory. Cultural inversion is explained by Ogbu in this manner:

> Cultural inversion is the tendency for members of one population, in this case involuntary minorities, to regard certain forms of behaviors, certain events, symbols and meanings as not appropriate for them because they are characteristic of members of another population (e.g., white Americans); at the same time, the minorities claim other (often the opposite) forms of behaviors, events, symbols and meanings as appropriate for them because these are not characteristic of white Americans. *Thus, what the minorities consider appropriate or even legitimate behaviors or attitudes for themselves are defined in opposition to the practices and preferences of white Americans.* (1987, 323, emphasis added)

Thus, for Deaf people, having a hearing loss is a core aspect of their identity and one to be closely held along with their language and values (Reagan 1985;

Padden and Humphries 1988; Kannapell 1993). This view runs directly counter to the perspective of the Hearing community, which holds hearing loss to be a negative, undesirable phenomenon and one that has the potential to exclude an individual from attaining or retaining a Hearing identity, from participating within Hearing society (which would be unfortunate in the Hearing worldview), or both. In other words, the different "center" (Padden and Humphries 1988) of the Deaf community holds deafness as the normative state of being while the possession of hearing is the marked condition. In the Deaf community, according to Padden and Humphries, a person who possesses a great deal of auditory capacity that enables him or her to function almost as a hearing person might be described as VERY-HARD-OF-HEARING whereas, within the Hearing world, a person who is described as "very hard of hearing" is an individual with a severe degree of hearing loss.

As one can see from this discussion, the very meaning of commonly held terms can differ widely depending on one's psychological and cultural orientation. However, to be Deaf or hard of hearing does not necessitate that one belong to a single political, cultural, or educational entity. One's status as a Deaf or hard of hearing individual is a function of audiological, sociocultural, and personal perceptions. The highly varying definitions of all three perceptions make it difficult to define an individual as belonging to any one of the categories of Hearing, Deaf, or hard of hearing.

EDUCATION OF THE HARD OF HEARING IN AMERICA

Education of deaf people in America began in 1817 when Thomas H. Gallaudet, a Protestant minister, and Laurent Clerc, a deaf man educated in France, established the first permanent school for the deaf in Hartford, Connecticut. Shortly thereafter, residential schools for the deaf quickly appeared in many states across America. At these schools for the deaf, hard of hearing individuals were often educated alongside their more profoundly deaf peers.

Before the early 20th century, hard of hearing individuals (and deaf people who had been born hearing) were referred to as "semi-mutes." Although most of these individuals were taught along with their profoundly deaf peers through sign language and fingerspelling under the "Combined System," which was developed by Edward Miner Gallaudet (Thomas Gallaudet's son), the hard of hearing (and some deaf) students also received additional instruction in speech production. Starting in the 1850s and 1860s, a movement began that pushed for the abolition of sign language and for deaf children to be instructed through speech alone (oralism). For an excellent exploration of the reasons for oralism's popularity and rise in acceptance, the reader is referred to Douglas Baynton's (1996) work.

The oralist movement was spearheaded by notables such as Alexander Graham Bell and Gardiner Greene Hubbard in the United States as well as others abroad such as the famous French physician Prosper Ménière and the Abbé Giulano Tarra from Italy. In the late 1870s, a series of conventions took place at which oralism was actively endorsed, and in 1880, this movement found its culmination at an international convention of educators of the deaf in Milan, Italy. At this convention (which had only one Deaf person in attendance) all of the 164 delegates, except for the five from the United States, voted to endorse oralism as the sole mode of instruction within schools for the deaf. Oralism came into primacy worldwide after the Milan convention, and most deaf and hard of hearing students were instructed through oral and auditory means alone. Although actively resisted in the United States, oralism soon took over also at the American schools for the deaf. Lane (1980) describes the swiftness of oralism's spread:

> There were 26 American institutions for the education of the deaf in 1867 and ASL was the language of instruction in all 26; by 1907, there were 139 schools for the deaf and ASL was allowed in none. (131)

According to anecdotal evidence within the Deaf community, educators of the deaf would often demonstrate the effectiveness of oral education by showcasing semi-mute students (without informing their audience of the background history of these students) as exemplars of what oral instruction could achieve (see Lane 1980, 1984). In addition, semi-mute and hard of hearing students were held up as models of oral communication for more profoundly deaf students to emulate. The comparison of hard of hearing students to deaf students was a naturally unfair one because these semi-mute or hard of hearing students possessed a natural advantage over their profoundly deaf peers in their ability to auditorily perceive some speech sounds or in their memory of how to speak, which they may have retained if they had been born hearing.

With the advent of electronic amplification in the early 20th century, the distinction between deaf and hard of hearing individuals began to emerge. Along with this differentiation and in conjunction with the push toward English-only, oral education (Lane 1980; Nover 1993), educators began placing increasing numbers of hard of hearing (and deaf) students in public school programs, a practice known as "mainstreaming." The impetus for mainstreaming gained extra force with the passage in the mid-1970s of Public Law 94–142, which was superseded in 1998 by P.L. 105–17. Since P.L. 94–142's passage, enrollments at many state schools for the deaf have significantly declined (Holden-Pitt 1997). Further, hard of hearing students are not encouraged to attend schools for the deaf, which is clearly indicated by the increase in enrollments at schools for the deaf of children with corresponding increases in severity of hearing loss (Holden-Pitt 1997).

At public schools, (and at some schools for the deaf) sign language and, especially, ASL is not considered to be a logical mode of communication for hard of hearing students because they are presumed to be capable of academic and social functioning through aural means alone. Consequently, hard of hearing students are frequently not exposed to any sign communication but are encouraged to develop their speech and auditory skills to promote a greater sense of identification and interaction with the Hearing world. Thus, hard of hearing people clearly have been and continue to be psychologically and physically isolated from the Deaf world. Branson and Miller (1993), working in Australia, assert that this psychological and physical isolation from the Deaf world ultimately teaches hard of hearing (and deaf) students to reject it (see also Woodward and Allen 1993).

DIFFICULTIES OF HARD OF HEARING INDIVIDUALS IN MAINSTREAMED SETTINGS

At first glance, one might easily conclude that hard of hearing individuals have more in common with hearing people than with deaf people because they can acquire speech and auditory skills to a greater degree than is possible for most deaf people. However, a great deal of empirical documentation points to deficiencies in the auditory and articulatory (speech) processes of hard of hearing children and adults that directly or indirectly translate into academic and social difficulties for this population (Davis 1990; Ross 1990) and that parallel the situation of more profoundly deaf children. Indeed, a number of studies have shown that, academically, hard of hearing students tend to lag two to three years behind their hearing peers (Ross, Brackett, and Maxon 1982; Brackett and Maxon 1986). Further, losses as mild as 15 dB to 25 dB (the point at which one can hear leaves rustling) can result in academic lags of more than a year, and the academic delay increases with greater degrees of hearing loss (Quigley and Thomure 1968). Although this academic delay is not as severe as has typically been found for severely and profoundly deaf children, it remains true that hard of hearing students experience academic difficulties in the regular school program as do severely and profoundly deaf children.

In addition, although hard of hearing people may possess the ability to rely on auditory processes alone for speech comprehension, they frequently report comprehension difficulties when they encounter extensive background noise or when the speaker is further away, does not articulate well, or uses a dialect different from that of the hard of hearing listener. The apparent inconsistency of hard of hearing students' responses to auditory stimuli (including speech) has led to a paradoxical social exclusion of these students by their hearing peers, who reported a higher social preference for their more profoundly deaf classmates (Elser 1959; Kennedy and Bruininks 1974; Kennedy et al. 1976; Ross 1990). That is, because hard of hearing students might respond to a hail or other speech event from one of their classmates under one set of auditory circumstances but not under another seemingly similar (to the Hearing student) situation, the Hearing student might perceive the hard of hearing student as being "moody" or as ignoring them, which decreases the desire to socialize with that person.

Despite the observations in the studies above that suggest Hearing students prefer to socialize with more profoundly deaf students than hard of hearing students, a pattern of relatively greater social isolation, not integration, is the reality for both deaf and hard of hearing students in "mainstreamed" (public school) settings. Under the "audist" (Lane 1992) paradigm, which emphasizes speech over sign, hard of hearing individuals and their teachers were discouraged from learning or using signs because this mode of communication was thought to inhibit the use of articulatory and auditory skills. Even now, some educators such as Duffy (1998) express concerns about the potentially detrimental value of signs for hard of hearing (and deaf) students, despite evidence to the contrary (Stuckless and Birch 1966; Israelite, Ewoldt, and Hoffmeister 1992; Daniels 1993; Strong and Prinz 1997) that suggests that exposure to signs, including ASL, does not hinder and may even help speech and English language development. Indeed, when exposed to signs after having relied solely on audition in their lives, many hard of hearing children and adults have expressed an appreciation for the broader opportunities for communication and socialization that signs provide for them (Moschella 1992; Grushkin 1996).

Rise of the American Deaf Community and Militantism

The idea has been fairly well established within the anthropological and Deaf-related literature that the American Deaf community exhibits characteristics (language, values, behaviors) validating the view of the Deaf as a cultural unit rather than as a subculture of deficient, "handicapped" individuals (Higgins 1980; Padden 1980; Reagan 1985; Padden and Humphries 1988; Kannapell 1993). Within this culture, audiological deafness and use of ASL are held as the primary prerequisites for "membership" within the community (Padden and Humphries 1988; Kannapell 1993).

The development of the American Deaf community can be directly traced to the establishment of schools for the deaf in America, starting with the American School for the Deaf in Hartford, Connecticut. These schools for the deaf provided a centralized location where large numbers of deaf individuals could come together and develop a language and social networks. The centralized aggregation of deaf students in schools is especially important for a "low incidence" condition such as deafness in which approximately one out of every 1,000 people are born deaf (Schein 1989). Without schools for the deaf, deaf individuals would be isolated from one another because most deaf children are born to Hearing parents who have no prior knowledge of deafness, and these families typically do not have any deaf neighbors in their immediate vicinity.

During a period that was fairly concurrent with the pivotal 1880 Milan Convention, members of the Deaf community established the National Association of the Deaf (NAD), which provided a base for advocacy for the educational, social, and financial rights of deaf people in America. NAD, fearing the loss of ASL in America as a result of oralist efforts, attempted to preserve signing through film in the early 20th century (Schuchman 1988; Weinrib 1994). In the 1960s, linguists, beginning with William Stokoe, began to recognize ASL as a full language in its own right rather than as a derivative of English or as a "poor substitute" for oral communication. The establishment of the NAD provided a means through which to empower the Deaf community, and the sense of empowerment rose with the recognition of ASL as a language.

This sense of empowerment reached a previously unknown peak in 1988, when Gallaudet University, the world's only liberal arts program for deaf and hard of hearing students (which had never before had a Deaf president), selected its seventh hearing president over two well-known Deaf candidates for the position. The University's students protested, shutting down the campus for a week until one of the Deaf candidates was appointed, in a movement now known as the "Deaf President Now" (DPN) protest. The following year, Gallaudet University hosted "Deaf Way," an international conference celebrating all things Deaf. These two events energized Deaf communities around the world, especially in America.

In addition, these two events fostered growth within a subset of the Deaf community, the "militant Deaf," who allegedly champion Deaf culture to the exclusion of Hearing people and Hearing culture, including their language, English (Bertling 1994; Caswell 2001). Although the reality may be that these militant Deaf are not as radically anti-Hearing as they are made out to be (especially in the rejection of English), it is important to understand that many Hearing (and some deaf) people perceive Deaf people as either belonging to or condoning the militant subset.

Some Deaf people's militancy is exacerbated by countertrends to the growth of Deaf culture that serve to isolate and "hearize" (Nover 1993) deaf individuals. As was discussed earlier, oralism and mainstreaming are two of these countertrends. Another countertrend is the attempt to transform ASL into a dialect of English (Lane 1980) through the use of signed English systems. These signed English systems, which use visual mechanisms for representing English morphology and syntax, are widely used in school programs for deaf and hard of hearing students in America despite growing evidence of their ineffectiveness in promoting English skills (Stokes and Menyuk 1975; Supalla 1991).

Another significant countertrend has been the development of assistive listening technology, especially the cochlear implant, which blends medical and amplification techniques to provide even profoundly deaf individuals some sense of hearing. The Deaf community has strongly protested the use of the implant, which is being used on a growing number of children with hearing losses, despite limited and mixed effectiveness. Their argument is that the implant serves only to continue the academic, communicative, and social isolation of deaf children.

The now-defunct television program for deaf and hard of hearing people, *Deaf Mosaic*, once broadcast a protest against the cochlear implant by French Deaf people, including one scene in which a Deaf leader took a sledgehammer to an implantation device. In addition, a student leader of the DPN movement has been quoted as desiring to "stick a pencil in [his] ear," should he ever become hearing, to maintain his identity as a Deaf person. Images and quotations such as these have only served to further the perception of the Deaf community's militancy. Hearing people with no prior understanding of Deaf culture and values are frequently shocked and scared by these images and often take these events on their face value as evidence of blind radicalism and rejection of Hearing people and their society.

CRITERIA FOR MEMBERSHIP IN THE DEAF COMMUNITY

The primary criteria for Deaf community membership have traditionally been to have a hearing loss and to use ASL (Padden and Humphries 1988; Kannapell 1993). However, the Deaf community is far from homogeneous; within its confines, one can find a wide range of types coming from an equally wide range of backgrounds. Although in most writings, the term *Deaf community* is used to refer to those within the community's "core," the Deaf community can encompass those who are relatively isolated from the core, for example, those deaf and hard of hearing people who refuse to use or have not had the opportunity to learn ASL.

The core members of the Deaf community have long been primarily defined as those who were congenitally deaf or deafened at an early age, attended a residential school for the deaf, and for some, were also born to Deaf parents. The Deaf community is also composed of individuals who were born deaf but were raised orally or attended public schools; hard of hearing people; and even some hearing people such as those who were born to deaf parents or maintain extensive social networks within the community (such as sign language interpreters). Some

of these individuals may enter the Deaf community through alternative enculturating sites such as a college for the deaf like Gallaudet University or through association with Deaf individuals at Deaf clubs or events (captioned movies, festivals,
outdoor activities, etc.).

SHIFTING ASSOCIATIONS AND STATUS

The degree of status that a Deaf person is given as a member of the Deaf community (judging from my experience in the Deaf community) appears to be influenced by a number of factors such as hearing status, age at which one learned to
sign, the extent to which one uses sign language and the degree of ASL present
in the person's signing, the quantity and quality of associations with Deaf people,
and the individual's own self-ascriptions or desires to be affiliated with the Deaf
community. For example, Padden and Humphries (1988) cite the case of a hard
of hearing person well-situated within the Deaf community who was described
by others as "deaf, but really hard of hearing" (51). Some individuals have had a
long-standing relationship with the Deaf community, yet have chosen to disasso-
ciate themselves from the community because of perceived injustices done to
them by other members or as a form of protest against the community's values
or militancy. These individuals may choose to identify themselves in other ways
than being Deaf to reinforce their stance as separate from the Deaf community.

Within the Deaf community, a somewhat pejorative sign is used to refer to an
individual who acts like or espouses ideas that are perceived as belonging to
Hearing people: THINK-HEARING. This sign, which incorporates a parametrical
change from the mouth to the forehead of the sign for HEARING-PERSON, literally
means "thinks like a Hearing person" (Padden and Humphries 1988). I have seen
Deaf people discount certain individuals as THINK-HEARING because they enjoyed
listening to music, referred to themselves as "hearing impaired" rather than as
"Deaf," or expressed the sentiment that Signed English is better than ASL for
communication or education. The true motives of a person labeled as THINK-
HEARING for socializing with the Deaf community subsequently come under some
suspicion, and the core members of the community reconsider whether that per-
son should be thought of as a member of the Deaf community. The sign THINK-
HEARING is the Deaf equivalent of the labels "Uncle Tom" or "Oreo" found in the
Black community. This suspicion of those who do not appear to conform entirely
to Deaf norms arises, in part, from historical relationships between Deaf and
Hearing people (see Lane 1992; Wrigley 1996) but, mainly, as a means of maintaining in-group cohesion, a means that also occurs in other minority groups such as
Native Americans and African Americans (Basso 1979; Higgins 1980; Fordham
and Ogbu 1986).

In other words, one's status within the Deaf community is not static; individuals can, over time, shift toward or away from the core, just as is the case for the
Lubovitcher Hasidim (Levy 1973) and other ethnic minority groups (see figure
6.1). That is, a person coming from outside or from the fringe areas of the in-
group may decide to actively pursue a greater degree of group membership and
may accomplish this deeper affiliation through intensive social interaction with
the group's core members and through an adoption of the values and behaviors
of the in-group. Within the Hasidim, for example, an informal and nonstatic con-

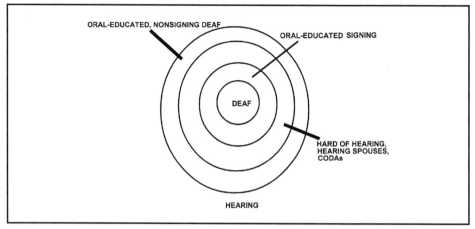

FIGURE 6.1 Schematic of relative relationships within the Deaf community

tinuum of classification appears to range from a core of Hasidim to a peripheral group of observant and nonobservant Jews who may or may not have accepted many of the cultural forms or rituals associated with Orthodox Judaism.

Like the Hasidim, an unspoken continuum exists for being Deaf, which has a core group of deaf people born to Deaf families at the center (Padden 1980; Erting 1982; Johnson and Erting 1989). Just outside of the core group are those who were born to Hearing parents but attended a residential school for the deaf and learned ASL early. Still further out are those deaf people who were educated in the public schools ("mainstreamed") but chose to identify with the Deaf community at some point in their lives, have learned sign language, and participate in the community's events. At the periphery are the orally trained deaf individuals, the hard of hearing people, and late-deafened adults who may identify more closely with Hearing people.

Like nonobservant Jews or non-Jews for the Hasidim, the oral deaf and hard of hearing people as well as Hearing people who wish to become a part of the Deaf community (e.g., through marriage or as an interpreter) may undergo the socialization process and become accepted community members, provided they conform to the values and behaviors of the Deaf community. The sites for enculturation of Deaf individuals have been found primarily within the schools for the deaf (Erting 1982) but also within Deaf clubs; Deaf organizations (NAD and its state affiliates as well as the National Fraternal Association of the Deaf); Deaf sporting groups, both informal and organized (World Recreational Association of the Deaf, U.S. Deaf Skiers Association, U.S. Athletic Association of the Deaf); and regular association with Deaf individuals in more informal settings.

THE HARD OF HEARING WITHIN THE DEAF COMMUNITY

Hard of hearing people have traditionally possessed a fringe status within the Deaf community (see figure 6.1) with the exception of those who have Deaf parents. Hard of hearing people with Deaf parents are usually fully accepted members of the community having grown up with the language and the cultural values and norms. The status of fringe membership emanates from a number of causes. One cause may be the presentation of hard of hearing individuals as models of oral communication to be emulated by profoundly deaf individuals, despite the inequity of auditory and oral communication skills. This inequity and exhibition of hard of hearing people as oral models may have led to understandable anger and rejection of these "favored individuals" by profoundly deaf people, rejection that came to be established as a cultural norm.

More importantly, hard of hearing people have traditionally been encouraged to and often do identify with Hearing values and culture through oral and mainstreamed education, as Branson and Miller (1993) have suggested. That is, hard of hearing people seem to choose to associate with Hearing people and are said to reject signs in favor of spoken communication, arguing that signed communication is not a necessary mode of communication for them. In addition, hard of hearing people, as a natural result of their auditory and communicative (through speech) capacities, frequently are quite capable of traveling in both worlds and are, therefore, suspect in their loyalties to Deaf culture and individuals (Higgins 1980; Padden and Humphries 1988). As Padden and Humphries (1988) state, "HARD-OF-HEARING people walk a thin line between being Deaf people who can be like hearing people and Deaf people who are too much like hearing people" (50).

This discussion does not mean to say that hard of hearing individuals are unconditionally rejected by Deaf people; on the contrary, hard of hearing individuals are occasionally asked to serve as informal interpreters for deaf people on certain impromptu occasions. At times, hard of hearing people have served as officers of Deaf organizations and clubs. However, as Padden and Humphries (1988) assert,

> [The hard of hearing] can be admired for their ability to seem like others [the Hearing] for specific purposes, but they are viewed with suspicion when they begin to display behaviors of the others [the Hearing] when there is no apparent need to, such as when there are no hearing people present. (50)

The dilemma of how to tread this fine line does not apply solely to hard of hearing people. Deaf people who have developed oral skills also have had to learn the cultural rules pertaining to when they might be "permitted" to use speech. One older Deaf adult informed me that these rules were learned at a young age at her residential school for the deaf when she would speak without signing to hearing adults and would receive minor ostracism, criticism, or insults as a result from her peers. I experienced a similar period of enculturation myself when I entered the Model Secondary School for the Deaf with minimal knowledge of signs. Until I attained a reasonable level of fluency, I experienced teasing and reduced social interaction among a broader set of peers, being labeled as "ORAL" with a classifier sign suggestive of an exaggerated, large set of lips flapping.

However, the two concepts—to be auditorily hard of hearing or to be culturally deaf and communicating through signs and speech—do not appear to be mutually exclusive. For example, Padden and Humphries (1988) make note of individuals, born to Deaf parents yet audiologically hard of hearing, who are well-accepted members of the Deaf community. Further, although their examples are relatively fewer, some hard of hearing individuals who had not previously been associated with the Deaf community have chosen to embrace a Deaf identity because of social and communicative difficulties in the Hearing world, so consequently, they socialize primarily within Deaf circles. Similarly, the hard of hearing students in my study, like other hard of hearing people elsewhere (Moschella 1992), have found that, instead of signing being a "problem," it is a "resource" (Ruiz 1988) that provides expanded social opportunities and clearer, unfettered communication. Thus, hard of hearing people could benefit from encouragement to associate and identify more closely with both Deaf people and Hearing people. The question that presents itself at this point is how can this sort of bicultural re-identification be promoted?

BEING HARD OF HEARING: AN ETHNIC PERSPECTIVE

When one accepts the perspective that the Deaf are a cultural or ethnic group, no great stretch of the imagination is required to envision hard of hearing individuals as being of "mixed ethnicity." Being, in part, Hearing and, in part, Deaf, they are analogous to those individuals who are born to parents of different races or ethnic backgrounds. That is, just as "mixed-race" children are not solely of one or the other ethnicity but share genetic and cultural aspects of both races, so too, hard of hearing people are neither deaf nor hearing but share characteristics of both.

In America during the era of slavery and segregation, a "one-drop" rule was adopted (however informally) under which an individual who possessed even one ancestor of African origin would be considered "Black," even if his or her physical characteristics revealed no traces of this ancestry (Zack 1993). Traditionally, mixed-race individuals have been pushed to identify solely with one of the races or cultures within their heritage to oblige institutionalized racism and to acquiesce to simplified bureaucratic documentation (such as census forms). However, in recent years, an increasing number of mixed-race individuals have resisted a forced choice, insisting that the various cultures or races in their backgrounds are equally valid and that to make a choice among them is misleading and potentially psychologically harmful for individuals of mixed heritage (Zack 1993; Courtney 1995; Leslie et al. 1995; Morganthau 1995).

Ironically, hard of hearing individuals also labor under a version of the one-drop rule. On one side, "audist" educators insist, as has been described earlier, that, because hard of hearing individuals have a significant amount of auditory capability, they must have more in common with Hearing people. However, on the other side, some Deaf people, experiencing a sense of militancy with respect to all things Deaf, have attempted to broaden the cultural and community base of the Deaf world by including at least some hard of hearing people within the ranks of the Deaf community. As one hard of hearing adult female informed me,

> I'm not really involved in the Deaf community. I just wanted a taste of what it feels like to say I'm Deaf. When I did . . . a lot of Deaf people would say "YES!," and then hard of hearing people would say "You're really hard of hearing!" Then, when I said to Deaf people that I'm hard of hearing, they resented that, saying "You're really Deaf!" That turned

me off. They did not really accept me as hard of hearing. But they accept me as Deaf, period.

Yet, even as hard of hearing people are encouraged to identify with the Deaf world, they are simultaneously rejected at some level by Deaf people when they engage in practices associated with Hearing people, for example, speaking (especially without signing) or listening to music. Another hard of hearing woman, culturally Deaf from a Deaf family, expresses some ambivalence and difficulty in reconciling her Hearing and Deaf selves:

I'm Deaf, yes. I sign fluent ASL, yes. But there are things like, I enjoy music, I like to hear, I like Hearing people, sometimes I talk with my voice and I enjoy that. But sometimes I feel that Deaf people . . . don't accept that. I feel, I feel they reject me, so sometimes I emphatically say "Yes I am Deaf, I'm just like you, I'm Deaf, I'm from the Deaf culture, but it just happens that I have those things." . . . Like for example, [I?] would sign music (remember back then that was so popular, signing music), and then Deaf militant people said . . ."Stop! Stop!" I felt, "No, it's not true [that Deaf people do not enjoy music]. I enjoy it, I think it's beautiful."

The first woman quoted above states that, when hard of hearing people engage in activities associated with Hearing people, they are then relegated to the status of THINK-HEARING. However, she expresses a desire to maintain a hard of hearing identity rather than a Deaf or Hearing identity:

I have [Deaf] coworkers who sometimes say "You hard of hearing people THINK-ORAL, THINK-HEARING." "Yes, I'm, hard of hearing." "[But] You're still Deaf, since you can't hear." "[Hey] Wait a minute. You say I'm THINK-HEARING, which?" So really, I, I can't say I'm Deaf period. I'm really hard of hearing.

Thus, hard of hearing individuals may appear to be condemned to a permanent state of psycho-sociocultural limbo: They are damned if they join the Hearing world and damned if they try to join the Deaf world. Indeed, Harvey (1989) warns of possible psychological harm to a hard of hearing (or deaf) individual who attempts to develop a "pseudo identity" as a Hearing person by attempting to "pass" (Goffman 1963) for Hearing. Harvey's warning has a reverse corollary: Perhaps, hard of hearing individuals cannot or should not attempt to pass for Deaf either. For a hard of hearing person to pass as Deaf would necessitate denying a part of his- or herself, a part that he or she may find pleasurable in some contexts. The dilemma of determining one's affiliations and place in the world has taken its toll on many hard of hearing individuals; Harvey (1989) reports that many hard of hearing patients enter therapy, claiming a sense of alienation and social rejection from others that leaves them socially isolated, withdrawn, and depressed, and that they often have problems with the abuse of drugs and alcohol.

Concepts of Bilingual-Bicultural Programming

Is this psycho-sociocultural limbo an inevitable result of being hard of hearing, a result that can never be changed? Currently, available evidence (Grushkin 1996) would indicate that this possibility is not necessarily so. One means of rectifying this situation lies in bilingual-bicultural (bi-bi) education, an approach that uses the two languages available to deaf and hard of hearing students, ASL and English, and that actively promotes the equality of the Deaf and Hearing cultures and communities. My study (Grushkin 1996) was conducted at the California School for the Deaf at Fremont (CSDF). CSDF uses a bi-bi approach, and the students are all exposed to an age-appropriate, cognitively challenging educational curriculum that is taken directly from the local school district, which is reputed to be one of the best in the area, if not in the state.

The introduction of educational material in sign language, in particular ASL, which is not a native language for most of the case study participants, does not appear to present a significant problem for comprehension. Indeed, for some classes such as physics and biology, the visual nature of signing appeared to further comprehension of complex topics such as the calculation of force and velocity or cellular biology because ASL classifiers and deixis (directionality) provide a visual representation of the concepts that, otherwise, are abstract written or spoken words (Grushkin 1996). The use of ASL is not perceived as a barrier to learning; quite to the contrary, the participants all expressed opinions to the effect that ASL was a more efficient medium for instruction and communication than signed English and even oral speech alone (168). Although some participants indicated a reliance on speechreading the "mouthing" (Davis 1989) of some signers, other signers who mouthed minimally or not at all did not appear to pose a problem in the participants' receptive language comprehension. As two of the participants demonstrated, hard of hearing students were certainly able to attain fairly good grades; indeed, all of the participants received passing grades.

The bi-bi program at CSDF engages the "maintenance model" in which the "native" language is encouraged, even as the second language is also promoted. Within this "additive" environment, the message is continually conveyed to the students that academic skills, including the development of written English, is imperative for their future success. In other words, whereas "transitional" models (in which students are quickly taught only in the majority language) deemphasize academics for language learning, the school's maintenance model does the reverse.

One can correctly reach the conclusion that, for hard of hearing individuals from public school backgrounds, bi-bi programming may be more correctly viewed as an "immersion" type of bilingual programming. Immersion bilingual education refers to the placement of children from majority language backgrounds in school programs where the minority (target) language is spoken a significant percentage of the time. A traditional bilingual immersion program is one that

> employs two languages, one of which is English, for the purposes of instruction and involves students who are native speakers of each of those languages. Both groups of students—limited English proficient (LEP) and

English proficient (EP)—are expected to become bilingual. They learn curricula through their own language and through the second language, become proficient in the second language, and continue to develop skills and proficiency in their native language. (New York State Education Department 1986, in Campbell and Lindholm 1987, 7)

Although several models have been developed to provide bilingual immersion education, several important aspects commonly contribute to its efficacy. First, the immersion component involves the placement of a percentage of language-majority speakers in an environment where the minority language is the primary language of instruction. Second, the majority language is taught as a curricular component for some portion of the day, usually one or two periods, as a "language arts" course. Third, the two languages are never mixed within an instructional period. This third element may be one that causes the most confusion about bi-bi programming.

One important influence on the efficacy of immersion programming is the issue of socioeconomic status. It is relatively well known that students of middle- and upper-class status tend to achieve academic levels higher than those of their working-class peers. Further, "transitional" bilingual programming is predominantly composed of students from immigrant families, which are usually of working-class status. Placement in these programs is often automatic. In contrast, immersion programming is almost always voluntary; students are usually placed in these programs at the behest of their parents, who want them to acquire fluency in a second (nondominant) language for some purpose. This desire for acquisition of a second language is typical of middle- and upper-class values, and students enrolled in immersion programs are predominantly middle-class and higher. In any case, the primary goal of these immersion programs is for students from both language groups to attain high levels of scholastic achievement in both languages, earlier and more efficient acquisition of English language skills, high self-esteem, and positive attitudes toward both languages and the communities they represent (Campbell and Lindholm 1987). Within these programs,

[i]t is . . . necessary for the students to develop linguistic and metalinguistic skills in both languages that will enable them to read academic texts, write acceptable essays and test responses, and be able to discuss subject-matter areas—mathematics, science and social studies in both languages. (Campbell and Lindholm 1987, 9)

It is clear from this discussion that for hard of hearing students, placement in bi-bi programs fits the "immersion" model. Students are enrolled at schools for the deaf, in concordance with the Individualized Education Plans, which are determined not only by the school district but by parents and students as well. For hard of hearing students, it would seem that parents who place their child in a signing environment recognize the additive benefit of a visual environment and language for their child. Hard of hearing students, with a fairly good command of English who also learn ASL, are well-situated to attain the linguistic and metalinguistic skills in both languages that Campbell and Lindholm underscore in the quotation above.

Bilingual immersion, or "two-way" bilingual programming, has been put into place in the United States and Canada. In Canada, English speakers are enrolled in French-speaking schools (Genesee 1984) while in the United States, a variety of immersion programs educate English speakers alongside speakers of one other language, including Spanish speakers (Campbell and Lindholm 1987; Lindholm 1988). Studies of these programs indicate that bilingual immersion has a positive effect on both groups of students. More specifically, Lindholm (1988) found that the students attained satisfactory achievement levels, despite being instructed predominantly in the second language (Spanish) for the English speakers and receiving minimal amounts of instruction in the second language (English) for the Spanish speakers. Swain and Lapkin (1991) suggested that, for majority-language children, whose first language is strongly reinforced by their environment and who have achieved a threshold level of performance in their second language, the tendency is for their first language performance to be enhanced. Finally, Genesee (1984) concluded that immersion programming is associated with positive social-psychological outcomes such as not experiencing a loss of ethnic identity with respect to one's home culture while developing a greater sense of similarity to the minority language speakers.

Bi-Bi Programming: Forging a "Mixed" Ethnicity?

The results of my study (Grushkin 1996) did support Genesee's (1984) findings that, for hard of hearing students, education through bi-bi programming does not result in any loss of identification with their Hearing background and enhances their sense of Deaf identification. These students also expressed highly positive attitudes toward ASL, which is also in keeping with Genesee's work. The identity that the students developed arose as an amalgam of their experiences in the Hearing and the Deaf worlds.

For the hard of hearing participants, hearing and speech remain an important part of their lives and their identity, despite being in an environment where the value of these abilities is diminished and even rendered irrelevant for their Deaf peers. Nevertheless, the hearing and speech abilities of these hard of hearing students are occasionally recognized and taken advantage of by students and, at times, faculty. For example, one participant recalled being used as an interpreter between his Deaf coach and an opposing Hearing team's coach at a basketball game. As long as hearing and speaking are not unduly "flaunted" in front of Deaf students, the hard of hearing students appeared to experience no overt stigmatization by their Deaf peers with respect to these audiological capacities. Despite being in an environment where the hard of hearing students might not use their speaking abilities for a large portion of time and receive only one session of speech therapy a week, their speech has been evaluated as very good, and no discernible deterioration in the quality of their speech has been reported.

For the participants, the ability to sign as well as to speak and hear offers hard of hearing students the opportunity to broaden the scope of their interactions with others. That is, whereas knowing spoken English alone would limit these students to developing relationships with only Hearing people, also knowing sign language allows them to form additional associations with Deaf and hard of hearing people. Further, the addition of signs to their linguistic repertoire extends the range of communicative options available to them when they are faced with situations in which they cannot understand their interlocutors through speech. Signing then, they assert, makes their daily lives easier in the educational and social arenas. Therefore, for these hard of hearing students, knowing ASL is a resource (Ruiz 1988).

In addition, the participants all displayed a well-developed understanding and use of the pragmatic strategies of signing such as attention getting, turn taking, and maintaining the privacy of signed communications. Perhaps the most significant pragmatic strategy developed is that of codeswitching, which occurs in bilinguals. The participants use signs with deaf peers and staff members and use their voices (whether in conjunction with signs or not) among themselves and with Hearing staff members. Rarely is an "inappropriate" mode used with the wrong person, indicating that the participants are well aware of their interactants and the communication modality (or modalities) that they prefer.

More important, some evidence indicates that to speak and sign at the same time serves the same function for hard of hearing individuals that signing ASL does for Deaf people: It serves as a symbol of their identity as hard of hearing people. Observation suggests that, at first, other students are understanding of the hard of hearing participants' signing efforts, even when they occasionally discontinue signing. However, after a period of time when the sense is that new signers have had sufficient exposure to achieve communicative competence, these other students significantly decrease their tolerance of these breaks, especially when the participants choose to use their voices with one another or with Hearing interactants instead of signing.

Regardless of those instances when the participants are chastised for not signing, the hard of hearing students as a group do not seem to be overtly discriminated against, especially when compared to hard of hearing students in the public schools. Rather, they appear to be well accepted by their peers, provided that they maintain the use of their signs, and this perception was confirmed by the participants themselves, who noted that their only difficulties with other students were directly related to signing (or more accurately, not signing). In addition, a number of hard of hearing students (from both Hearing and Deaf families) at the school have become well-liked, popular, and even leaders among their peers.

Being at a school for the deaf that has a bi-bi philosophy has not precluded the participants from forming or maintaining friendships with Hearing children in their home communities. However, because of their present circumstances, most find their friendships to be predominantly with other deaf and hard of hearing children. Some critics of deaf education such as Evans (1975), Evans and Falk (1986), and Bertling (1994) have criticized schools for the deaf, especially residential schools, on the grounds that they unduly shelter their charges, failing to prepare them for independent, productive life outside their grounds. However, at this school for the deaf, though the students do lead a fairly structured life, students' activities are relatively free of restrictions.

Although most of the participants enjoy and even look forward to residential living, only one expressed any feelings of restriction or dissatisfaction engendered by living apart from his family. Indeed, in that one case, the separation from his family, to whom he is extremely close emotionally, is what this student objects to and not the idea of residential living itself. The structure of residential living, however, is looked on positively by the participants as a sort of preparation for future living such as in a college dormitory or apartment house with several housemates.

Finally, the participants all appeared to be developing some sense of identity and their place in the world, which is developmentally appropriate as adolescents. The identity that they develop arises as an amalgam of their experiences in the Hearing and the Deaf worlds. None of the participants seemed to reject their membership in the Hearing society, but the degree to which they embrace the company of Deaf people varied. Following Holcomb's (1997) framework, the four hard of hearing student participants in my dissertation research each appeared to be developing a sense of identity and biculturalism that lies on a continuum of preferences. For the first student, a Hearing-dominant identity is most likely whereas, for the second, a Deaf-dominant identity is probable. The one female student, although from a Deaf family, espouses a desire for a balanced identity, although she likely will be, like her friend, Deaf-dominant. The fourth student's perception that he will primarily associate with Hearing people in the future because of his career interests is belied by his appreciation of the Deaf environment in which he finds himself. Quite possibly, this student, although potentially working primarily with Hearing people on a daily basis, will come to maintain associations with Deaf people in his personal time, as many in the Deaf community do.

Hard of hearing individuals have long been thought to rightfully belong to the Hearing society because of their predominantly Hearing parentage and their abilities to speak and hear. Indeed, they do differ from Deaf people in the extent to which they value the use of their voices, audition, and contact with Hearing people. However, this study demonstrated that hard of hearing children and adults do experience many of the same difficulties in schooling and life that their profoundly deaf peers encounter. Therefore, to some extent, hard of hearing individuals may also be considered to be rightfully belonging to the Deaf world. In fact, some of the participants mentioned feeling that they belonged to "two worlds." One gave indications that she subscribes to this "dual ethnicity" hypothesis, however unconsciously, when she stated "I have a little bit of both [Hearing and Deaf] in me."

In other words, the hard of hearing students in this study appear to perceive the school for the deaf as their Least Restrictive Environment (LRE). Although most, if not all, states around the country have interpreted the LRE to be the public school, the original intent of this clause in Public Law 94–142 was for the child to be placed in the environment in which learning is most readily accomplished (Siegel 1994). Even though the wording of the law does not actually specify the environment, the spirit of the LRE would suggest that this setting is the environment in which the child is able to learn at all levels—academic as well as social and emotional. That is, learning for all children, hearing or deaf, occurs not only within the classroom but also in daily, nonacademic interactions with their peers and teachers in the halls, lunchrooms, and playgrounds. Clearly, these students have access to a quality education. However, in their positive perceptions of their social relationships and ease of communication at this school, they are indicating that this aspect, too, is an important part of their lives, one that would be lacking or, at least, not as readily attained in the public schools, which was confirmed by their recollections.

HARD OF HEARING: A THIRD CULTURE?

The findings of my study are not anomalous: In Sweden and Denmark, where bi-bi education has been in place for at least ten years, similar results have been found. Shawn Mahshie (1995) reported that mainstreaming efforts in these two European countries have resulted in patterns of social, academic, and linguistic frustration for hard of hearing children similar to those that have been reported in the United States and elsewhere. However, the results have not been uniform; different results have been obtained, depending on the method of instruction and placement of the hard of hearing students, according to Mahshie (1995) and Bagga-Gupta and Domfors (this volume). Nevertheless, in these two countries, hard of hearing people have become increasingly politicized, allying their national organization of hard of hearing adults with their National Association of the Deaf and the National Parents Organization in the fight to achieve social and educational policy changes. Young hard of hearing people in Sweden and Denmark are beginning to assert that they have been "denied (through lack of knowledge of sign language and lack of opportunities for interaction) the right to the support and socialization of the Deaf Community" (Mahshie 1995, 152). Further, Mahshie sees hard of hearing people in these countries developing a cultural identity of their own.

In fact, hard of hearing individuals in Sweden apparently are attempting to develop a "third culture," one that is allied with both the Deaf and the Hearing communities. This possibility was raised by MJ Bienvenu, a well-known Deaf activist, albeit while discussing a different group of people within the Deaf community (sign language interpreters):

> Being bi-cultural means knowing how to move comfortably between two distinct cultures. Third culture is special in that it represents the possibility of coming to a halfway point, making contact with members of the other culture, but maintaining all the while one's identity as a member of one's first culture. (Bienvenu 1987, 1)

Whether a "third culture" of hard of hearing people will develop in the United States is open to debate. For political and social reasons, the reactions to this idea vary. The participants of my dissertation study, who represent the future of the hard of hearing segment of the Deaf community, were evenly split on this issue. Two felt that a hard of hearing culture would arise, although they had no conception of what such a culture would look like. In contrast, the other two did not see a need for a hard of hearing culture, but each had different reasons. One, from a Deaf family, denied the possibility on the basis of affiliation with the Deaf community:

> I don't think it is necessary to have a third culture. What for? Hearing people, Deaf people, hard of hearing are "in the middle." But in my opinion, most percentage of hard of hearing people prefer the Deaf world than the Hearing world because the Hearing world tends to reject them while the Deaf don't. Sometimes, some do . . . but all? I doubt it.

In direct contrast, the other, from a Hearing family, based his opinion on the ties that hard of hearing people have with Hearing people:

> I feel hard of hearing people will combine with Hearing people. I feel that because many hard of hearing people go to Hearing schools. True, a few come to Fremont, they join the Deaf [community]. But . . . most of the hard of hearing can join the Hearing.

This split also was seen among hard of hearing adults. Ms. E., a hard of hearing African American woman, thinks there is, or will be, a hard of hearing culture:

> I think they have it, but it's never been noticed. I think hard of hearing people . . . have not really come out the way . . . I see Deaf see them. But I think they've come out the way hard of hearing people see them. Will there be a hard of hearing culture? Yes.

In comparison, Ms. H., a hard of hearing woman from a Deaf family, thinks a hard of hearing culture could arise but fears the consequences:

> I've thought maybe we should have a group, a support group for hard of hearing people who live in the Deaf world. Especially there. Hard of hearing people in the . . . Hearing world . . . hard of hearing have SHHH [Self-Help for Hard of Hearing people], they have ALDA [Association of Late-Deafened Americans] . . . but for some reason SHHH and ALDA is not exactly what we need. . . . But I think "wow," to create another group, to create more divisions, I don't want to see that. I think the way we can help hard of hearing people understand Deaf people, their culture, the Deaf culture [is] to accept that and to educate Deaf people to understand that there are certain things about them that they appreciate, and to leave them alone [about it].

Only time will tell whether hard of hearing people will form a cultural unit in their own right as a "third culture" or will be accepted members of the Deaf community, representing the diversity that is possible. Regardless, it is certain that bi-bi education will (or should) play a key role in the eventual creation of the hard of hearing identity, whatever it may become. This identity will come about, given the increasing numbers of hard of hearing children educated in bi-bi schools and the eventual need of the hard of hearing community (as well as that of the larger society) to decide whether or not the bi-bi environment represents a viable educational setting for them. It is significant that in Sweden, a national organization of hard of hearing adults is lobbying for the rights of hard of hearing people to affiliate with the Deaf community in education and society. However, as Ms. H. indicates, SHHH, that organization's closest counterpart in the United States, is more orally aligned and unlikely to advocate for similar reforms. Nevertheless, just as the National Association of the Deaf was instrumental in the creation and recognition of the Deaf community as a cultural and political unit (Van Cleve and Crouch 1989), so too will hard of hearing people require an equivalent means of organizing, should they desire to restructure how the educational system and society perceives them.

CONCLUSIONS

Can we conclude that bi-bi programming is a viable educational option for hard of hearing children, especially in the area of promoting a stable sense of identity? Certainly, bi-bi programming does not appear to do any harm, and it does provide many benefits that are not (and often cannot) be experienced in the public schools. Further, in the long term, bi-bi programming may even prove to be beneficial for this population. The bi-bi framework does appear capable of encompassing those who are hard of hearing. There is no need to significantly reformulate the bi-bi philosophy to accommodate hard of hearing people; however, bi-bi schools might be wise to specifically incorporate hard of hearing students within their curricula and services.

Today, hard of hearing people appear fated to be "culturally marginal" (Glickman 1986), or without a secure sense of self and identity. Given the potential psychosocial consequences of cultural marginality as described by Goffman (1963) and Harvey (1989), how can a hard of hearing person avoid or be helped to avoid this area of difficulty? Schools and parents can consider the lessons learned by interracial parents and can adopt several strategies. First, attempts should be made to stimulate the children's interest and pride in their nondominant heritage (Benson 1981) or, in this case, in their Deaf identity. Second, the advantage of having exposure to two different cultures and perspectives should be stressed. The values and traditions of both cultures should be communicated to these children (Motoyoshi 1990).

Moreover, an important element of biculturality is the need for positive attitudes and acceptance of both cultures. Within the Deaf community, as stated earlier, the trend has been to militantly reject Hearing values and to insist that one can be Deaf only if one adheres strictly to Deaf behaviors, language usage, and thought patterns. However, as Mottez (1990), Cohen (1994), and Turner (1994) suggest, one can be Deaf in multiple ways, just as one can, in multiple ways, be a member of many cultural and ethnic minorities. For instance, Preston (1994) observes that, although oral (nonsigning) deaf people have not traditionally been viewed as being Deaf, they can be considered to be members of the Deaf community. Further, he makes a case for hearing children of Deaf parents being members of the Deaf community, noting that these individuals frequently think of themselves as Deaf—more so than do oral deaf people.

Montgomery (1994) suggests that membership in the Deaf community be defined by an "LAA," or "Lowest Admissible Admit" (259). This concept, he claims, eliminates the "Deaf/Not Deaf" dichotomy, replacing it with a map of "relative belonging." Montgomery's conception is consonant with that of Levy's (1973) representation of the Lubovitcher Hasidim in the sense that the Lubovitcher group has ties to one another but is not a homogeneous group with identical values and ways of being.

Bagga-Gupta (1999) has suggested the idea (similar to my conception of hard of hearing as a "mixed ethnicity") that hard of hearing people be viewed as possessing a "composite" identity: one that consists of multiple, yet equally shared identities. She argues that everybody in the world has a set of composite identities that include combinations such as husband and father, daughter and sister, Black and White, Deaf and Hearing, and so forth. Each of these identities overlaps others, and none essentially possesses a status significantly higher than any other. Thus, according to Sangeeta Bagga-Gupta during a conversation in November 1997, the use of the word *composite* places a positive emphasis on the concept of multiple levels of identification in contrast to the term *mixed*, which can have negative connotations. In effect, the frameworks supplied by Bagga-Gupta (1999), Montgomery (1994), and myself (Grushkin 1996) all offer a potentially useful means of visualizing and incorporating hard of hearing people and other subgroups within the Deaf community. However, research along these lines needs to be conducted to develop an understanding, both inside the Deaf community and out, of the multiple ways in which one can be Deaf and hard of hearing. Results of this research may show that we can truly speak of hard of hearing people as having the "best of both worlds" rather than being "lost between two worlds."

NOTES

1.   The word *deaf* is conventionally capitalized to denote a cultural orientation to deaf people and their community. When uncapitalized, the same word refers to a purely audiological perspective. The word *hearing* is similarly capitalized or uncapitalized in this chapter to refer to a cultural or audiological perspective, although this second treatment is not conventional.

2.   The trend is becoming increasingly obvious that groups of disabled people are rejecting the "handicapped" label, stating that societal conditions are what create a handicap. See Shapiro (1993) for an excellent discussion of this issue. It should also be noted that Deaf people have long felt that they are not handicapped because they have always been equally able to perform any job that did not require oral communication (Higgins 1980; Padden and Humphries 1988; Jacobs 1989).

REFERENCES

Bagga-Gupta, Sangeeta. 1999. Tecken i kommunikation och identitet: Specialskolan och vardagsdeltagande (Signs in communication and identity: Special schools and everyday participation). In *Möten: Vänbok till Roger Säljö* (Meetings: In honor of Roger Säljö), ed. Ullabeth Sätterlund Larsson, Kerstin Bergkvist, and Per Linell, 111–39. Linköping, Sweden: Linköping University.

Basso, Keith H. 1979. *Portraits of "The Whiteman": Linguistic play and cultural symbols among the Western Apache.* Cambridge, Mass.: Cambridge University Press.

Baynton, Douglas. 1996. *Forbidden signs: American culture and the campaign against sign language.* Chicago: University of Chicago Press.

Benson, Susan. 1981. *Ambiguous ethnicity.* London: Cambridge University Press.

Bertling, Tom. 1994. *A child sacrificed.* Wilsonville, Oreg.: Kodiak Media Group.

Bienvenu, Martina J. 1987. The third culture: Working together. *Journal of Interpretation* 4:1–12.

Brackett, Diane, and Antonia Maxon. 1986. Service delivery alternatives for the mainstreamed hearing impaired child. *Language, Speech and Hearing Services in Schools* 17:115–25.

Branson, Jan, and Don Miller. 1993. Sign language, the deaf and the epistemic violence of mainstreaming. *Language and Education* 7 (1):21–41.

Campbell, Russell N., and Kathryn J. Lindholm. 1987. *Conservation of language resources.* Los Angeles: University of California, Educational Resources Information Center. Educational Report No. 5. ERIC, ED 287 309.

Caswell, Paulette. 2001. Hidden curricula, pseudoscience, phonemic language deprivation, and cultural change in international and intercultural education: Historiographic, epidemiological, and variable-based analyses of outcome measures for deaf and hard of hearing students. Ph.D. diss., University of Southern California.

Cohen, Leah Hager. 1994. *Train go sorry: Inside a deaf world.* Boston: Houghton Mifflin.

Courtney, Brian A. 1995. Freedom from choice. *Newsweek,* 13 February, p. 16.

Daniels, Marilyn. 1993. ASL as a factor in acquiring English. *Sign Language Studies* 78:23–29.

Davis, Jeffrey. E. 1989. Distinguishing language contact phenomena in ASL interpreting. In *The sociolinguistics of the deaf community,* ed. Ceil Lucas, 85–102. San Diego: Academic Press.

Davis, Julia, ed. 1990. *Our forgotten children: Hard-of-hearing pupils in the schools.* 2d ed. Bethesda, Md.: Self-Help for Hard of Hearing People.

Duffy, John K. 1998. Teach English to deaf. *New York Times,* 18 March, p. A18.

Elser, R. P. 1959. The social position of hearing handicapped children in the regular grades. *Exceptional Children* 25:305–9.

Emerson, Robert, Rachel Fretz, and Linda Shaw. 1995. *Writing ethnographic fieldnotes.* Chicago: University of Chicago Press.

Erting, Carol. 1982. Deafness, communication and social identity: An anthropological analysis of interaction among parents, teachers and deaf children in a preschool. Ph.D. diss., The American University, Washington, D.C.

Evans, A. Donald. 1975. Experiential deprivation: Unresolved factor in the impoverished socialization of deaf school children in residence. *American Annals of the Deaf* 120 (6):545–52.

Evans, A. Donald, and William Falk. 1986. *Learning to be deaf.* New York: Mouton de Gruyter.

Fordham, Signithia, and John Ogbu. 1986. Black students' school success: Coping with the "burden of acting white." *The Urban Review* 18 (3):176–206.

Genesee, Fred. 1984. Beyond bilingualism: Social psychological studies of French immersion programs in Canada. *Canadian Journal of Behavioral Science* 16 (4):338–52.

Glickman, Neil. 1986. Cultural identity, deafness and mental health. *Journal of Rehabilitation of the Deaf* 20 (2):1–10.

Goffman, Erving. 1963. *Stigma: Notes on the management of spoiled identity.* New York: Simon & Schuster.

Grushkin, Donald A. 1996. Academic, linguistic, social and identity development in hard-of-hearing adolescents educated within an ASL/English bilingual/bicultural educational setting for deaf and hard-of-hearing students. Ph.D. diss., University of Arizona.

Hammersley, Martyn, and Paul Atkinson. 1983. *Ethnography: Principles in practice.* London: Routledge.

Harvey, Michael A. 1989. *Psychotherapy with deaf and hard-of-hearing persons: A systemic model.* Hillsdale, N.J.: Erlbaum.

Higgins, Paul C. 1980. *Outsiders in a hearing world: A sociology of deafness.* Beverly Hills: Sage.

Holcomb, Thomas K. 1997. Development of deaf bicultural identity. *American Annals of the Deaf* 142 (2):89–92.

Holden-Pitt, Lisa. 1997. A look at residential school placement patterns for students from deaf- and hearing-parented families: A ten-year perspective. *American Annals of the Deaf* 142 (2):108–14.

Israelite, Neita, Carolyn Ewoldt, and Robert Hoffmeister. 1992. *Bilingual/bicultural education for deaf and hard-of-hearing students: A review of the literature on the effects of native sign language on majority language acquisition.* Toronto: Ministry of Education.

Jacobs, Leo M. 1989. *A deaf adult speaks out.* 3d ed. Washington, D.C: Gallaudet University Press.

Johnson, Robert E., and Carol Erting. 1989. Ethnicity and socialization in a classroom for deaf children. In *The sociolinguistics of the deaf community,* ed. Ceil Lucas, 41–84. San Diego: Academic Press.

Kannapell, Barbara. 1993. *Language choice—identity choice.* Burtonsville, Md.: Linstok Press.

Kennedy, Patricia, and Robert H. Bruininks. 1974. Social status of hearing-impaired children in regular classrooms. *Exceptional Children* 40 (5):336–42.

Kennedy, Patricia, Winifred Northcott, Robert McCauley, and Susan M. Williams. 1976. Longitudinal sociometric and cross-sectional data on mainstreaming hearing impaired children: Implications for preschool programming. *Volta Review* 78 (2):71–81.

Lane, Harlan. 1980. A chronology of the oppression of sign language in France and in the United States. In *Recent perspectives on American Sign Language,* ed. Harlan Lane and François Grosjean, 119–61. Hillsdale, N.J.: Erlbaum.

———. 1984. *When the mind hears: A history of the deaf.* New York: Random House.

———. 1992. *The mask of benevolence: Disabling the deaf community.* New York: Knopf Press.

Leslie, Connie, Regina Elam, Allison Samuels, and Danzy Senna. 1995. The loving generation: Biracial children seek their own place. *Newsweek,* 13 February, p. 72.

Levine, Lawrence W. 1977. *Black culture and black consciousness: Afro-American folk thought from slavery to freedom.* Oxford: Oxford University Press.

Levitan, Linda. 1993. What do others call us? And what do we call ourselves? *Deaf Life* (May):18–29.

Levy, Sydelle. 1973. Shifting patterns of ethnic identification among the Hassidim. In *The new ethnicity: Perspectives from ethnology,* ed. John W. Bennett, 25–49. St. Paul, Minn.: West Publishing.

Lindholm, Kathryn. 1988. *The Edison Elementary School bilingual immersion program: Student progress after one year of implementation.* Report No. 9. Los Angeles: University of California, Educational Resources Information Center.

Mahshie, Shawn Neal. 1995. *Educating deaf children bilingually.* Washington, D.C.: Gallaudet University Press.

Montgomery, George. 1994. My culture is superior to your culture: A digression on status and the culture-vulture. *Sign Language Studies* 84:251–64.

Morganthau, Tom. 1995. What color is black? *Newsweek,* 13 February, pp. 63–65.

Moschella, Janet. 1992. The experience of growing up deaf or hard of hearing: Implications of sign language versus oral rearing on identity development and emotional well-being. Ph.D. diss., Antioch College, New Hampshire.

Motoyoshi, Michelle M. 1990. The experience of mixed-race people: Some thoughts and theories. *Journal of Ethnic Studies* 18 (2):77–94.

Mottez, Bernard. 1990. Deaf identity. *Sign Language Studies* 68:195–216.

New York State Education Department. 1986. *Applications for new grants for two-way bilingual education programs.* Albany, N.Y.: Office of State Printing.

Nover, Stephen. 1993. Our voices, our vision: Politics of deaf education. Paper presented at the CAID/CEASD Convention, Baltimore, Md., June 28, 1993.

Ogbu, John. U. 1987. Variability in minority school performance: A problem in search of an explanation. *Anthropology and Education Quarterly* 18 (4):312–34.

Padden, Carol. 1980. The deaf community and the culture of deaf people. In *Sign language and the deaf community: Essays in honor of William C. Stokoe,* ed. Charlotte Baker and Robbin Battison, 89–104. Silver Spring, Md.: National Association of the Deaf.

Padden, Carol, and Tom Humphries. 1988. *Deaf in America: Voices from a culture.* Cambridge, Mass.: Harvard University Press.

P.L. 105–17 (111Stat.37; 20 USC 1400 et seq.).

Preston, Paul. 1994. *Mother father deaf: Living between sound and silence*. Cambridge, Mass.: Harvard University Press.

Quigley, Stephen, and F. Eugene Thomure. 1968. *Some effects of a hearing impairment on school performance*. Urbana: University of Illinois, Institute of Research on Exceptional Children. Typescript.

Reagan, Timothy. 1985. The deaf as a linguistic minority: Educational considerations. *Harvard Educational Review* 55 (3):265–77.

Rosen, Roslyn. 1980. *Appropriate educational placements for hearing impaired children*. Reston, Va.: Educational Resources Information Center Clearinghouse on Handicapped and Gifted Children. ERIC, ED 197 578.

Ross, Mark. 1990. Definitions and descriptions. In *Our forgotten children: Hard-of-hearing pupils in the schools*, ed. Julia Davis, 3–17. Bethesda, Md.: Self-Help for Hard-of-Hearing People.

Ross, Mark, Diane Brackett, and Antonia Maxon. 1982. *Hard-of-hearing children in regular schools*. Englewood Cliffs, N.J.: Prentice-Hall.

Ross, Mark, and Donald R. Calvert. 1967. The semantics of deafness. *Volta Review* 69 (10):644–49.

Ruiz, Richard. 1988. Orientations in language planning. In *Language diversity: Problem or resource?* ed. Sandra McKay and Sau-Ling C. Wong, 3–25. Boston: Heinle & Heinle.

Schein, Jerome D. 1989. *At home among strangers: Exploring the deaf community in the United States*. Washington, D.C.: Gallaudet University Press.

Schuchman, John S. 1988. *Hollywood speaks: Deafness and the film entertainment industry*. Urbana: University of Illinois Press.

Shapiro, Joseph P. 1993. *No pity: People with disabilities forging a new Civil Rights movement*. New York: Times Books.

Siegel, Lawrence. 1994. *Least restrictive environment: The paradox of inclusion*. Horsham, Pa.: LRP Publications.

Spradley, James P. 1980. *Participant observation*. Fort Worth, Tex.: Holt, Rinehart & Winston.

Stokes, W., and Paula Menyuk. 1975. A proposal for the investigation of the acquisition of American Sign Language and Signed English by deaf and hearing children enrolled in integrated nursery school programs. Boston University. Typescript.

Strong, Michael, and Philip Prinz. 1997. A study of the relationship between American Sign Language and English literacy. *Journal of Deaf Studies and Deaf Education* 2 (1):37–46.

Stuckless, E. Ross, and Jack W. Birch. 1966. The influence of early manual communication on the linguistic development of deaf children. *American Annals of the Deaf* 111 (2):452–60.

Supalla, Samuel. 1991. Manually coded English: The modality question in signed language development. In *Theoretical issues in sign language research*, ed. Patricia Siple and Susan Fischer, vol. 2, 85–109. Chicago: University of Chicago Press.

Swain, Merrill, and Sharon Lapkin. 1991. Additive bilingualism and French immersion education: The roles of language proficiency and literacy. In *Bilingualism, multiculturalism, and second language learning: The McGill Conference in Honour of Wallace E. Lambert*, ed. Allan G. Reynolds, 203–16. Hillsdale, N.J.: Erlbaum.

Turner, Graham H. 1994. How is deaf culture? Toward a revised notion of a fundamental concept. *Sign Language Studies* 83:103–26.

Van Cleve, John V., and Barry A. Crouch. 1989. *A place of their own: Creating the deaf community in America*. Washington, D.C.: Gallaudet University Press.

Weinrib, Melinda. 1994. A study of the minority status of independent films in the deaf community: Implications for Deaf Studies curriculum development. Master's thesis, University of Arizona.

Witcher, Betty. 1974. She's not deaf, she's hard of hearing. *Volta Review* 76 (7):428–35.
Wrigley, Owen. 1996. *The politics of deafness*. Washington, D.C.: Gallaudet University Press.
Woodward, James, and Thomas Allen. 1993. Models of deafness compared: A sociolinguis-
    tic study of deaf and hard of hearing teachers. *Sign Language Studies* 79:113–25.
Zack, Naomi. 1993. *Race and mixed race*. Philadelphia: Temple University Press.

7 | Sociolinguistic Dynamics in American Deaf Communities: Peer Groups versus Families

Ceil Lucas and Susan Schatz

The importance of the peer group in shaping and determining sociolinguistic behavior has long been noted in studies of spoken languages (see Labov 1972; Milroy 1987; Eckert 1989). The role of the peer group is particularly important in Deaf communities, especially given the fact that no more than 10% of deaf children are born to deaf parents. Consequently, most deaf children do not have native access to the spoken language of their hearing parents. Although the peer group plays a pivotal role in both spoken language and sign language communities, some sharp areas of contrast do exist.

Although the peer group exerts a strong influence in spoken language communities, the language used in the family setting or by caretakers is always present and audiologically available to the children as a competing model. One might say that the situation in Deaf communities parallels the situation found in some spoken language bilingual communities in which parents use one language, possibly a minority language, and the children opt for the majority language. However, the situation in Deaf communities still would seem to be unique: Whereas the parents and children in a bilingual spoken language situation all have audiological access to the various languages (i.e., they can hear them) and choose one or another for sociolinguistic reasons, deaf children do not have similar access to the spoken language of their parents. Although many hearing parents of deaf children are now learning to sign, many still do not sign a majority of the time. The result is that, from earliest childhood, deaf children often communicate with their families by a variety of means, including home sign systems, talking (which the child may be able to produce but not hear), fingerspelling, and writing. In contrast, natural sign language is used in children's deaf peer groups. It is this language used with school friends that most often becomes the deaf individual's primary means of communication for life.

Residential schools for deaf children have traditionally served as crucibles for the acquisition of American Sign Language (ASL), and a variety of social organizations such as local deaf clubs and sports groups have important language maintenance functions. Lane, Hoffmeister, and Bahan (1996) explain:

> Sports rapidly become a vehicle of acculturation for the Deaf child, a shared experience, a source of Deaf pride, and an avenue for understanding customs and values in the DEAF-WORLD. . . . Athletics . . . also serve linguistic and political functions. ASL is a truly national language, in part because of the co-mingling of Deaf people in the residential schools, in the clubs and in regional and national athletics. (131)

By considering the functions of families from a sociolinguistic standpoint, we might better frame the discussion. First, a family provides the child with a native model of language structure that reflects the family's sociolinguistic reality, including factors such as geographic region, ethnicity, and socioeconomic status. Second, the family provides a model of appropriate language use, including how to use language in social interactions. Finally, the family provides an avenue for the development of metalinguistic awareness. In the context of family language use, children develop awareness of what their society perceives to be appropriate and inappropriate language use along with the means to talk about this awareness.

Deaf children of hearing parents, however, often do not share a common language with their parents and do not acquire their first language from them. The question becomes the following: How and where are the sociolinguistic functions that normally occur within a family carried out in the lives of these deaf children? The goal of this chapter is to explore this question by considering data from a six-year project (June 1994–July 2000) on sociolinguistic variation in ASL funded by the National Science Foundation.

RELATED RESEARCH

The research most relevant to the present study has to do with (a) peer interaction among deaf children and (b) the nature of communication in hearing families with a deaf child. With respect to peer interaction, many scholars have recognized the importance of the residential school for deaf children as the site of socialization into the Deaf world (Wright 1969; Markowicz and Woodward 1978; Padden and Humphries 1988; Supalla 1994; Reilly 1995). In addition, they have recognized the fact that this socialization is managed by peers, both in terms of language teaching and the transmission of cultural values and behaviors. Generally, newcomers to a residential school rapidly acquire what may be their first language from the older students, and as Supalla (1994) points out, "this unique language learning and maintenance takes place in the dormitory and playground, not in the classroom" (586). Reilly (1995) argues that

> this outcome occurs whether or not teachers know the sign language, and often they do not. Since language learning both involves and enables the transmission of worldly content, a substantive teaching-learning process

among children is implied. . . . The social relations are so strong and satisfying that they maintain their life-long bonds in a signing, deaf adult community. (18)

As Reilly (1995) points out, the observations by other scholars about the nature of peer interaction in residential schools are based on outcomes and not on firsthand studies of the interaction itself. In fact, Reilly's work is the one notable exception to this pattern. He provides a detailed picture of the peer interaction in a residential school for deaf children in Thailand and a simply remarkable description of the strategies that the older children have devised to ensure that the younger children acquire a natural sign language (Thai Sign Language), norms for appropriate social behavior, and world knowledge. These strategies are all carried out independently of the formal educational activities required by the school.

Reilly also describes the children's interaction with their families, particularly the linguistic isolation of deaf children within hearing families. These situations usually do not involve any shared means of communication, and as one child stated, "I came back to school a few days early because there's no one I can talk to at home. Here [at the residential school] I have my friends and we have lots of things to talk about" (1995, 91).

Other researchers have examined the use of language in hearing families with deaf children. Greenberg (1980) reported that, among the hearing parents of deaf children, only one parent in ten could communicate with his or her deaf child (see also Swisher and Thompson 1985). The situation in hearing families with deaf children is in contrast to the situation encountered by deaf children in deaf families in which the family shares a language, namely, natural sign language. Lane, Hoffmeister, and Bahan (1996) state:

On the one hand, Deaf parents are likely to have close rapport with their Deaf child, fluent communication, high expectations, and a well-founded positive outlook. On the other, fearful and frustrated hearing parents may not be able to communicate substantively with their Deaf child, who, in turn, is frustrated and tantrum-prone. (40)

THE DATA

The data on which this chapter is based come from a six-year study on sociolinguistic variation in ASL. The project is summarized in figure 7.1 (for a full description of the project and its findings, see Lucas, Bayley, and Valli 2001).

As figure 7.1 shows, the overall goal of the project was a description of sociolinguistic variation in ASL based on data from a broad spectrum of communities. ASL users were allowed to converse informally in small groups. Following these conversations, a subset of each group was interviewed in depth by the deaf researchers about language use and interaction patterns. In addition, each participant was asked to provide written information on his or her background, including information about age, education, and occupation as well as information about use of language with teachers, families, peers, coworkers, and strangers. As the researchers reviewed this written information and viewed the

LENGTH OF PROJECT:

A six-year project on sociolinguistic variation in ASL, funded by the National Science Foundation (June 1, 1994–July 31, 2000).

OVERVIEW OF DATA COLLECTION:

SITES

1. Staunton, Virginia

2. Frederick, Maryland

3. Boston, Massachusetts

4. New Orleans, Louisiana

5. Fremont, California/San Jose, California

6. Kansas City, Missouri/Olathe, Kansas

7. Bellingham, Washington

GROUPS

Twelve groups in Massachusetts, Louisiana, California, and Missouri; six groups in Virginia, Maryland, and Bellingham, WA (only white groups). A total of 204 American Sign Language signers. Each group consisted of 2–6 signers.

Black Groups		White Groups	
Middle Class	Working Class	Middle Class	Working Class
15–25	15–25	15–25	15–25
26–54	26–54	26–54	26–54
55–up	55–up	55–up	55–up

OVERALL GOAL OF THE PROJECT:

A description of phonological, morphosyntactic, and lexical variation in ASL as well as the correlation of variation with external factors such as age, region, gender, ethnicity, and socioeconomic status.

FIGURE 7.1. The project at a glance

videotapes of each interview, they began to notice sharp contrasts between the participants' reported use of language with their families and their reported use of language with their peers.

This observation inspired us to take a closer look at the patterns. As figure 7.1 also shows, data were collected in seven sites around the United States. In this chapter, we focus on the data from Boston and New Orleans. These two sites were chosen because of their obvious geographical contrast. In both sites, we examine the language use patterns for both black and white signers in three age groups (15–25, 26–54, and 55–up) and at two economic levels, working-class and middle-class. The language use patterns reported by a total of 64 signers in 22 groups will be described. All of the signers being discussed were exposed to ASL as children in either residential or day programs.

THE PATTERNS OF LANGUAGE USE

Table 7.1 shows the patterns of language use for the Boston groups. No black deaf families were included in the sample, so all interaction by the black signers is with hearing families, and we see that, with one exception, no ASL is used by the participants with their hearing families. (Note that we were unable to identify any individuals in the black, middle-class, 55–up category to take part in the study, either for Boston or New Orleans.) Communication with hearing family members takes place through spoken and written English, fingerspelling, contact signing (also known as Pidgin Sign English, or PSE, in the deaf community), and in two cases, gestures. We found no really remarkable differences correlating with socio-economic status or age. The one difference of note is the use of ASL with the mother by one middle-class participant in the 15–25 age group. The contrast between language use with family members and with deaf friends—in the latter case, universal use of ASL—is striking. Some form of English is also used with hearing friends, again, in contrast to the use of ASL with deaf friends.

The patterns with the white Boston signers are very similar: They almost exclusively use some form of English with hearing family members and almost exclusively use ASL with deaf friends. Once again, one middle-class participant in the 55–up group uses ASL with her deaf sons. Among the white signers, we also see language use in deaf families that is exclusively ASL.

We turn now to the New Orleans signers, whose language use is shown in table 7.2. With the black signers, we see once again the sharp contrast between language use with family members and with friends. Language use with hearing family members includes writing, speaking, and fingerspelling. In only one case does a participant report using signs with a sibling. Once again, ASL is used in a deaf family, and ASL is used universally with deaf friends while, with one exception, some form of English is used with hearing friends.

We see similar patterns with the white signers: They use some form of spoken English with hearing family members and ASL in deaf families. One working-class participant in the 15–25 age group reports using some signs with her mother and sister. In one deaf family, the parents were raised orally and insisted on the use of spoken English when the participant was young, but the family now uses ASL. Only three participants reported language use with hearing friends (some form of English in all three cases), and all reported ASL use with deaf friends.

TABLE 7.1   The Boston Data

| | | Black Participants | | | | | |
| | | Working Class | | | Middle Class | | |
		15–25 *n* = 2	26–54 *n* = 3	55–up *n* = 1	15–25 *n* = 2	26–54 *n* = 3	55–up
Language used with families	Hearing	1. S/WE, fs w/ youngest brother 2. S/WE	1. WE, fs w/ mother 2. S/WE 3. PSE, WE, gestures	1. S/WE	1. S/WE 2. ASL w/ mother only	1. Gestures, WE 2. SE, few signs w/mother 3. SE, some fs	n/a
	Deaf	2. Fs	2. Signs				n/a
Language used with friends	Hearing			1. S/WE	1. SE, fs, some signs	1. Signs (taught) 2. SE	
	Deaf	1. ASL 2. ASL	1. ASL 2. ASL 3. ASL, PSE, gestures	1. ASL	1. ASL 2. ASL	1. ASL 2. ASL 3. ASL	

White Participants

		Working Class			Middle Class		
		15–25 n = 2	26–54 n = 3	55–up n = 2	15–25 n = 2	26–54 n = 3	55–up n = 3
Language used with families	Hearing	1. S/WE, MCE, ASL	1. SE w/parents; PSE, FS w/ sisters 2. SE 3. SE		1. SE, PSE 2. ASL, SE	3. SE, gestures, home signs w/sibling	1. SE 2. SE w/parents 3. SE?
	Deaf	1. ASL w/sister 2. ASL w/sister		1. ASL, MCE 2. ASL		1. ASL 2. ASL 3. ASL w/deaf parents	2. ASL w/deaf parents
Language used with friends	Hearing	1. S/WE		1. SE 2. SE	1. WE		1. S/WE 2. SE
	Deaf	1. ASL 2. ASL 3. ASL	1. ASL 2. ASL, CS, MCE 3. ASL	1. ASL 2. ASL	1. ASL 2. ASL	1. ASL 2. ASL 3. ASL	1. ASL 2. ASL 3. ASL/MCE

Note: SE = Spoken English, WE = written English, S/WE = spoken and written English, fs = fingerspelling, MCE = manually coded English, PSE = Pidgin Sign English

TABLE 7.2   The New Orleans Data

| | | Black Participants | | | | | |
| | | *Working Class* | | | *Middle Class* | | |
		15–25 $n = 2$	26–54 $n = 3$	55–up $n = 3$	15–25 $n = 2$	26–54 $n = 3$	55–up
Language used with families	Hearing	1. SE, fs 2. SE/siblings sign	1. WE, speechread 2. SE, fs 3. SE, fs	1. SE 2. S/WE 3. WE, fs	1. SE w/parents 2. SE	1. SE 2. SE	
	Deaf				1. ASL w/deaf siblings	3. ASL	
Language used with friends	Hearing	1. Some signs w/ hearing	1. fs 2. SE	1. WE 2. WE/PSE	1. SE 2. WE	1. S/WE 2. WE	
	Deaf	1. ASL 2. ASL	1. ASL 2. ASL 3. ASL	1. ASL/PSE 2. ASL 3. ASL	1. ASL 2. ASL	1. ASL 2. ASL 3. ASL	

White Participants

		Working Class			*Middle Class*		
		15–25 n = 2	26–54 n = 2	55–up n = 2	15–25 n = 1	26–54 n = 2	55–up n = 3
Language used with families	Hearing	1. SE, some signs w/sister and mother	1. WE, fs, home signs	1. SE 2. S/WE w/ hearing; ASL w/deaf cousin		1. SE, fs	1. SE 2. S/WE 3. SE?
		2. ASL (2 deaf uncles)					
	Deaf		2. ASL		1. ASL	2. SE early age/ ASL later age	
Language used with friends	Hearing	1. fs			1. WE		1. SE 2. SE
	Deaf	1. ASL 2. ASL	1. ASL 2. ASL	1. ASL 2. ASL	1. ASL	1. ASL 2. ASL/PSE	1. ASL 2. ASL 3. ASL

Note: SE = Spoken English, WE = written English, S/WE = spoken and written English, fs = fingerspelling, MCE = manually coded English, PSE = Pidgin Sign English

Summary of Findings

The findings from the analysis of language use by deaf participants with their families and with their friends can be summarized as follows:

- Use of some form of English with hearing families, across the board, regardless of region, age, ethnicity, or socioeconomic status

- Very little signing with hearing family members; some signing with siblings in New Orleans

- ASL use in deaf families, across the board

- Use of ASL and some English with deaf friends

- Use of English with hearing friends; in one case, use of signs

- Some signing in both 15–25 middle-class groups, but not in the 26–54 and 55–up middle-class groups—a possible reflection of recent changes in educational policy

- Fingerspelling with family members in New Orleans, but not in Boston

This summary underlines the stark contrast in how communication is accomplished in hearing families with deaf children, in deaf families, with one's deaf peers, and with one's hearing peers. The overwhelming majority of participants in this study report using some form of English with their hearing family members and peers and ASL with their deaf friends. Most deaf children do not have useable access to spoken English, and the use of writing and fingerspelling, even for the transmission of simple messages, is extremely laborious. It is hard to escape the conclusion that deep, meaningful communication of the kind that ensures the child's relatively unfettered socialization is simply not taking place between the deaf child and his or her hearing family members.

Because children with Deaf peer groups do have complete access to a visual means of communication, in this case ASL, deep and meaningful communication clearly can take place in interaction with peers. It is no surprise that the acquisition of a native language and socialization into the world often take place in the deaf child's peer group instead of in the deaf child's family.

Implications of the Study

Earlier, we outlined the sociolinguistic functions of the family. These functions assume the presence of a shared code of communication, a code for which the adult members of the family provide a native model for the child. In situations such as the ones we see in Boston and New Orleans in which (a) deaf children and adults communicate with their family members through a code to which they do not have complete access and (b) deaf children and adults communicate with their peers through a code to which they have complete access, the obvious implication is that the sociolinguistic functions usually accomplished by the family are being accomplished by the peer group. Thus, the peer group provides the native model of language structure and of appropriate contextual use as well as helps develop the child's metalinguistic awareness.

In a hearing family with a deaf child in which the hearing family members do not use a natural sign language to communicate with the deaf child, the sociolinguistic function of providing a native model of language structure cannot be fulfilled. It cannot be fulfilled for either the natural sign language or for what most likely will become the child's second language, English. Communication methods such as using a spoken language that the child cannot hear, writing notes, and fingerspelling cannot provide a deaf child a useful foundation in English. In contrast, repeated observations confirm that the deaf children from deaf families in which ASL is used have strong English skills (Lane, Hoffmeister, and Bahan 1996). This language acquisition occurs mainly because the deaf children in these families acquire their first language natively and with it, a cognitive sense of what a language is; the next step to competence in written (and, in some cases, spoken) English is easily taken.

By providing a native model of a sign language, the parents and caretakers provide a beginning model for general language learning that can then be built on when learning English in educational settings. For the deaf child in a hearing family, however, from a sociolinguistic standpoint, the peer group often becomes the family. This observation is supported both by numerous anecdotal accounts and by studies in the United States and elsewhere. Reilly's work in Thailand, for example, clearly shows the centrality of the peer group for language acquisition and socialization in deaf communities.

A related implication is that, in addition to providing the site for language acquisition, the peer group also becomes central in the transmission of world knowledge, again, because of the availability of a language to which the deaf child has complete access. Furthermore, the centrality of the peer group has implications for language variation and change in sign languages. In spoken language situations in which parents and children share a common language, patterns of language variation and change are often observed to be cross-generational. Variation and change may also be cross-generational in deaf communities, but the interesting difference is that it will necessarily be across generations of peers and not across generations of individuals related by blood and kinship. The effects of this difference have yet to be researched.

Finally, the study throws light on what should happen if the hearing families of deaf children are to fulfill their sociolinguistic functions—those functions that are already fulfilled by hearing families with hearing children and deaf families with deaf children. What should happen is simply that the models of language structure and metalinguistic awareness have to be provided to the deaf child through a language that he or she can understand, a natural sign language. In the comparison by Lane, Hoffmeister, and Bahan (1996) of hearing and deaf families cited earlier, the authors point out that

> it is the same child in both family situations. So the root of the problem cannot be the Deaf child. Rather it must lie with the parents. It lies indeed with the hearing parents' inability to expose their Deaf child to a natural language without taking special measures. (40–41, italics in original)

But as recent and ongoing changes in deaf education are showing (and as they are reflected possibly in our data, in the middle-class 15–25 groups), parents are capable of learning a natural sign language and of therefore developing communication with their children that is as meaningful as the communication between hearing children and hearing parents or between deaf children and deaf parents. Clearly, the key to making this communication happen is to educate the parents of deaf children about the family's sociolinguistic functions and about how these functions are to be carried out in a family with a deaf child. This education of the parents of deaf children is being undertaken in a variety of programs both in the United States and abroad, and it leaves us with hope that deaf children will enjoy meaningful communication with both their families and their deaf peers.

ACKNOWLEDGMENTS

This paper was originally presented at the Sociolinguistic Symposium 11, Cardiff, Wales, September 1996, in a session called "The Sociolinguistics of Signed Languages." The authors are grateful to Jayne McKenzie for the preparation of this manuscript.

REFERENCES

Eckert, Penny. 1989. *Jocks and burnouts*. New York: Teachers College Press.

Greenberg, Mark T. 1980. Hearing families with deaf children: Stress and functioning related to communication method. *American Annals of the Deaf* 125:1063–71.

Labov, William. 1972. *Language in the inner city*. Philadelphia: University of Pennsylvania Press.

Lane, Harlan, Robert Hoffmeister, and Ben Bahan. 1996. *A journey into the Deaf-world*. San Diego: DawnSign Press.

Lucas, Ceil, Robert Bayley, and Clayton Valli. 2001. *Sociolinguistic variation in ASL*. Sociolinguistics in Deaf Communities, no. 7. Washington, D.C.: Gallaudet University Press.

Markowicz, Harry, and James Woodward. 1978. Language and the maintenance of ethnic boundaries in the deaf community. *Communication and Cognition* 11:29–38.

Milroy, Leslie. 1987. *Language and social networks*. 2d ed. Cambridge, Mass.: Blackwell.

Padden, Carol, and Tom Humphries. 1988. *Deaf in America: Voices from a culture*. Cambridge, Mass.: Harvard University Press.

Reilly, Charles. 1995. A deaf way of education: Interaction among children in a Thai boarding school. Ph.D. diss., University of Maryland.

Supalla, Sam. 1994. Equality in educational opportunities: The deaf version. In *The Deaf Way: Perspectives from the International Conference on Deaf Culture*, ed. C. J. Erting, R. C. Johnson, D. L. Smith and B. D. Snider, 584–92. Washington, D.C.: Gallaudet University Press.

Swisher, Virginia, and Marie Thompson. 1985. Mothers learning Simultaneous Communication: The dimensions of the task. *American Annals of the Deaf* 130:212–17.

Wright, David. 1969. *Deafness*. New York: Stein & Day.

8 School Language and Shifts in Irish Deaf Identity

Barbara LeMaster

What it means to be Deaf in the Republic of Ireland has been changing over the years (LeMaster 1990; Matthews 1996; Burns 1998). Similarly, what the term *Irish Sign Language* (ISL) refers to has also been changing (LeMaster 2002b). The sociolinguistic expression of Deafness in Ireland is completely embedded in a particularly Irish way of life. To understand both pathological "deaf" and sociocultural "Deaf" identities (or simultaneous "d/Deaf" identities) of people living in Dublin, one needs to consider the historical role of residential school language policies and various d/Deaf social movements within Ireland over time.[1]

THEORY, METHODS, AND THE RESEARCHER'S ROLE IN THE COMMUNITY

As an American conducting research in Ireland, I began my work through the lens of American understandings of d/Deaf group formation. What I found was a rhetoric of Deafness that was expressed in ways familiar to the U.S. situation yet was conveyed through unfamiliar linguistic means. For a number of years, the United States has been fond of describing a Deaf community that uses sign varieties in hegemonic, dichotomous, diglossic (Ferguson 1959) ways, a community in which English varieties of signing are used with outsiders and American Sign Language (ASL) is used among in-group members (Stokoe 1969–1970; Markowicz and Woodward 1978; Padden 1980). Many early researchers linked the primacy of language use to deaf/Deaf group formation and cohesion in the United States (Stokoe 1960; Jacobs 1972; Woodward 1972; Padden and Markowicz 1975; Padden 1980; LeMaster 1983; Padden and Humphries 1988).

This body of research uncovered how ASL often serves as a signal of Deaf culture membership, exclusion of outsiders, or both. Those who could not use ASL would have trouble claiming a Deaf identity and being accepted as a member by other Deaf culture members. Although the American situation has often been presented in dichotomous ways as though the concept "d/Deaf versus hearing" people represents real and clearly bounded groups, the situation is actually much more complex as more recent scholarship suggests (Aramburo 1989; Lucas 1989;

153

Lucas and Valli 1992; De Garcia 1995; Ramsey 1997; Metzger 2000; Lucas, Bayley, and Valli 2001; see also Woodward 1976; Shroyer and Shroyer 1984). The appropriate use of ASL plays a vital role in the expression of American Deaf identity nonetheless. Considering the great complexity among American Deaf people's signing, one realizes that the notion of a "Deaf community" is in many ways an imagined reality (Anderson 1983) as Nakamura points out in chapter 11 of this volume, and this imagined reality is always culturally situated.[2]

When I began my research in Dublin in the 1980s, deaf people talked about themselves in terms similar to those used within the U.S. Deaf communities. Although the term *Deaf culture* was not as prevalent in community rhetoric during the early days of my research, the dichotomous view that distinguished "real Deaf" people (alluding to a cultural attribute) from people who are "just deaf" (in the pathological sense) still influenced how Deaf people talked about one another. This idea of legitimate Deaf status was tied to perceptions of skill in ISL (LeMaster 1998).

However, although the rhetoric used in Ireland seemed to mirror the dichotomous American view that ASL (or in this case, ISL) was linked to Deaf identity and that the use of signed versions of English was linked with outsiders, the language practices of the Irish did not seem to match their rhetoric in two ways. First, English-based signing with mouthing was often used during discussions about political Deafness (whether the addressees were deaf or hearing). Second, generation and gender were prominent factors in language and identity negotiations among the Irish more so than distinctions between Deaf and hearing (LeMaster 1990; McDonnell and Saunders 1993; Matthews 1996; Burns 1998; Ó Baoill and Matthews 2000; LeMaster 2002b).

The community's more senior members signed without lip movements and would be more likely to use ISL with hearing people. In contrast, during the 1980s, the younger members of the community often spoke or, at least, used English lip movements with their signing and were more likely to use English-influenced signing with hearing people. Yet, the younger Irish Deaf people were the ones who talked about how they were more culturally Deaf and used more ISL than the older people. Each group would say that the other group did not use ISL or did not use "good" ISL. Yet, clearly, both groups used ISL according to the language conventions of their generation.

From my American perspective, this dichotomy—older folks not being Deaf and younger folks being more Deaf (according to younger folks, mostly)—did not parallel American descriptions of being Deaf (Padden and Markowicz 1975; Stokoe 1969–1970; Woodward 1973a, 1973b). Unlike the American situation, the speaking and more English-influenced signers were the younger and more politically Deaf members of the community whereas the nonspeaking, signing members of the community were the more politically conservative, more senior members and were more accepting of hearing people into the group. Clearly, linguistic expressions of identity and even ideas about identity are embedded in local culture.

The research for this chapter was conducted between 1984 and 1988 in Dublin and then again in the summer of 2000. When in Dublin, I lived with Anne and Laurence Coogan, two leaders in the Dublin Deaf community. My research methods included extensive ethnographic observation, structured and unstructured interviews, examination of archival written and film data, and collection of elicited and naturally occurring linguistic data. In addition to living with people who used sign language on a daily basis, I worked with four key consultants (two women and two men) and various institutions such as the schools for the deaf, the Dublin Deaf Centre, the National Association of Deaf People (NADP), the Irish Deaf Society (IDS), the St. Joseph's House for Adult Deaf and Deaf-Blind facility, the Irish Sign Language Teachers' Association, Trinity College Dublin (TCD), Institiúid Teangeolaíochta Éireann (ITE), and others.[3] I spent a lot of time visiting d/Deaf people in their homes. I also spent time with parents of deaf children and the deaf children themselves. For more information about specific methods used in the most extensive phases of field research, see LeMaster (1990).

Many changes had taken place within the Irish Deaf community between 1988 and the summer of 2000. Although no certified professional interpreters served the community in 1988 and no interpreter agency had been established in Ireland at that time, by the year 2000, several certified interpreters were working through interpreting agencies. Clearly, interpreting has become a valued profession in Ireland. Similarly, through the training of sign language teachers, the teaching of ISL has become more professionalized and more available. The Sign Language Teachers' Association (whose members taught classes at the club) branched out to teach sign language in many places throughout Ireland, and the IDS began teaching sign language classes at Trinity College and elsewhere.

In addition, much more information was available by 2000 for and about the Irish Deaf community. Beginning in the fall of 1988, a television program about Irish Deaf people was broadcast in sign language with male and female hosts (who primarily used the male form of signing).[4] Today, signers regularly present news segments on television. The NADP and the Sign Language Association of Ireland (SLAI) sponsored a dictionary project conceived of and directed by Deaf people (*Sign On* 1992). The Linguistics Institute of Ireland, which has conducted studies of spoken and written language since the 1960s, began linguistic projects on ISL directed by Patrick Matthews, a Deaf man. Through this project, two books have been published on the community and the language (Matthews 1996; Ó Baoill and Matthews 2000). Irish people such as Edward Crean (1997), the father of a Deaf son, are also writing about their own experiences. The dictionary of Irish Sign Language, first printed in 1979, was revised and reprinted in 1996 (Foran 1996). The IDS has produced several videotapes on ISL and is amassing an impressive library of video and print publications about their community and language. Trinity College Dublin has just opened a Deaf Centre, which hired its own director and Deaf teaching staff. Deafness is becoming a viable commodity in Ireland, and thus, more Deaf people have been able to participate in the public construction of their own identity and language.[5]

The Effects of Educational Language Policies

Ireland has a long and rich signing tradition. The main schools for the deaf were signing schools until the 1940s, long after the Milan Conference of 1880 had convinced other European countries to adopt oralism. Educational language policies have had profound effects on current Irish Deaf identities. Particularly important is what has happened since the introduction of oralism in 1946. My contention is that the differences in notions of identity between older and younger community members in Ireland stem from school language policies that required using either sign or oralism. When carried out, these language policies to use sign and, later, oralism each sent strong messages about deafness being either a relatively normal or abnormal condition.

Scholars of education have argued that denying children's culture and language can lead to oppositional stances within the majority language and culture (Ogbu 1987; Ogbu and Simons 1998). They have also argued that treating minority children's primary culture and language as valid and introducing them to other cultures and languages in an additive way leads to higher integration of these children into the majority culture and greater facility with the majority language (Cummins 1986).

Applying these ideas to the Irish example, then, members of the younger, oral generation would be more likely to become militant advocates of a strong Deaf community and Deaf identity and more likely to adopt an oppositional stance toward the hearing majority. This is what I assert happened as a result of the change to exclusive oralism in lieu of sign for most students at the schools described below. Exclusive oralism denies the need of the deaf body for easily accessible visual communication and underscores deficiencies rather than maximizes strengths of deaf children. Signing, in contrast, enables and empowers deaf children to communicate freely because it is the most natural form of communication for their deaf bodies. If deafness is treated as one of the many normal societal variants for the human condition, then deaf people will excel in language and in their participation within a predominantly hearing society.

I argue that imposed, exclusive oral communication for deaf children sends a message to the children and to others in the society that deafness is an abnormal variant of the human condition that requires accommodation to others (see also McDonnell and Saunders 1993). As a result of this daily denial of their deafness through the use of imposed, exclusive oralism and through their continuous struggle with one of the most fundamental aspects of their daily life—communication—deaf people as a group will more likely develop an oppositional relationship with nondeaf others and with deaf others who function well in the hearing world as Ogbu (1987) and Ogbu and Simons (1998) suggest happens for other language minority groups. Oralism per se does not lead to an oppositional stance; instead, the imposition of oralism rather than the choice of the individual to use oralism is what leads to opposition.

SIGNING AT THE CABRA SCHOOLS

In 1846, an all-girls' school called St. Mary's School for Deaf Girls was established in the Cabra section of Dublin. Approximately ten years later in 1857, the boys' school, St. Joseph's School for Deaf Boys, was opened. Because the schools are located in the Cabra section of Dublin, they are referred to colloquially as the "Cabra schools." The focal purpose of the Cabra schools was to teach Catholic deaf children to be sufficiently literate in the English language so they could receive the sacraments and thereby "be saved" (O'Dowd 1955). Without these two new Catholic schools, the schools available to deaf children in Ireland were generally Protestant-run schools that would not teach Catholic deaf children about the sacraments and their importance.

What sets the Cabra schools apart from most other deaf residential schools throughout history is the way in which English literacy was taught. It was taught through the use of sign language in a school community where both hearing and deaf people signed. No interactions were in spoken language (LeMaster 1990; Griffey 1994; Crean 1997).

The language policies at the Cabra residential schools have had a huge impact on Irish ideologies of deafness in the Republic of Ireland. For the first 100 years, sign language was used exclusively at the schools, and they were world-renowned for their English literacy success.

Both of the Cabra schools used sign language as the primary means for face-to-face communication inside and outside of the classroom from the mid-1800s until the middle of the 20th century (LeMaster 1990; LeMaster and Dwyer 1991; LeMaster 1997; see figure 8.1). The language policy to use sign language on campus is not unique to these two schools, but how the policy was carried out is. Hearing people used sign language on the campuses not only with deaf people but also with one another. At other residential deaf schools, when sign language is used, hearing teachers generally sign when they believe a deaf person is "listening," but will otherwise speak to another hearing person without sign. At the Cabra schools, hearing teachers did not speak to one another—ever (Sister Nicholas Griffey, taped personal communication, 1986).[6] The teachers referred to them-

Saint Mary's School for Deaf Girls during the Period 1846–1946	Saint Joseph's School for Deaf Boys during the Period 1855–1957	General Irish Society
• Principal means of communication: Signed language derived from French pedagogical signs; indigenous signs	• Principal means of communication: Signed Language derived from French pedagogical signs; indigenous signs	• Deafness relatively accepted by society; deaf people enjoy "legitimate" (if somewhat circumscribed) positions in Dublin society
• Signed language used by students, teachers, visitors	• Signed language used by students, teachers, visitors	• Burden on hearing people to bridge communication gaps
• Linguistic community relatively isolated from boy's school	• Linguistic community relatively isolated from girl's school	

Figure 8.1. The influence of the educational language policy in Dublin's Cabra Schools for the Deaf to use ISL in classrooms for all face-to-face communication

selves as living in a "silent" community where no one used spoken language. The people I interviewed in the 1980s did not know why these communities operated as "silent" communities, just that they did.

At these schools, hearing residents not only signed to one another but also served as interpreters for any hearing, nonsigning visitor. Therefore, the deaf people living at these schools had access to everything that was said both inside and outside of the classroom—as long as they could see the communication. The importance of this widespread use of sign language to the development of d/ Deaf identity is that it created a relatively normal communicative environment for deaf people. The message at these residential schools was clear: deaf people are normal people who use a visual-gestural language, and hearing people must accommodate their communicative needs.

During the time that sign language was used exclusively at the Cabra schools, the schools were owned by the Catholic Church. The residential girls' school was located at the sequestered Dominican Sisters' convent. Within walking distance was the residential boys' school, which was administered by the Christian Brothers who also lived on site. Although the majority of the teachers at that time were from these clerical orders and were hearing, a few of the exceptional deaf students eventually became teachers at the schools and, generally, continued to live on campus.

Another language policy that had a profound effect on the Deaf community was the policy to ensure that every deaf student became proficient in English literacy. Although children were accepted to the schools regardless of their family's religious orientation, the primary purpose of English literacy was to ensure that deaf children would be able to receive the Catholic sacraments. This religious focus had a collateral benefit. The focus to teach competent literacy skills led educators to use sign language as the medium of instruction. Educators also wrote their own textbooks to include mention of deaf people as normal members of Irish society (LeMaster 1990, 78). As a result of these educators' various pedagogical literacy efforts, Irish deaf children acquired extraordinary English skills. In fact, the schools became known for their amazing success with English literacy education.[7]

The sign and English language policies at the schools had at least two effects on deaf identity. The first involves a societal view of deafness as a relatively normal condition, which reinforced this understanding among deaf people themselves. This did not mean that deaf people were not considered to be deaf. Instead, deaf people were viewed as being able to participate in society. Yes, they were still considered to be disabled, but they were people who fit into the fabric of society as deaf people. Most important, deaf people were not required to mask their deafness. Instead, hearing people who did not know sign language were expected to use written English with deaf people or to use an interpreter when on school grounds or when interpreters were otherwise available. (At the time sign language was used at the schools, there were few, if any, interpreters outside of the Cabra schools and some churches.) I do not mean to imply that deaf people did not feel deaf in a predominantly hearing society; they did. Instead, I am arguing that the expectation of the greater society for deaf people to show their deafness in their communication with others—to either sign or write—affects

how deaf people—as deaf people—view themselves as a normal part of Irish society.

After recent conversations with Deaf Irish people, I understand that deafness
was perhaps not as normalized as I had described in my earlier writings. Rather
than willingly accommodate deaf people's communicative needs, hearing people
apparently engaged in writing with deaf people somewhat reluctantly—only
when they felt it was necessary. Hearing people sometimes used more convenient
means available to them to communicate with deaf people, such as writing in the
air. Also, not all hearing employers were willing to take the time to write to employees or fully explain themselves through the written word, which caused re-
sentment on both sides. Nonetheless, what is unique to Ireland is the initial
socialization experience at the residential schools where deafness was treated relatively normally in terms of the kinds of communication channels expected to be
used within the school by both deaf and hearing people. This accommodation in
the schools was significant.

However, this school policy did not always promote harmony among deaf
students. Instead, the school policy to use sign language had a probably unexpected and divisive effect. The emergence of gender signs associated with the two
schools served to divide deaf people from one another by gender. In short, because the two schools functioned as though they were separate islands, two very
different sign vocabularies emerged at the gender-segregated schools. These differences have been detailed elsewhere (see LeMaster and Foran 1987; LeMaster
1990; LeMaster and Dwyer 1991; LeMaster 1997, 2000; see also Crean 1997, 41;
Burns 1998; Ó Baoill and Matthews 2000). Although the solution for communicating between the sexes has been that women adopt the male signs instead of their
own, research has also shown that this adoption is not complete. The female
forms have not been entirely abandoned. So how has the existence of school-
generated gender signs affected d/Deaf identity in this Irish community? It produced an age-graded effect. Those who attended residential school when sign
language was used (or on the heels of it) know and, in most cases, use these
gendered variations. For older Irish d/Deaf people, then, gender became something that needed to be negotiated through language use. Younger signers face a
different set of challenges.

Change from Sign Language to Oral Education

The next significant effect of the Cabra educational language policies came in the
change from exclusive use of sign language to exclusive use of oralism (lip- or
speechreading and speaking) in the mid-20th century (see figure 8.2). Former Deaf
Cabra students were in favor of adding oralism to their curriculum, according to
Sister Nicholas Griffey during a taped interview in 1986. Sister Nicholas explained
that Deaf workers would go to England when no work was available in Ireland,
which was, and still is, typical for anyone, hearing or deaf. Once in England, they
were held to the British societal expectations of deaf people to accommodate to
hearing norms through the use of speechreading and speaking. Because British
employers expected British Deaf people to be able to speak and speechread, they
were reportedly unwilling to write notes between themselves and their Irish Deaf
employees. Instead, British Deaf people were used as interpreters. Imagine that

Saint Mary's School for Deaf Girls during the Period 1946–Present	Saint Joseph's School for Deaf Boys during the Period 1957–Present	General Irish Society
• Principal means of communication: Oralism (method of speaking and speech-reading)	• Principal means of communication: Oralism (method of speaking and speech-reading)	• Societal stigma against the use of sign language
• Oral methods used by students, teachers, visitors (except in manual section of school)	• Oral methods used by students, teachers, visitors (except in manual section of school)	• Burden on deaf people to bridge communication gaps
• Children segregated by hearing abilities and oral abilities	• Children segregated by hearing abilities and oral abilities	
• Girls' school now has social events with boys' school	• Boys' school now has social events with girls' school	

FIGURE 8.2. The influence of educational language policy in Dublin's Cabra Schools for the Deaf on the use of oralism in classrooms for all face-to-face communication

situation: British Deaf people had to speechread the employer, then sign to the Irish Deaf person (after deciding whether to use British or Irish Sign Language), then the Irish Deaf person would sign back to the British Deaf person who would speak on behalf of the Irish Deaf person. Sister Nicholas also reported that Irish people felt disadvantaged in this kind of situation. Although Irish Deaf people felt they had an advantage in terms of their high literacy skills, they disliked having to use British Deaf people as interpreters. During a taped interview Sister Nicholas explained that because of this perceived disadvantage, Deaf Irish adults asked the schools to add oralism to the curriculum. They did not ask, however, to have sign language removed.

In the same interview, Sister Nicholas said that, because Deaf people requested oralism be added to the curriculum, she went to Holland to learn how to do that (but see Griffey 1994). In Holland, she learned to exclude sign language when using oralism with deaf people. She also explained that the reason signs and oralism could not be used simultaneously was because deaf people would look at the signs and not at the lips. For this reason, sign language was strictly excluded from use at the girls' school when oralism was introduced in 1946. Because the boys' school was run by a different order, the Christian Brothers, it did not institute the oral language policy until 1957, at about the time that the Department of Education took over financial responsibility for both schools.

Although not verified by any official person, my perception was that the boys' school was not as strictly oral as the girls' school during my first two visits in 1984–1985 and 1986 but was certainly exclusively oral during my visit in 1988. Yet by the year 2000, sign was being used again in a limited way among oral children, and now in 2002, ISL-using Deaf teachers are working at a newly opened pre-school on the campus.

During my first visit in 1984–1985, the boys' school allowed Deaf adults to come onto campus where I videotaped their production of gendered signs. In 1986, I witnessed several teachers signing to boys in front of the school when their attempts to speak to them failed. However, by 1988, I saw no evidence of sign used at the school with the exception of the multiply handicapped unit at the school, and the Christian Brothers I had known who could sign had been transferred out of the school.

Until very recently, only two general exceptions to the "no sign" policy had been allowed officially at the two schools. Multiply disabled children and nonoral deaf children had been allowed to sign. The nonoral deaf children had been allowed to sign at school only if they were transferred to the multiply handicapped section with parental permission. Yet deaf adults and some parents of deaf children told me that parental permission to transfer from the oral part of the school to the manual part had not often been granted. For these parents of deaf children, the manual part of the school took on a stigma of "oral failure" for their child and an implication to the outside world that their child had multiple disabilities. As with most parents who do not have sufficient evidence to the contrary, these parents reported to me that they felt they were making the best decision for their deaf children by leaving them in an oral program. Oralism, the parents said, would better prepare their child for mainstream life among hearing people after graduation.

To better contextualize both of the schools during the change from sign language to oralism, it is essential to point out other changes that were occurring simultaneously.

1. The Department of Education took over financial administration of the schools, which led to most non-university-certified deaf teachers leaving the school or being transferred to work in the multiply handicapped manual section of the school.
2. Hearing teachers who could sign were transferred out of the schools, and new, nonsigning hearing teachers were brought in.
3. Deaf, signing employees were asked not to sign in front of the oral deaf children.
4. Children were increasingly segregated by hearing abilities. More and more, students with residual hearing, students with profound loss, and manual students were not allowed to have social times together.
5. In at least one case, oral and manual siblings were instructed to go through interpreters at home rather than talk directly to each other.
6. In another case, deaf oral children were instructed to use their oral mother as

an interpreter to talk to their manual father and to a sibling who was not in an oral school program.

7. School curriculum was expanded to include college preparatory courses while English literacy skills greatly declined.
8. Few oral deaf children had good access to standard versions of sign language, so many new forms of sign emerged from both schools.
9. Many other deaf schools emerged in different locations within the Republic, some using the "total communication" approach. Therefore, the two Cabra schools, while still the largest in the Republic, no longer produced long-reaching effects as they had done before.

Yet, as mentioned earlier, the current language situation at the schools is undergoing further changes. At the girls' school, the very first deaf woman has been promoted to an administrative position. This person is Maura Buckley, who is bilingual in ASL and ISL and equally competent in spoken and written English. The boys' school is using more signing among some deaf students, although those signs do not always match the vocabulary of native ISL users (according to stories told to me by these students). Finally, as mentioned above, a preschool that will use ISL has been established on the grounds of the boys' school.

Effects of Oral Education on d/Deaf Identity

So what effect did the change of school policy from exclusive sign to exclusive oralism have on a d/Deaf identity? First and most critically, by requiring deaf children to speechread and speak as their only options for face-to-face communication and by not allowing them to sign in school, children were asked to mask their deafness. Although many deaf people may want to have the option of being able to lipread and speak when they choose to do so, requiring children to rely on oral strategies as their only method of face-to-face communication sends them a message that being deaf is not okay. In this sense, speaking and speechreading is not an additive component to their education. It is not one of the many ways that they may choose to communicate. Instead, oralism in these situations is instituted to replace sign language. In this kind of situation where the natural language of children is forbidden, a stigma develops (as Cummins 1986 argues for other similar language-minority situations).

Many of these deaf children became aware of how much hearing they had, worried about whether or not they could hear on the phone, and became concerned about the intelligibility of their speech. This kind of language socialization experience occurred for both girls and boys. For most of the students at these schools, their acquisition of sign language occurred covertly through informal networks. As happens in so many oral educational situations, children invented signs when they did not have access to currently existing signs. After graduation, they found a wider variety of signs in use among their age group, and many of their signs differed from the signs used by the older, sign-only generation (see LeMaster 1990). This younger cohort is no longer concerned with gender differences but, instead, is concerned with oppositional and hegemonic deaf-versus-hearing issues.

EXPRESSION AND POLITICIZATION OF D/DEAF IDENTITIES IN COMMUNITY GROUPS

The adult Deaf community has members from both the sign and oral periods in Irish Deaf education. Although several organizations of and for deaf people have been established in the area during the 1980s and today, from my perspective, three organizations have been central in the social and political lives of the adults with whom I worked (see LeMaster 1990). They are the Dublin Deaf Centre (their Deaf club) where the Dublin Deaf Association (DDA) resides, the NADP, and the IDS.

THE DEAF CLUB AND THE DUBLIN DEAF ASSOCIATION

At the time of my most intensive field research during the 1980s, the Dublin Deaf Centre was the central public place where deaf people gathered (see Crean 1997, 75). The DDA is the largest and oldest deaf association in Ireland (see http://www.deafbase.com). It comprises self-managed sports as well as social and cultural clubs that are both nonpolitical and nondenominational. When the club was in Rathmines in the center of Dublin, it offered a wide range of activities, including sign language classes. Also located at the club were the Community Information Centre for the Deaf (National Social Services Board), Irish Deaf Sports Association (a national and international group), and offices for the NADP social worker, club leaders, and the Catholic Institute for the Deaf (CID). I cannot underscore enough the importance of this club. It was well used by d/Deaf people of all ages and, perhaps equally important, by all Deaf political affiliations. In other words, Deaf people who had competing agendas for how Irish deafness should (or should not) become politicized within Dublin all used the same Deaf club.

My attending the social nights at the club became important in my research. As is typical for Deaf people around the world (see Hall 1991 for a U.S. example), d/Deaf people of all ages convened at the centralized deaf club in Dublin. They interacted with one another even though some of them were monodialectal users of oralism, some spoke or mouthed and speechread while using sign language, and others signed without lip movement. When I was there in the 1980s, most of the leaders were male and signed without lip movement. The younger leaders generally grew up oral, learning sign covertly or acquiring sign as adults. The signs used by the younger and older generations were not always the same, so they struggled to understand one another. Yet, they all made the effort to try to understand one another's signing.

However, during the 1980s, the club moved from Rathmines to a beautiful facility north of city's center. It is fair to say that fewer people attend the club now than during the 1980s, preferring to meet elsewhere in age-group cohorts, generally at pubs throughout the city. Yet, the club still provides a place for people to meet, especially in large groups. Yearly meetings of organizations are held in the club's large auditorium, as are special lectures and other activities requiring space for large groups. Scheduled activities such as the seniors' luncheons on Tuesdays continue at the club. Community members conducting research on sign language and related issues also use space at the club. So although the club is perhaps not attracting as large a crowd on social nights as it once did, it is still an important part of the community.

NATIONAL ASSOCIATION OF DEAF PEOPLE

Another important organization was and is the NADP. In the 1980s, it housed the only social worker for deaf people in the Republic of Ireland. Until 1986, this social worker was the only person in the office who knew how to sign. The structure of the NADP included deaf and hearing adults on the board of directors, who represented prominent society members and less well recognized people.

The structure of the NADP and its history as the state-sanctioned organization serving Irish deaf needs (until the late 1990s) gave it an advantage over any other deaf organization in Ireland, particularly the newly formed IDS, which was newly established at the time I was there in the 1980s. Given that the NADP Board had prominent society members, the organization had been favored in the past by the Irish government with respect to governmental funding for projects related to deafness. In 1986, the chairman of the Irish NADP was the Honorable Niall McCarthy, a judge who served on an Irish court equivalent to the U.S. Supreme Court.[8] McCarthy was instrumental in hiring staff members who could sign such as the chief executive, Niall Keane. When I returned in 1988, the new on-site staff at NADP could sign. Also during the 1980s, the new projects funded by the NADP were largely those designed, executed, and performed by Deaf people themselves.

According to the NADP Web site (http://www.iol.ie/~nad/nad-homepage .html), which provides a statement of purpose and a range of other information, their mission is to

- Promote the right of every deaf person to enjoy an equality of opportunity in all aspects of life, and to develop full independence and citizenship.

- Promote the right of parents of deaf children to enjoy access to the full range of appropriate supports and services, and to take an active role in their child's education and development.

- And plan to fulfill this mission
  - through advocacy for equal opportunities.
  - through development of direct services.
  - through encouraging the development of services by others.

- Deaf people are full members of society.

- They have equal rights, should be afforded equal respect and must be able to exercise equal opportunities.

- Deaf people have the right to equality of access to information and full participation in society.

- In providing services, full account must be taken of deaf people and other consumers, their experiences, their values, their rights and their opinions.

The NADP continues to serve as an umbrella service organization for deaf people and their families, offering a wide variety of services to help deaf people manage their lives.

The Irish Deaf Society

The IDS began as the Deaf Action Group in 1981, the International Year of the Disabled Person. According to my fieldwork interviews, Stan Foran and Anne Coogan were among the original founders of the Deaf Action Group, which was originally formed to bring to the Irish people's attention the needs and strengths of d/Deaf people. Feeling that they had met their original goals, Foran and Coogan had stopped their association with the organization by the time I had arrived in 1984. New leadership took over the Deaf Action Group and resurrected it as the IDS in 1983.

In the 1980s, the IDS clearly vied for official recognition within Ireland. With new leadership, the IDS competed with the NADP for recognition by the government and others as the primary representative group of Irish Deaf people, and sought to gain greater prominence within Ireland. The state seemed to be greatly reluctant to replace the NADP, a long-standing organization that had the support of established d/Deaf leaders. In contrast to the ties that the NADP had with the Irish government and because the NADP received great financial and social support from various established philanthropists, the newly established IDS organization was still considered to be fledgling within Ireland at that time.

Although the IDS had not yet gained prominence within Ireland during the 1980s, it had captured the attention of many Deaf youth. IDS had also positioned itself in the world as Ireland's representative to the World Federation of the Deaf (WFD) and the Euroaction Working Group in the European Union. By the summer of 2000, the IDS had clearly gained the respect of many Irish d/Deaf people and had gained the recognition of the Irish government. The IDS had successfully competed for a £600,000+ grant from the government to study adult literacy among Deaf people. The IDS had also worked with Trinity College Dublin to establish a Deaf Centre and had worked with the government and St. Joseph's school to have an ISL-using preschool opened on the grounds of St. Joseph's School for Deaf Boys and to have it staffed by Deaf teachers.

The IDS Web site (http://indigo.ie/~ids/) posts their mission statement:

> The Irish Deaf Society as Ireland's National Association OF the Deaf, strives to highlight the societal needs of all sections in the Deaf community, advocates the human rights of the Deaf through empowerment and . . . equal access in all aspects of life endowed by the full Irish citizenship. The empowerment and equality shall be through upholding the status of Irish Sign Language and its related culture and norms.

During my fieldwork in the 1980s, IDS was clearly positioning itself as a culturally Deaf organization by promoting itself as an organization run by Deaf people for the interests of Deaf people. The goals of the IDS reminded me of the goals of American Deaf people in the 1970s when they were asserting their rights to govern themselves and were working toward greater recognition and acceptance of ASL both within their own community and more broadly.

However, the Irish situation, though familiar to me from my experience in the United States, was also unfamiliar. The presentation of Deaf culture was uniquely

Irish, which differed in interesting ways from what I knew in America. For me, a conundrum in the 1980s was that the membership of the IDS seemed to include more oralists (who signed while mouthing) than signers (who did not mouth while signing). In the United States, the strongest advocates for Deaf culture did not speak and sign simultaneously but required ASL both in public and in situations in which ASL had previously not been used. From my perspective, the strongest spokesperson for the IDS during the 1980s was a very intelligent, charismatic woman who had attended St. Mary's school at the time it was oral. She had married a nonoralist signer, was completely bilingual in ISL and English, and was a very competent speechreader. What puzzled me was that, in most of her interactions with hearing people that I had observed, she would speak and speechread rather than sign—even when talking about Deaf culture and ISL issues. She became, in a sense, the quintessential cultural broker who could function effectively in a hearing world and a Deaf world, and she was representing the Deaf political cultural position.

The reason so many IDS members in the 1980s held an oralist orientation was probably because the IDS seemed to attract more young d/Deaf people than older d/Deaf people at that time. These younger Deaf members had attended the Cabra schools when they used the oral-only language policy. Once, in talking with a younger IDS person, he chastised me for not talking or mouthing English words while I was signing; I had been signing without speaking English. I had become accustomed to signing without mouthing in Ireland with older, nonoral Irish signers. When interacting with politically active, culturally Deaf Irish people, I automatically switched to the signing style I most associated with that political stance in America. But in Ireland, that approach was not what was expected at the time. Cultural Deafness in the 1980s, according to my perception, did not conform to my understanding of language use among politicized cultural Deaf people in the United States. Although the Deaf political rhetoric used in Ireland was familiar to me, the use of mouthing English while signing in this context was not as familiar. As a linguistic anthropologist, I found this cultural difference fascinating.

The leadership of the IDS has changed since the 1980s, and the IDS is now a much more ISL-focused organization. In my most recent visit during the summer of 2000, I found the IDS to be a growing and vital organization. Although its members use a variety of language styles that are consistent with language norms of the community, the IDS promotes ISL, and the leaders, who are all Deaf, use it, especially during public functions.[9] The new IDS leadership is rather young for such a powerful organization. Most of the leaders are in their 20s or 30s. From my discussions with older d/Deaf people, the new IDS organization has gained their confidence, and many of the older generation have taken membership in the IDS.

The several meetings and social gatherings of the IDS that I attended in the summer of 2000 were all conducted in ISL. When non-ISL signers were present or expected to be present, interpreters were provided. IDS has also produced videotapes to teach ISL to others. The organization is politically active, and its members have fought diligently to have ISL used both in the homes of deaf children and in schools. The IDS is currently fighting for national recognition of ISL as the legitimate first language of Irish Deaf people.[10]

Influences from Other Deaf Communities on Irish Deaf Identity

One of the most significant factors contributing to ever changing d/Deaf ideologies in this Dublin Deaf community is the influence of outside communities. Irish d/Deaf people have read literature and met with people from many nations, and they have learned how d/Deaf identities are constructed elsewhere. There has been a strong connection between Ireland and Gallaudet University that has led to student exchanges and other collaborations. But perhaps what is most immediately important to the community is that Irish Deaf people have been able to interact with other Deaf people in the European Union. Travel and conference monies have been made available to Irish Deaf people that have enabled many to learn firsthand about d/Deaf experiences elsewhere and to share their own experiences with others.

Within this more European and sometimes more international context, the relationship of d/Deaf identity to language type and variety has entered into discussions of the Irish d/Deaf identity. These discussions occur particularly among younger d/Deaf people, those who had attended school when oralism was the primary method of classroom communication. These "oralists" now talk about the necessity to differentiate between ISL and versions of signed English. Although they are able to sign both ISL and English-based signing styles, this group is more likely to use English-based language with non-ISL signers, which is a completely natural linguistic accommodation made by bilingual people. And it is more generally the younger bilinguals in this community who claim Deaf cultural identity.

The older, "signing" generation takes little part in this kind of public discourse about Deaf ethnicity and ISL. These more senior members of the community are the people who used sign without mouthing in school, who learned to distinguish between "proper" signing (Signed English) as they call it and deaf signing (ISL). They still use both versions of sign in public discourse and often refer to the "proper" signs as the "correct" signs for use in public settings because those were signs that had been acquired at school (see LeMaster 2002). And yet, although more senior members are aware of d/Deaf identity issues, few take part in public discourse about Deaf ethnicity as it may be linked to signing practices. The leaders from this older age group are often more concerned with the process of publishing information about their language in the form of ISL films and videotapes, dictionaries, and children's books as well as with the publication of previously handwritten documents about sign (Foran 1994; Foran 1996; Buckley 1998; and David Breslin's privately held films and videotapes).

The differences between the generations and their attitudes toward ISL, signed English and oralism as well as whether or not they identify themselves as culturally Deaf can be explained by linking school language policies and practices to d/Deaf socialization (LeMaster 1990; LeMaster 2002b). The older, signing generation grew up during a time when deafness was acknowledged at school and when sign language was accepted as a normal part of being deaf. This generation has excellent literacy skills, giving them a means to interact with nonsigning hearing people and a key to English language resources. The important aspect of their life stories is that, by being expected to learn sign language and written English—

both forms of visual communication well suited to deafness—these deaf people were not expected, either by society or by themselves, to deny their deafness.

The younger deaf people, on the other hand, have largely experienced societal rejection of their deafness through the use of oralism in the schools and the prohibition of signing. Every act of oralism reminded them that they were required to accommodate hearing people's communicative needs and deny their deafness (LeMaster 1990). In this context, deafness is not viewed as normal but as a disability that is further stigmatized if they choose to use sign language, which visibly marks the disability. This group of people—who were ostracized through oralism because of their deafness—are the people who embrace the literature on Deaf ethnicity and values that mark the differences between deaf and hearing people, and they are the people who give validity to the d/Deaf experience.

I am not arguing that Deaf culture emerges only in this context. Indeed, the argument is that if deafness is denied by exclusively using oralism, by replacing the use of sign language rather than adding to their knowledge of sign, then the message sent to deaf children is that they need to mask their deafness and deny who they are. This is not about the use of oralism per se but, rather, about the imposition of exclusive oralism that supplants sign language as a mandate rather than a choice for deaf people. This situation is similar to so many other situations of language minority children who are required to deny and replace their native languages by exclusively adopting a majority language. In these cases, as in this Irish case, oppositional identities often emerge (see Cummins 1986; Ogbu 1987; Ogbu and Simmons 1998). In this Irish case, an oppositional Deaf identity emerged among the children who were raised with exclusive oralism practices that supplanted sign language. Although the sentiments of a Deaf identity in opposition to a majority hearing population mirror the U.S. situation in many ways, the linguistic markers of this identity differed dramatically during the 1980s. However, on my return in 2000, the scene was more familiar to what I have known in the United States. I saw many more similar uses of ISL linked to expressions of a Deaf cultural identity, yet, they were clearly still not identical to the U.S. situation. How Irish people mark their political Deaf identities is uniquely Irish.

What is constant among d/Deaf people in Ireland is a strong sense of affiliation with one another. A sense of Deaf culture and Deaf community exists whether the main form of communication is sign without voice or mouthing with accompanying signing. What is remarkable, however, is that, within less than 50 years, a series of dramatic changes have occurred within the composition of the community, and the expression of their d/Deaf identity has changed. Deafness went from a relatively unmarked, relatively accepted status to a more highly marked, disabled status. Gender identity went from being a focal point to being largely unimportant within a very short period. The change in educational language policy was an important contributor to this identity shift, but the discourses about deafness held in other parts of Europe, in the United States, and elsewhere were also important. These factors led to the increased recognition of "Deafness" as a distinctive identity attribute among this younger group of Irish Deaf people.

WHAT CAN BE GAINED FROM CROSS-CULTURAL STUDIES?

One goal of oral education is to mainstream deaf children into the broader, hearing society. Because the majority of deaf children are born to hearing parents who have no experience with deafness before the birth of their deaf child, the parents generally favor oralism. These hearing parents would certainly prefer their children to use language as they do (in the oral channel). The use of speech and speechreading masks the condition of deafness, an otherwise invisible handicap. Deaf children who use oralism may look like other children who are not deaf. Also, they will be using the same mode of communication that their future employers, teachers, government leaders, and others will most likely use.

Yet, as in all situations of oral education, sign language still persists within Deaf communities—even in "purely" oral schools. Sign language survives because monochannel oralism is too difficult for the daily communication needs of most deaf people and because deaf people cannot achieve the hearing identity that is often so fervently sought after by many hearing parents and educators through the use of exclusive oralism with deaf children. The frustrations experienced through oral communication remind deaf people of their deafness in almost every interaction. It emphasizes precisely the limitation of deafness: the inability to hear. Even though deaf people may try to adopt the communication strategies of hearing people, they can never become hearing people; in short, they cannot adopt a hearing identity. It is not accessible to them while they live in a deaf body. When society forces deaf people to use oralism at the exclusion of sign language, deaf people will often reject oralism to release themselves from society's pressure to adopt the inaccessible hearing identity.

Why, then, is oralism maintained in the linguistic repertoire of younger signers in the Dublin Deaf community who champion Deaf identity? The answer is simple. The ability to speak and speechread, though not without its costs, can be an asset when interacting with the majority hearing and speaking population—as long as it is just one of the many tools Deaf people may choose to use at will. It is primarily this orally schooled group of Deaf people who have championed Deaf rights and who now seek official, governmental recognition of their natural sign language, ISL. How all members of this Dublin Deaf community use language variation in their negotiations of political agendas and selfhood are uniquely Irish.

Further investigation is needed to better understand how Deaf identities are culturally situated. From this cross-cultural example, we learn that expressions of Deaf culture are not universal and may not even be uniform within the same deaf community (which is true also for the American situation). We would benefit from ethnographic studies that explore the cultural situatedness of Deaf identity.

Notes

1.   Consistent with American conventions, the lowercase *d* in *deaf* is used to represent biological or pathological deafness, and the capital *D* in *Deaf* connotes social deafness. Use of *d/Deaf* represents both of these ideas simultaneously.

2.   For an interesting discussion of Deaf ethnicity, see Johnson and Erting's 1984 and 1989 discussions and LeMaster's modification to this idea in 1990. Johnson and Erting developed their argument for Deaf ethnicity through use of anthropological scholarship, notably, Barth (1969), Cohen (1974), Isajiw (1974), and Fishman (1977).

3.   My consent forms guaranteed anonymity, so I cannot provide names of consultants at this time.

4.   Predominantly women born before 1930 and men born before 1945 acquired

gendered forms of sign (a male and a female version) from the Dublin residential schools for the deaf (see LeMaster 1990).

5.   I will not discuss this idea of "deafness as a commodity" here but have presented it at the 97th meeting of the American Anthropological Association, November 1999, in a paper titled "Language Movements in Deaf Ireland" and again in a public lecture titled "Changes in Irish Sign Language" that was given in Ireland at the Deaf Club, and finally at the International Gender and Language Association in England in 2002. I am working on this idea for future publication.

6.   Sister Nicholas, a Dominican Sister, worked at the school when sign language was used and was the primary force behind the conversion to an oralist program (LeMaster 1990).

7.   In a meeting with representatives from a local school district, I was told that deaf students in the United States still graduate with a reading level of second to fourth grade.

8.   Sadly, Niall McCarthy and his wife, Barbara, were killed in a head-on collision on a holiday trip to France.

9.   The chairperson, vice chairperson, honorable secretary, and honorable treasurer are, respectively, Kevin Stanley, Eddie Redmond, John Bosco Conama, and Eilish Bradley (see http://indigo.ie/~ids/boardmbrspic.htm). The directors are Patricia Breen, Charles Grehan, Susan O'Reilly, Noel Ball, Brian Crean, Michelle Quinn-Campbell, and Larry Stanley.

10.   For more information about the IDS organization and scope of their projects, see their website (http://indigo.ie/~ids/).

REFERENCES

Anderson, Benedict. 1983. *Imagined communities: Reflections on the origin and spread of nationalism.* London: Verso.

Aramburo, Aaron. 1989. Sociolinguistic aspects of the black deaf community. In *The sociolinguistics of the deaf community*, ed. Ceil Lucas, 103–19. San Diego: Academic Press.

Barth, Fredrik, ed. 1969. *Ethnic groups and boundaries.* Boston: Little, Brown.

Buckley, Hugh. 1998. *Sign it: An illustrated A to Z guide to fingerspelling.* Dublin: Dublin Deaf Association and Sign Language Association of Ireland.

Burns, Sarah E. 1998. Ireland's second minority language. In *Pinky extension and eye gaze: Language use in deaf communities*, ed. Ceil Lucas, 233–73. Washington, D.C.: Gallaudet University Press.

Cohen, Abner. 1974. Introduction: The lesson of ethnicity. In *Urban ethnicity*, ed. Abner Cohen, ix–xxiv. London: Tavistock Publications.

Crean, Edward J. 1997. *Breaking the silence: The education of the deaf in Ireland 1816–1996.* Dublin: Irish Deaf Society Publications.

Cummins, J. 1986. Empowering minority students: A framework for intervention. *Harvard Educational Review* 56 (1):18–36.

De García, Barbara Gerner. 1995. Communication and language use in Spanish-speaking families with deaf children. In *Sociolinguistics in deaf communities*, ed. C. Lucas, 221–54. Washington, D.C.: Gallaudet University Press.

Ferguson, Charles. 1959. Diglossia. *Word* 15:325–40.

Fishman, Joshua. 1977. Language and ethnicity. In *Language, ethnicity, and intergroup relations*, ed. Howard Giles. New York: Academic Press.

Foran, Christopher. 1994. *Transcript of the 1847 manuscript Irish Sign Language Dictionary.* Dublin: Dublin Deaf Association.

Foran, Stanislaus. 1996. *The Irish Sign Language.* Rev. ed. Dublin: National Association for Deaf People.

Griffey, Nicholas O. P. 1994. *From silence to speech: 50 years with the deaf.* Dublin: Dominican Publications.

Hall, Stephanie. 1991. Door into American: Folklore in an American deaf social club. *Sign Language Studies* 73:421–29.

Isajiw, Wsevolod. 1974. Definitions of ethnicity. *Ethnicity* 1:111–24.

Jacobs, Leo. 1972. *A deaf adult speaks out.* Washington, D.C.: Gallaudet College Press.

Johnson, Robert, and Carol Erting. 1984. Linguistic socialization in the context of emergent deaf ethnicity. Working Papers in Anthropology, Wenner-Gren Foundation, New York.

———. 1989. Ethnicity and socialization in a classroom for deaf children. In *The sociolinguistics of American Sign Language,* ed. Ceil Lucas, 41–84. New York: Academic Press.

LeMaster, Barbara. 1983. Marking ethnic identity in signed conversations. Master's thesis, University of California, Los Angeles.

———. 1990. The maintenance and loss of female and male signs in the Dublin deaf community. Ph.D. diss., University of California, Los Angeles.

———. 1997. Sex differences in Irish Sign Language. In *The life of language: Papers in linguistics in honor of William Bright,* ed. Jane Hill, P. J. Mistry, and Lyle Campbell, 67–85. Berlin: Mouton de Gruyter.

———. 1998. Irish deaf identity. *Sign Language Communication Studies: The Quarterly of the Japan Institute for Sign Language Studies* 29:12–19.

———. 1999. Language movements in Deaf Ireland. Paper presented at the 97th Annual Meeting of the American Anthropological Association, Chicago, Ill.

———. 2000a. Changes in Irish Sign Language. Paper presented at the St. Joseph's Deaf Centre, Dublin, Ireland.

———. 2000b. Reappropriation of gendered Irish Sign Language in one family. *Visual Anthropology Review* 15 (2):1–15.

———2002a. The political economy of community discourses shaping the role of gendered Irish Sign Language over time. Paper presented at the International Gender and Language Association, England.

———. 2002b. What difference does difference make? Negotiating gender and generation in Irish Sign Language. In *Gendered practices in language,* ed. S. Benor, M. Rose, D. Sharma, J. Sweetland, and Q. Zhang, 309–38. Stanford: CSLI Publications.

LeMaster, Barbara, and John Dwyer. 1991. Knowing and using female and male signs in Dublin. *Sign Language Studies* 73:361–96.

LeMaster, Barbara, and Stanislaus Foran. 1987. The Irish Sign Language. *The Gallaudet encyclopedia of deaf people and deafness,* ed. John V. Van Cleve, vol. 2, 82–84. New York: McGraw-Hill.

Lucas, Ceil, ed. 1989. *The sociolinguistics of the deaf community.* San Diego: Academic Press.

Lucas, Ceil, and Clayton Valli. 1992. *Language contact in the American deaf community.* San Diego: Academic Press.

Lucas, Ceil, Robert Bayley, and Clayton Valli. 2001. *Sociolinguistic variation in American Sign Language.* Washington, D.C.: Gallaudet University Press.

Markowicz, Harry, and James Woodward. 1978. Language and the maintenance of ethnic boundaries in the deaf community. *Communication and Cognition* 11:29–38.

Matthews, Patrick A. 1996. *Survey report: History of education, language and culture.* Vol. 1 of *The Irish deaf community.* Dublin: Institiúid Teangeolaíochta Éireann.

McDonnell, Patrick, and Helena Saunders. 1993. Sit on your hands: Strategies to prevent signing. In *Looking back: A reader on the history of deaf communities and their sign languages,* ed. Renate Fischer and Harlan Lane, 255–60. Hamburg: Signum.

Metzger, Melanie, ed. 2000. *Bilingualism and identity in deaf communities.* Washington, D.C.: Gallaudet University Press.

Ó Baoill, Dónall P., and Patrick A. Matthews. 2000. *The structure of Irish Sign Language*. Vol. 2 of *The Irish deaf community*. Dublin: Institiúid Teangeolaíochta Éireann.

O'Dowd, Michael. 1955. The history of the Catholic schools for the deaf, Cabra. Master's thesis, University College, Dublin.

Ogbu, John. 1987. Ethnoecology of urban schooling. In *Cities of the United States: Studies in urban anthropology*, ed. Leith Mullings, 255–78. New York: Columbia University Press.

Ogbu, John, and Herbert D. Simons. 1998. Voluntary and involuntary minorities: A cultural-ecological theory of school performance with some implications for education. *Anthropology and Education Quarterly* 29 (2):155–88.

Padden, Carol. 1980. The deaf community and the culture of deaf people. In *Sign language and the deaf community*, ed. Charlotte Baker and Robbin Battison, 89–104. Silver Spring, Md.: National Association of the Deaf.

Padden, Carol, and Harry Markowicz. 1975. Crossing cultural group boundaries into the deaf community. Paper presented at the Conference on Culture and Communication, Temple University, Philadelphia, March.

Padden, Carol, and Tom Humphries. 1988. *Deaf in America: Voices from a culture*. Cambridge, Mass.: Harvard University Press.

Ramsey, Claire L. 1997. *Deaf children in public schools: Placement, context, and consequences*. Washington, D.C.: Gallaudet University Press.

Shroyer, Edgar H., and Susan P. Shroyer. 1984. *Signs across America*. Washington, D.C.: Gallaudet College Press.

Sign on: Basic signs used by Irish deaf people. 1992. Dublin: National Association of the Deaf and Sign Language Tutors Association of Ireland.

Stokoe, William C. 1960. *Sign language structure: An outline of the visual communication systems of the American deaf*. Silver Spring, Md.: Linstok Press.

———. 1969–1970. Sign language diglossia. *Studies in Linguistics* 21:27–41.

Woodward, James. 1972. Implications for sociolinguistic research among the Deaf. *Sign Language Studies* 1:1–7.

———. 1973a. Language continuum, a different point of view. *Sign Language Studies* 2:81–83.

———. 1973b. Some observations on sociolinguistic variation and American Sign Language. *Kansas Journal of Sociology* 9 (2):191–200.

———. 1976. Black southern signing. *Language in Society* 5 (2):211–18.

9 | *Surdos Venceremos:* The Rise of the Brazilian Deaf Community

Norine Berenz

This account of the Brazilian Deaf community and its language is necessarily localized in time and space and does not pretend to do justice to the richness and variety of the community or the language. A look at a map shows that Brazil is a vast landmass, extending over three climatic zones from north to south and, at its broadest, stretching from the Atlantic almost to the Pacific. Here, diversity is the norm, not the exception. Most of the country's citizens live along the Atlantic littoral; the great reaches of the sparsely populated interior are more tenuously connected to the nation and its interests.

The north is tropical jungle, with a population that is typically of Indian and European descent to varying degrees. The northeast is hot but dry, with a population that is mostly of African and European descent. The south is more temperate in climate, with a population more European in ancestry, its numbers swollen by those fleeing World War II and its aftermath, although in more recent decades, migration from the less industrialized, less prosperous north and northeast has gone some distance to changing the "face" of the region.[1] The other, and earlier, non-European addition to the region's population is largely centered in São Paulo, the country's major industrial and commercial city. São Paulo boasts a population of Japanese descent, established in the early 1900s following the Russo-Japanese war, and now claims to be the largest urban concentration of Japanese people outside Tokyo (here more accurately, "Japanese Brazilians," given that they are Brazilian by birth as well as by cultural adaptation).

THE ROLE OF RIO

If São Paulo is Brazil's economic muscle, then Rio de Janeiro, the capital from colonial times to the 1950s, is its cultural heart.[2] People from elsewhere challenge the hegemony of the *cariocas* (Rio residents born and bred) for a place on the narrow strip of land between the sea and the mountains. Deaf people, too, come to Rio from all over the country, forming perhaps the most vibrant and certainly the most visionary segment of the national Deaf community. Although I visited deaf people in Recife in the northeast, in Belo Horizonte in the central region, and in São Paulo, Curitiba, and Porto Alegre in the south, Rio's Deaf community provides the bulk of the data on which this chapter is based.[3]

A number of factors significantly affect the relationship between local Deaf communities and a truly national Deaf community. Unlike the United States, Brazil has no real equivalent of the National Association of the Deaf with its century-old tradition of broad-based advocacy that regularly brings together deaf people and familiarizes all participants with the regional particularities of language and socio-historico-political situation. Brazil has a long-established Deaf national sports association, but its mission and constituency are narrower than that of typical Deaf advocacy-based organizations. Moreover, Brazil never had a network of residential schools where large numbers of deaf children could have enjoyed early and intensive (if perhaps officially prohibited) exposure to sign language and Deaf culture let alone a Gallaudet University with a student population drawn from nearly all regional communities.

Unlike many European countries, Brazil's territorial vastness makes travel difficult and expensive, beyond the reach of ordinary deaf people. These limits on social interaction among members of the various local Deaf communities in countries such as Brazil may mean that an effective national Deaf community is more a hope than a reality. In Brazil, an effective national Deaf community is nascent; its development depends on the fostering of a Deaf social identity anchored in a championing of the sign language. If there is a site, however, where the seed of an effective national Deaf community could grow, it is Rio de Janeiro.

SETTING, TOPIC, AND ETHNOGRAPHER

The locality most important to the story I am about to tell is Rio, and the time most important is the first half of the 1990s. I had the good fortune to witness a major shift in the notion of what an ideal deaf person should be—from a conception of the model deaf person as one fluent in Portuguese to one who is a fluent and skillful signer. If we can extend the d/Deaf-distinction (in which *deaf* refers to hearing loss and *Deaf* to culture or social identity) to encompass the idea that the deaf person is not only culturally Deaf but also explicitly recognizes, actively embraces, and even celebrates a Deaf social identity, this would best capture the paradigmatic shift in consciousness I am reporting.[4]

Before going on, let me establish a convention to refer to the sign language. As will be discussed later, the language of the Brazilian Deaf community is known by several names. The preference of members of the community with whom I worked most closely is Língua de Sinais Brasileira, or LSB. For this reason, I will adopt the name LSB for purposes of the present discussion. The reader should understand that the use of the label LSB is a convenience.

I should also identify myself, the ethnographer, because I am neither Brazilian nor deaf. In 1983, I was introduced to LSB by Brazilian linguist Lucinda Ferreira Brito, who asked me to help prepare for English-language publication a number of manuscripts reporting her research on the sign languages of Brazil.[5] In 1985 and again in 1986, I spent six weeks meeting deaf people in various regions of Brazil. From fall 1991 to spring 1992, I worked with a second-generation deaf Brazilian signer, joined occasionally by her brother, also deaf, both residing in the United States. I then spent 10 months in Brazil in 1992 and the year August 1993 to August 1994. From March 1995 to January 1996, I hosted a native Deaf Brazilian signer in the United States.

In Brazil, the medium of communication was, of necessity, either Portuguese, LSB, or a combination of the two; few hearing and no deaf Brazilians with whom I interacted in everyday activities had sufficient knowledge of English to make it a reliable means of communication. The native Deaf Brazilian signer with whom I worked intensively and extensively was bilingual in LSB and ASL, but had little mastery of Portuguese. I had little mastery of ASL. It is primarily to him that I owe my LSB and to the shopkeepers, bus drivers, and co-residents of my apartment building that I owe my Portuguese.[6] Although I would not claim full fluency in either Portuguese or LSB, my skills in each allowed me to satisfactorily carry on both my professional work and my personal life.

SIGN LANGUAGE AND DEAF SOCIAL IDENTITY

Ella Lentz, a Deaf American poet, actor, and educator, once advised Maria Massone, a visiting Argentine Sign Language (LSA) linguist, to encourage and support deaf people's efforts to gain recognition for LSA through its use in art forms—as is done, for example, in the United States by the National Theater of the Deaf—rather than by initially pushing for its recognition in the educational and governmental spheres.[7] The wisdom of this advice lay not only in the utility of opening hearing people's eyes to the eloquence and sophistication possible in signed discourse as a means of gaining their support for later educational and political initiatives but also, and perhaps more crucially, in raising awareness within the Deaf community itself as a way of resolving the conflict between intense feelings of affection and shame that many deaf people have for their sign language.

A parallel might be drawn with the African American community, which in the 1960s sought self-affirmation through cultural items such as hairstyle (Afros, dreadlocks, and cornrows), clothing and decoration (dashikis and leather amulets), and personal naming drawing on African traditions ("Kwame" for a boy born on a Saturday). The Black-Is-Beautiful movement succeeded in broadening standards of beauty by vigorously rejecting long-standing negative imputations imposed on the community from outside.

Negative imputations for a Deaf social identity, imposed from outside, focus on sign language rather than on physical type or region of origin because deafness levels these other distinctions to a considerable degree. The results in terms of a love-hate relationship with the source of stigma can be the same in Deaf communities as in other stigmatized groups. The importance of language for social identity is well-established (Blom and Gumperz 1972; Gumperz 1982; Thiong'o 1986; and others). No less among signers than speakers, the linguistic means of communication index the social identity and social relations being enacted in any situation.

Conflicting feelings were apparent in the attitude to LSB of many members of the Brazilian Deaf community. The impression that LSB was parasitic or inferior to Portuguese found expression in members' assessments of each other. The paradigmatic shift in consciousness from a Portuguese-skilled deaf person to an LSB-skilled Deaf person is inextricably linked to a shift in the perceived status of LSB vis-à-vis Portuguese.

A Brief History of the Brazilian Deaf Community

The research project that brought me to Brazil was not ethnographic in focus but ethnographic in method. That is, I sought to elucidate a grammatical system (namely, person deixis), for which I found previous analyses of similar systems in a number of sign languages problematic, by contextualizing the system within broader conversational practice (Berenz 1996). I neither invented nor elicited relevant forms but, rather, observed them in spontaneous conversation. The historical account I will present was in part pieced together from those conversations.[8]

Some of the historical material presented below was collected as part of a curriculum development project to which I contributed, modeled on the ASL curriculum *Signing Naturally* (Smith, Lentz, and Mikos 1988), which includes a number of pieces on American Deaf history and culture. There is to date no compendium of historical information on the Brazilian Deaf community similar to Jack Gannon's work on the American Deaf community, *Deaf Heritage* (1981). Until the 1990s, there was no Brazilian counterpart to the NAD's journal *Silent Worker*, which documents important moments in early American Deaf community history. Efforts to compile historical information by Otaviano de Menezes Bastos, a deaf sign language teacher who met with Gannon to discuss the project when Otaviano visited Gallaudet in 1989, were frustrated initially by the inaccessibility of written sources, as well as an inability to enlist the cooperation of members of the community in coming forward with their recollections and memorabilia.[9] As is the case for many Deaf communities, our knowledge of the history of the Brazilian Deaf community and of the development of LSB is incomplete.[10]

Early History[11]

Early reports to the colonial government state that there was a high incidence of deafness, although official efforts made at the time to confirm this claim were unsuccessful. Whatever the truth may be, by the mid-1800s, it came to the emperor's attention that there were substantial numbers of deaf boys in the streets of Rio de Janeiro whose disruptive behavior was drawing public notice. It was determined that a school should be established where these boys could receive instruction and their energies could be constructively channeled. The mandate of the school was to provide the boys with skills that would be of service to the emperor.

To this end, a deaf teacher from Paris, Padre Huet (some records list his given name as Eduardo, others as Ernesto) established the first government-supported school for the deaf in Brazil in 1857, originally called the Instituto Imperial de Surdo-Mudos (Imperial Institute of Deaf-Mutes) and now called the Instituto Nacional de Educação de Surdos (National Institute for the Education of the Deaf, INES).[12] The original site of the school was in the city's downtown area, but within a few years it moved to its present location in a quieter though still very urban neighborhood called Laranjeiras. A sprawling pink stucco building with flag-stone-paved courtyard and tree-shaded grounds, INES is more than just the oldest and largest deaf school in the country; it is the cultural center of the Brazilian Deaf community.

For more than a century, INES was primarily a residential school.[13] Students came from all over Brazil with a variety of idiosyncratic sign systems that they had been using among their families and friends. Once at INES, they encountered in the dorms, corridors, and grounds of the school, perhaps in the classrooms as well, the sign language that was developing out of the meeting of Huet's Old French Sign Language with whatever signs and communicative conventions already existed in the sign system(s) Brazilian deaf people were using before 1857. The students encountered this creole sign language and they likely helped to shape it.[14] Returning to their home regions, they spread the language throughout much of Brazil. INES has also long had a teacher training program, so it is possible that hearing teachers picked up the sign language and disseminated it to their schools.

Deaf Education in Brazil

In Brazil as elsewhere, the school setting is a route of access to the Deaf community. As already noted, Brazil never had an extensive network of specialized, deaf residential schools. INES was the school for deaf boys, and in 1929 an order of Catholic nuns established a school for deaf girls, Santa Terezinha, in São Paulo.[15] In recent decades, both of these schools have turned to day school programs serving both boys and girls, as provision is now more frequently made to educate deaf children closer to their homes. A third important locus of deaf education is Concórdia in Porto Alegre. Founded in the 1970s with the support of an American Lutheran philanthropic organization, Concórdia's programs are strongly influenced by American trends.[16]

Schooling for deaf children seems to be a haphazard mix of official indifference and personal interest. Deaf education is primarily a local matter. When there are deaf children in sufficient numbers, a special classroom may be set up to accommodate them in a publicly funded school. Other schools have been established by religious organizations. Alternatively, a wealthy and influential parent of a deaf child sometimes founds a school to provide an educational setting for the child, which then would serve other local deaf children as well. Not uncommonly, deaf children sit out their schooling in hearing classrooms or simply do not attend school.

Educational policy seems to have been eclectic in the early days. Whatever may have been the Portuguese emperor's reason for inviting a French educator to set up a school in Brazil, we can assume that Padre Huet introduced the French "manual" method. Following the 1880 Milan Conference, hearing Brazilian educators traveled to Europe to gather information on the new "oral" method. They returned to Brazil to argue for a pragmatic version of oralism. That is, they suggested that oralism be employed in the education of those children for whom it was deemed suitable. I did not find archival records documenting how this policy became pedagogical practice in the post-Milan era; however, in the mid-1980s and into the 1990s, when I visited a number of schools for the deaf, the classroom practice was in the main oralist, with or without recourse to electronic amplifica-

tion. The mode of instruction was not determined by the individual child's aptitude for a method but by the pedagogical philosophy and linguistic preferences
of the teacher or the school.

MODERN HISTORY OF THE DEAF COMMUNITY

Rio de Janeiro owes its status as the de facto capital of the Brazilian Deaf world
in large measure to the presence of INES. However, Rio is also home to the Universidade Federal do Rio de Janeiro (UFRJ), where in the late 1980s sign language
classes were first offered through a public university and continue to be held on
a regular basis.[17] It is in Rio where FENEIS (Federação Nacional para a Educação
e Integração dos Surdos), the national deaf advocacy organization, was founded
in 1987 and is headquartered. And it was there on the beach at Copacabana that
the vision of members of the Compania Surda de Teatro, a local deaf theater
group, having given rise to the grassroots movement *Surdos Venceremos* (We Deaf
Will Overcome), was realized as the first large-scale, public demonstration to demand language rights for deaf people.

 Brazil provides constitutional guarantees to its native peoples with respect to
language rights; *Surdos Venceremos* sought to have those guarantees extended to
the Deaf community. The major purpose of the demonstration was to win official
recognition for LSB as a medium of instruction in deaf schools and as a language
supported by the government, specifically in the provision of interpreting services. The September 1994 march drew a crowd of more than 1,000, deaf and
hearing people, including representatives of public and private schools that serve
deaf children. Groups of deaf workers marched under banners naming their employers and demanding official recognition of LSB. Representatives of various
political parties also attended and proclaimed their support. The march was
videotaped, and copies were distributed to Deaf organizations in other locales,
along with a call to action eloquently articulated by several Deaf activists (Nelson
Pimenta de Castro, Silas Queiroz, and Carlos Alberto Gómes) in which they proposed that such demonstrations be replicated throughout the country until the
policymakers in Brasilia took heed.[18]

 This march, then, marks a milestone in the emergence of the Deaf community's sense of being a minority linguistic and cultural group within the larger Brazilian society. Once previously, students at INES had held a demonstration that
sought language rights, but its potential to influence the public consciousness and
conscience was muted by the fact that the demonstration was confined to the
school grounds. The march along Copacabana was both a broader-based and a
more public statement. The Copacabana march is, however, the climax of the story
for which the "complicating action" is the gradual process through which the
Deaf community came to define itself as a linguistic and cultural minority population within the Brazilian body politic.

LANGUAGE AND THE REINVENTION OF THE DEAF COMMUNITY[19]

The first step of this definition process dates to 1987 when two visionary and able
deaf people, Ana Regina de Souza e Campelo and João Carlos Carreira Alves,
attended a national conference of the disabled held in Rio at which they were

elected to represent the Deaf community. Inspired by the conference, they determined to set up a national organization for Deaf advocacy.

Ana Regina learned that there was a moribund organization that had been founded by a hearing teacher who was formerly at INES and was now retired, from whom Ana Regina was able to obtain the documents necessary to reestablish the entity. One of the first acts of the reborn organization was a rechristening. The organization had been called the Federação Nacional para a Educação e Integração de Deficientes Auditivos (National Federation for the Education and Integration of the Hearing-Impaired), or FENEIDA. Although its mission remained focused on education and integration, the medicalized term *deficientes auditivos*, a euphemism emphasizing what the deaf lack vis-à-vis the hearing, was replaced by the word *surdos* (deaf), an ethnonym for the social group.[20] Thus, FENEIDA became FENEIS, and deaf Brazilians entered the national arena of social activism under their own banner.

THE INTRODUCTION OF A SIGN LANGUAGE COMPONENT TO FENEIS's MISSION

Deaf leaders realized that the success of their advocacy efforts depended in large measure on the quality of sign-to-Portuguese interpretation. Yet few hearing Brazilians had sufficient sign skills to bring an adequate level of competence and professionalism to the demanding task. There was no ready pool of adult children of Deaf parents waiting to assume the role of interpreter.[21] Early on, many interpreters came from the ranks of evangelists whose interest in the sign language was as a vehicle for proselytizing rather than as a means for facilitating Deaf-hearing interaction generally and Deaf empowerment ultimately. To redress the lack of qualified professional interpreters, Fernando Valverde, upon succeeding Ana Regina as president of FENEIS, organized sign language courses that were open to the public.

The teachers in those early days were Ana Regina, João Carlos, Fernando, and a few others. Demand for classes grew when not only interpreters but also other professionals who serve the Deaf community (among them, teachers, speech therapists, and counselors) sought this means to improve communication between themselves and their deaf students and clients. Increasingly as well, families with a deaf member recognized the need to take on some of the responsibility for intrafamilial communication rather than impose the burden solely on the deaf member. FENEIS then put out the call to deaf signers to become teachers.

Among the first to answer that call was a young man named Roberto Robson. He was perhaps the first FENEIS instructor to bring "deep" LSB with full sign language grammar and facial expressions into the classroom. His contribution is all the more remarkable because he had only shortly before gained an appreciation for LSB. Audiologically hard of hearing, he had in his school days become painfully aware of the contempt with which his (hearing) teachers viewed signing. Roberto, in turn, was active in encouraging other young deaf people to join the FENEIS sign language teaching staff.[22]

To prepare instructors, Fernando saw a need to establish the legitimacy of the sign language as separate from yet equal to Portuguese. To this end, he presented a comparison of lexical and grammatical conventions that set the two apart. He also urged the instructors to call their language *língua de sinais* (sign language) instead of *mímica* (mimicry), the Portuguese name in common use at the time. *Mímica* conveys the sense of an imitation or copy of some object or action, more of a theatrical performance than a linguistic one. Fernando wanted to convince LSB instructors of both the autonomy of the sign language from the spoken language and the equivalence of the two with respect to linguistic status.

WHAT'S IN A NAME?

The choice of name is itself a political act. Fernando was, in fact, making a more radical claim than the English translation of *língua* reveals. In Portuguese, there are two words, *língua* and *linguagem*, which both translate to English as "language." *Língua* is properly used only for exemplars of true languages: *língua portuguesa*, *língua inglesa*, and so on. *Linguagem* is "language" with a capital L—language in the sense of the general cognitive ability for creating, acquiring, and using linguistic systems that we credit only to our own species, the general conceptual construct that subsumes the peculiarities of particular instances of *língua*. However, *linguagem* also applies to the systems of communication used by birds, bees, computer hackers, and the like.

The Portuguese Name in the Local Context

A dictionary of Brazilian signs (Oates 1983) bears the title *Linguagem das mãos* (Language of the Hands) and refers in its preface to the *linguagem-mímica*. A second volume (Hoemann, Oates, and Hoemann [1981] 1984), an anthology of articles treating some linguistic and social aspects, is entitled *Linguagem de sinais do Brasil*. Although these early works contributed in important ways to bringing attention to the study of the language, as much within the Deaf community as without, the implication is that this sign language is not *língua*, "true language." My own experience was that nearly all hearing people I spoke with on the subject said "*linguagem de sinais*," even if I had just said "*língua de sinais*," likely attributing our different choice of terms to my ignorance of the finer points of Portuguese rather than their ignorance of the linguistic status of the sign language. Implicit in Fernando's choice of name, then, is the claim that LSB is a proper exemplar of *língua* and not simply *linguagem* in the sense of generalized communication system.

The Portuguese Name in the Wider Context

Of course, *língua de sinais* is not precise enough when the language must be identified beyond Brazil's own borders, as is increasingly the case, in the context of international meetings and academic scholarship. Although there has been some discussion of the matter, the Deaf community has not agreed on a common term. Two candidates are Língua de Sinais dos Centros Urbanos do Brasil (LSCB) and LIBRAS, a blend of the words *Língua Brasileira de Sinais*. These two labels were each offered by hearing professionals. The former was suggested by Lucinda Ferreira Brito, as the first linguist to work extensively on sign language in Brazil. Her research also brought her into contact with a second, unrelated sign language used among the Urubu-Kaapor, an indigenous group living in the Brazilian Amazon. This language she designated *Língua de Sinais do Urubu-Kaapor* (LSKB).[23] The fact that there exists in Brazil this other sign language is little known among the urban deaf and, even when known, has little direct impact on them. Primarily for this reason, the name LSCB and its English translation have never been used outside the academic context of research and writing. The second term, *LIBRAS*, was coined by Marta Ciccone, a speech therapist and educator. This name has gained wide acceptance among deaf people to the extent that its fingerspelled form shows evidence of nativization into the sign language system; that is, the forms of the individual letters are no longer clearly delineated and the transitions between them are subsumed into a characteristic movement (see Padden 1991 for a discussion of ASL fingerspelling and loan signs). [24]

Sign Name

Fernando's concern about the name of the sign language was actually with respect to how it should be rendered in Portuguese. In terms of the sign language itself, there is a sign that can be glossed SIGN-LANGUAGE:[25] two spread hands held upright, facing each other at chest height, move forward from the signer's body making alternating circles in two vertical planes several inches apart, one on either side of the midline of the body. That this sign is a noun and, therefore, a possible name is likely because it differs from another sign that could be glossed TO-USE-SIGN-LANGUAGE, which modifies the form already described by adding the internal movement of a finger wiggle. These signs differ from their ASL counterparts, and the ASL signs differ from the fingerspelling ASL-fs.[26] SIGN-LANGUAGE unmodified means the Brazilian Deaf community's sign language. This is in keeping with the practice common to populations with limited contact with other languages whose name for their own language is simply the word for "language," "talk," or "tongue" in that language.

SIGN-LANGUAGE can refer to other sign languages, in which case the compound sign PORTUGUESE + SIGN-LANGUAGE specifies Brazil's sign language (and, for example, either ENGLISH or AMERICAN specifies the sign language of the United States). It should not be deduced from the glossing convention that Brazil's sign language is related to Portugal's sign language or to that of other Portuguese-speaking locales (or that ASL is related to the sign languages of England or to other English-speaking locales). Familial relationships for sign languages are matters for empirical investigation. Moreover, given that I have observed some Brazilian deaf people who are native in the sign language using the sign PORTUGUESE with a meaning closer to "spoken language" rather than to "Portuguese," the semantics of the sign glossed this way may differ significantly from the semantics of the Portuguese word (*português*) that is the source for the gloss.

Encoding the Distinction between LSB and Portuguese

In LSB lexicon and conversational practice, LSB is distinguished from Portuguese. The LSB sign glossed NAME means "the Portuguese word for X," where X stands for a concept. The appropriate response to a query made with this sign is a fingerspelling of the relevant Portuguese word. There is another, formationally unrelated sign glossed NAMESIGN, which is used to elicit the sign for a concept. For example, the Portuguese word meaning "sad" is fingerspelled T-R-I-S-T-E; the sign for this concept is made at the signer's chin by thumbtip contact of the Y-hand, a handshape that is in no way motivated by the Portuguese word.[27]

Community Consensus Versus Practical, Political, and Scholarly Exigencies

The choice of a Portuguese name has been further complicated by efforts to gain official recognition for the sign language under the name LIBRAS. Although all support the campaign, it was undertaken before consensus on the name emerged from the Deaf community. The process has been co-opted in part by the needs of researchers to name the object of their study in funding proposals and in the dissemination of findings and analyses. Still, the fact that the Deaf community is debating the issue is strong evidence that it has recognized the linguistic status of its means of communication as being real language and has assumed the right to name it.

Although only time will tell which of the above or, perhaps, some other term becomes the name of choice of the community as a whole, the name *Língua de Sinais Brasileira* is truer to the name in the sign language itself.[28] It is perhaps in keeping with current political consciousness to render a translation of names of ethnic groups and their languages as closely as possible to the source language.

HEIGHTENED ROLE OF LANGUAGE IN DEAF SOCIAL IDENTITY

Perhaps even more than for other minority groups, language plays a defining role in the Deaf community because, for deaf people, communication is rarely a given. Rather, it must be won at considerable expenditure of focused effort. The members of the community are united neither by physical type or by region of origin of themselves or their families (loosely speaking, race or ethnicity), nor by residence within a bounded locale or social class, and often fall into low-income groups because of restrictions on employment, real or imagined, attributed to hearing loss. Rather, deaf people are united by their communicative experience in crucial areas of everyday life such as familial relations, education, and employment histories. That experience is generally marked by subtle and not-so-subtle forms of oppression imposed by the hearing majority.[29] The current interest in language issues among deaf people is evidence of an awakening consciousness within the Deaf community. The paradigmatic shift in Deaf consciousness is the move from valuing fluency in Portuguese to valuing fluency in LSB.

CONTACT SIGNING[30]

Recently, among some Deaf people, the name LIBRAS has come to identify a simplified variant of the sign language, a kind of "foreigner talk." This variant is an accommodation to Portuguese-speakers that attempts to alter the language to make it more accessible for them. In this way, it resembles American systems like SEE (Signing Exact English, Seeing Essential English).[31] While SEE is imposed on deaf students by well-meaning educators, usually hearing, LIBRAS in this narrower sense of the simplified variant is imposed on hearing students by well-meaning instructors, usually deaf. Often, the instructors are themselves late learners of the sign language. Because of an assumption that sign language instructors should know Portuguese, many of the long-time deaf instructors have had considerable exposure to Portuguese. They are, then, Portuguese-dominant bilinguals or semi-bilinguals, considering that they often have only partial, primarily lexical, knowledge of the two languages. Either consciously or unconsciously, they have incorporated neologisms and nonnative grammatical structures into the form of the sign language that they teach to hearing people. The variant shows a number of features that set it apart from the form that deaf people use among themselves.[32]

To demonstrate the difference between the two forms, I offer here a few examples of neologisms and Portuguese-influenced grammatical structures. Regarding the former, two strategies are employed to create substitutes for fingerspelled loan signs because the general assumption is that hearing people cannot fingerspell, either receptively or productively.[33] The first strategy relies on complexes of signs, for example, HISTORY + OLD + VISIT-TO-SEE + HOUSE instead of MUSEU-fs (museum), CHEESE + ROUND-FLAT-OBJECT instead of PIZZA-fs. This is not to say that LSB does not have compounds natively but, rather, that this mechanism for creating new signs is used to invent signs specifically for use in language contact situations. The second strategy substitutes initialized signs, for example, [S-hand held upright in front of the body rotates slightly twice] in place of SOGRA-fs (mother-in-law), which begins with the upright S-hand, then rotates smoothly inward as the medial letters are rapidly articulated to the final A-hand position. An example of a nonnative grammatical structure is the use of a lexical intensifier MUCH in a verb phrase rather than the modulation of the verb for intensive aspect. Another example is a simplified use of space to indicate subject-object relations, as well as a reduction in the use of classifiers.[34] Like other contact languages, the form of the neologisms and the use of nonnative grammatical structures vary across signers and even across utterances of a single signer.

Nelson Pimenta de Castro, a fluent Deaf native signer, first raised this practice of accommodation to the perceived expectations of hearing people as a pedagogical issue and continues to argue forcefully against the teaching of the "foreigner variant" of LSB. Nelson is representative of a new generation of sign language teachers who are carrying Fernando's efforts to a higher level of linguistic sophistication. As coordinator of a research group that developed the first nationally distributed teaching materials for the language (Pimenta de Castro et al. 1994b), Nelson moved teaching practice away from its dependence on Portuguese.

THE NEED FOR AN LSB-CENTERED CURRICULUM

Until the materials developed by Nelson's group became available in late 1994, most sign language instructors were teaching sign-for-word correspondences from lists of Portuguese words, usually grouped by part of speech (verb, noun, adjective, and such) or by semantic domain (family, food, animals, and such). The especially creative instructor might provide a number of example sentences containing the target item in order to familiarize students with the semantic range of the sign, which could differ significantly from the Portuguese word that provides the source of the sign gloss. Example sentences may also have provided a glimpse at the sign language's grammar, which is typologically distinct from that of Portuguese. Exemplified or not, these differences were often left unremarked, so the Portuguese-dominant learner was not sensitized to semantic and syntactic specificities of the sign language.

This Portuguese-based teaching methodology was woefully inadequate, and the students did not learn the language. Especially disappointing was student performance with respect to comprehension. In contrast to the more typical second-language learning situation, receptive skills lagged far behind productive skills. Even the better professional interpreters had great difficulty interpreting from LSB to Portuguese. The less-skilled could neither understand most deaf signers nor produce Portuguese to LSB interpretation that was readily comprehensible to deaf people.

On several occasions at which I was present, deaf people with sufficiently intelligible speech had to take over interpretation of sign to speech while people with sufficient residual hearing or superior speechreading skills had to take over interpretation from speech to sign, even in the case of regional meetings of FENEIS and national symposia on disability for which we can assume the best interpreters were provided. Recognition of the implications of this situation for the Deaf community led Nelson to offer a course targeted to interpreters (Pimenta de Castro et al. 1994a), whose number included the reader for the signed television news broadcast.

In the new, conversation-based approach, lessons were designed around typical interactional routines. When I left Brazil in 1994, it was too early to claim student outcomes to be consistently superior, but the impression I had in the classroom was that both receptive and productive skills were markedly improved. Aside from gains for students, the conversation-based approach to teaching empowers deaf teachers because it underscores the autonomy of LSB from Portuguese and, thus, gives substance to the claims Fernando set forth.[35]

THE MODEL DEAF PERSON

Until recently and in some quarters even now, fluency in Portuguese, in both its spoken and written forms, was seen as an important, perhaps the most important, measure of an intelligent and successful deaf person. This opinion was held not only by hearing Brazilians but also by members of the Deaf community. Although full fluency in Portuguese was rarely achieved, the closer a deaf person approximated that ideal, the more respected he or she was likely to be. Even deaf people whose primary means of communication was LSB and whose own Portuguese skills were minimal held this opinion.

A PORTUGUESE-CENTERED DEAF IDENTITY

Evidence that the elevation of Portuguese over LSB was quite general can be seen in the fact that the largest Deaf social club in Rio, Alvarado, was originally established as a meeting place for deaf people to practice their Portuguese skills. Other evidence comes from statements of deaf individuals. A telling incident involves an officer of a deaf organization with a national constituency, a fluent signer whom I never heard voice Portuguese and whose written Portuguese skills were only modest. His LSB was so native that the interpreters engaged for the organization's general assembly were unable to interpret it, usually an indication that the signing is not at the signed-Portuguese end of the dialect continuum. Yet, while assessing an LSB-fluent appointee to a position for which LSB-fluency should have been the primary qualification, the officer remarked derisively, "He has no brain." The person who reported this comment to me understood it to have its basis in the candidate's limited Portuguese skills.

The appointee himself complained to me many times that his efficacy in the position was hampered by the lack of respect in which he was held by some of the officers and functionaries because of his level of control of Portuguese. The situation deteriorated to the point where he tendered his resignation. With the rethinking that followed the introduction of the conversation-based LSB teaching methods, he was subsequently reinstated and, for the most part, enjoyed his colleagues' support.

Another example was reported to me by a teacher at INES. We were discussing a particularly bright deaf man, a graduate of the school, whose work was making an important contribution to the community. This man was bilingual in LSB and ASL but had low Portuguese skills. The teacher confided in me that her colleagues who had been his teachers were incredulous about his accomplishment. To my, "Why so?" she answered, "They thought him very limited." Evidently, the fact that the teachers and their student did not share a language obscured his potential for academic achievement. Presently, the deaf man is employed at the school as an LSB instructor. Among his students may be some of his former teachers, who now recognize not only the intellectual ability of this particular deaf person but also, and more importantly, the key that LSB provides to unlocking the abilities of their current students.

A third example comes from a discussion with a long-time deaf LSB teacher about requisite skills for teachers of LSB. The teacher asserted that knowledge of Portuguese was essential. My attempt to draw a parallel with the hypothetical case of me being an adequate teacher of English, despite my limited Portuguese skills, could not persuade her. Without Portuguese, she reasoned, an LSB teacher would not know the signs' names. I tried to show that an articulation of the sign was equivalent to an articulation of the word. I did this by drawing attention to my hand movements for the sign and my mouth movements for the word. Then I tried to show that an "orthographic" representation of the sign could also be equivalent to an orthographic representation of the word.[36] For this demonstration, I notated the same sign in Stokoe notation as found in *The Dictionary of American Sign Language* (Stokoe, Casterline, and Croneberg 1976) and compared that to the written Portuguese word. She was unmoved.

My interlocutor was deaf from birth, had married within the Deaf community, and had at one time been president of a Deaf club in which she continued to be active. Her social relations outside her hearing family were almost exclusively with deaf people. Such a biography might be expected to produce a Deaf-centered worldview. Yet, at least as far as language was concerned, she held a strong Portuguese-centered position.

This view was quite prevalent in the Deaf community and was reinforced by hearing professionals, providers of a variety of social services to deaf people who tended to prefer Portuguese-fluent LSB teachers over those with strong LSB skills.

The refusal of a prestigious private deaf school to hire an LSB-fluent physical education teacher because he lacked sufficient command of Portuguese is a case in point. That this teacher succeeded in finding employment in a school for hearing children only increases the irony. That his hearing students were picking up LSB increases the frustration of those who understand the loss it is for deaf children to grow up without a language model for the only kind of language they can acquire natively.

With the introduction of the conversation-based teaching methodology, much needed change may be in progress. Workshops held throughout the country are well attended. To most effectively use the new materials, the instructor needs not only native or near-native fluency in LSB but also a clear sense of the cultural values and social conventions of the Deaf community. The more forward-thinking Deaf leaders recognize the limitations of the Portuguese-based teaching methodology, and with that has come a reassessment of what it means to be deaf—not a "broken" hearing person, but a member of a linguistic group with a rich and unique cultural heritage.

AN LSB-CENTERED DEAF IDENTITY

The deaf person has been defined as "not hearing" or, sometimes, as "not hearing and not speaking."[37] Even the sign for *deaf* originates in a point to the ear and the mouth, as if these organs were the most central to Deaf identity. The LSB sign glossed SURDO has this form (as does the ASL cognate sign). It is, however, an ethnonym; it cannot be translated "deaf-mute." Evidence that it is an ethnonym comes from the comparison of SURDO with another sign [R-hand taps ear], which translates as "can't hear" or "didn't hear." Bahan (1989b) shifts the focus to the visual, where deaf people are not disabled but, often, quite remarkably abled.[38] Padden and Humphries (1988) argue persuasively that the Deaf world is a vision-centered world.

Yet the symbols traditionally associated with deaf people have often been hearing-centered. An example is the logo of the newsletter of FENEIS, an ear with a bar through it (see figure 9.1a). In contrast to this logo, the group Surdos Venceremos chose a logo showing two hands breaking a chain that binds Brazil with the name of the group written across the breadth of the country. The *S* of *Surdos* and the *V* of *Venceremos* are the handshapes of the manual alphabet (see figure 9.1b). This sequence, s-v, provided a dynamic, visual rallying "cheer" as the throngs of marchers passed along the Copacabana beach. FENEIS has a new logo that shows the sign for FENEIS (the index fingers and thumbs of the two hands linked) spanning the map of Brazil (see figure 9.1c). The logo symbolizes a Brazil where deaf people have joined together to pursue their common goals.

With this change of symbols, the Deaf community celebrates its strength. It has come to own its language in both name and substance. This has been made possible by the shift away from an identity as "broken" hearing people and an orientation toward the model deaf person as being the embodiment of Deaf language and cultural values. This shift has awakened deaf people to a new awareness of LSB. Deaf poets and storytellers are now producing original work where, previously, they shared only translations from Portuguese. The translations tended to be quite literal, so most of the Portuguese words but little of the emo-

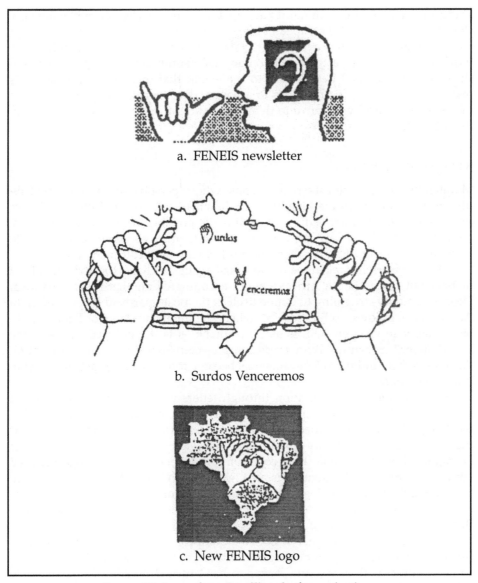

a. FENEIS newsletter

b. Surdos Venceremos

c. New FENEIS logo

FIGURE 9.1 Logos from Brazilian deaf organizations

tional essence came across. The new work brings to the audience the evocative power of literary uses of language to transcend the everyday and imagine different worlds. I am told that deaf school children at the Centro Educacional dos Surdos (the site of a good deal of my fieldwork in 1994), having been recently introduced to the American Deaf literary genre of ABC stories, now compete among themselves for the best original creation.

A BRAVE NEW WORLD

A different world worth imagining might be one in which deaf children are educated by means of a language that is readily accessible to them and in which deaf adults are included in meaningful participation in many areas of public life now closed to them for lack of competent interpreting services. Deaf people have kept their sign languages alive against the odds and in spite of the counterefforts or indifference of the majority population and its institutions. The rights of citizenship have been denied deaf people to the extent that their full participation is restricted by the failure of polities to accommodate their language needs. With the estimable worldwide move to democratization, these restrictions call for redress in Brazil and elsewhere.

KEEPING IN CONTACT

Maintaining contact with the many people whose personal stories have contributed to the moment in the history of the Brazilian Deaf community that I have described in this account is difficult, so it is not possible to confirm that the momentum of the shift to an LSB-centered social identity continues to build. I do know that the goals of Surdos Venceremos have not been fully achieved.

My own work has taken me not to Brazil again, as I had expected when I left in 1994, but first to South Africa, where I encountered another nascent national Deaf community struggling to define itself in the post-apartheid dispensation. In August 2000, I moved to Puerto Rico, where the linguistic status of Puerto Rican Sign Language vis-à-vis ASL is as problematic as is the political status of the island under U.S. control. With a research project in South Africa and opportunities for one here in Puerto Rico, time has become more of an obstacle to travel to Brazil than money.

Long-distance communication through letters is not a satisfactory solution because LSB does not have an orthography. An exchange of video-recorded "letters" helps, but access to video cameras and recorders is not always reliable. Portuguese literacy is necessary for conventional letter writing, yet a low level of Portuguese literacy is, ironically, a common consequence of a Portuguese-oriented educational practice. Portuguese is also necessary to take advantage of modern telecommunication technology. In addition, telecommunication devices for the deaf, relay services, fax machines, and e-mail are not as widely available to deaf Brazilians as they are to deaf Americans.

Until recently, Ana Regina de Souza e Campelo, one of the founders of FENEIS and still in the vanguard of her community, was one of the few deaf Brazilians I know with e-mail access, and it was to her I turned initially to update some information in this chapter. Now I can witness the advances of the community in the successes of Nelson Pimenta de Castro, whose political, artistic, and commercial activities are on his Web site (http://www.lsbvideo.co.br).

As for the shift in the notion of the model deaf person, suffice it to say that, although it has not been completed, the prospects are brighter in the new millennium than at any other time in the history of deaf people in Brazil and perhaps elsewhere.

ACKNOWLEDGMENTS

Information in this chapter draws on research supported by the Wenner-Gren Foundation for Anthropological Research (#5454), the National Science Foundation (#DBS-9214764), and Tinker Foundation travel grants. The writing of this chapter was supported by a Richard Carley Hunt Fellowship from Wenner-Gren (#6151). An earlier version of this work appeared in Douglas A. Kibbee's *Language Legislation and Linguistic Rights* (Berenz 1998).

NOTES

1. In 1992 when I visited Rio Grande do Sul, Brazil's southernmost state, newspapers were full of discussion, evidently quite serious, of secession by the three southern and richest states, the intent being to stem the flow of migrants into the region and the flow of capital (in the form of taxes to the federal government) out of the region.

2. The move inland to the newly constructed Brasilia was the realization of a plan first envisioned more than 100 years earlier by the Portuguese emperor when he sought escape from Napoleon by taking refuge in Brazil. Dom Pedro feared that Rio's geographical position on the sea made it vulnerable to attack. A second motive for the move was to strengthen Brazil's hold on its vast interior.

3. I do not mean to dismiss the many Deaf activists in these cities and regions but, rather, to say that Rio's Deaf community enjoys a larger concentration of Deaf activists than may be found elsewhere. The reasons for this will become apparent in the following sections.

4. This distinction in consciousness is captured in ASL by the pair of neologisms HEARING-IN-THE-HEAD and DEAF-IN-THE-HEAD in which the locations of the signs HEARING and DEAF are replaced by the forehead location.

5. At that time, Ferreira Brito's research included the São Paulo variety and a variety used by the Urubu-Kaapor. The latter is independent of and unrelated to the several regional varieties here subsumed under the label LSB.

6. I studied Portuguese at the University of California at Berkeley for some years but count my in-country experience as the real site of Portuguese acquisition. Exposure to ASL and to the American Deaf community during three semesters of study at Vista College in Berkeley in the early 1980s was important preparation for encountering LSB and the Brazilian Deaf community, although the languages are mutually unintelligible and the communities are, of course, different. I hope both my Portuguese and my ASL teachers will forgive me for not being a more apt student.

7. This encounter took place at the home of University of California at Berkeley psycholinguist Dan Slobin in November 1994, during a meeting of the UCB-based Sign Language Research Group.

8. I used the conversation analytic method advocated by John Gumperz, which allows for review of the analysis with participants (Gumperz and Berenz 1993). These conversations about language were also a valuable source of historical information.

9. It is common practice in Brazil to refer to individuals by personal name in subsequent mentions because there is no hard-and-fast rule with respect to which of several family names a particular individual must use. I follow that practice in this chapter. The explanation of the practice, which was striking in its divergence from my American expectations, was provided by Diane Grosklaus, an American translator who has resided in Brazil since the 1970s. Her expertise as a "culture broker" in this and other matters was invaluable.

10. In November 1998, Otaviano reported that his project was nearing completion. At last report (November 2001), it was still unavailable.

11. Historical information comes from 19th-century documents archived at the National Institute of the Deaf (INES), except as noted. I owe a debt to Emeli Marques C. Leite, a hearing teacher at INES and the mother of a deaf son, for bringing the materials to my

attention. Emeli was perhaps the first teacher in INES's modern history to use sign language in the classroom and was surely the most ardent in support of its use at the school. Her classroom practice and her political stance for Deaf empowerment were at odds with the practice and politics of most of her colleagues.

12. Smith Stark (1990) reports that this was the first school for the deaf in all of Latin America.

13. According to an excerpt from the Comissão de Levantamento Histórico do INES (1990), after Padre Huet's arrival in 1855, he began instructing two deaf pupils: a 12-year-old girl and a 10-year-old boy. However, at the founding of INES as a residential school in 1857, the student population was limited to boys. INES only began admitting girls in the latter half of the 20th century as it became a day school program.

14. Although I found no records detailing the emergence of LSB, we may suppose the process to have been similar to that of Nicaraguan Sign Language discussed in A. Senghas (1995), Kegl, Senghas, and Coppola (1999), and R. Senghas (chapter 14).

15. Santa Terezinha admitted a few boys as day students.

16. Both Santa Terezinha and Concórdia are private schools.

17. The first UFRJ instructor was José Roberto Cruz, a second-generation deaf signer who was Lucinda Ferreira Brito's tutor and informant in São Paulo and who continued in these capacities for some time after Lucinda joined the UFRJ faculty in 1987. Lucinda arranged for José Roberto to give classes at UFRJ. The lessons the two developed were passed on to José Roberto's successor, Myrna S. Monteiro, who was the instructor when I attended URFJ classes in the early 1990s.

18. This video distribution was the second effort at raising the Deaf community consciousness using video to get the message out. Earlier in 1994, Nelson and Sérgio Marmora de Andrade, who was at the time vice president of FENEIS, produced and distributed a video in which they reported their experiences in Deaf communities in the United States and Sweden respectively, where support for broad implementation of the respective sign language is strong.

19. The information on the early years of FENEIS comes from João Carlos Carreira Alves and Emeli Marques C. Leite.

20. Of course, both labels, *deficientes auditivos* and *surdos*, are Portuguese words. An explanation of the ethnonym in LSB can be found in the section titled "An LSB-Centered Deaf Identity" in this chapter, along with a brief discussion of the sign FENEIS.

21. An exception to this was Luciana Pais, whose career as an interpreter on a national television news program ended when she refused to shift from LSB to SimCom, the simultaneous production of signs and spoken words, which results in a distortion of both languages of input to the point of unintelligibility for many deaf viewers.

22. The deaths of both Roberto Robson and José Roberto Cruz in 1995 were a great loss to the LSB teaching and research mission. The occurrence of deaths such as theirs attributable, in part, to the inaccessibility of health information to deaf people is a serious failure of public health and strong evidence of the necessity of disseminating information in LSB.

23. The first linguist to describe this sign language was an American, Jim Kakumasu, who was supported by the Summer Institute of Linguistics to work on spoken Kaapor. Kakumasu published only a single piece of work on signing among the Kaapor (1968). Interestingly, his Portuguese-Kaapor dictionary (1988) includes no entry for *deaf*.

24. Fingerspelling uses the Brazilian manual alphabet, a set of handshapes each of which represents a letter of the Brazilian Portuguese alphabet.

25. Signs are represented by the closest English gloss written in small capitals. Where a multiword gloss is required to represent a single sign's meaning, the words are connected by hyphens. The "+" connects glosses for a compound sign. Fingerspelled loan

signs are glossed with the Portuguese word that is the source of the sign and the flag "-fs." Where necessary, an English translation is provided.

26. See also Padden and Humphries (1988) on the various labels for the sign language of American Deaf people. Kegl, Senghas, and Coppola (1999) discuss the process that the Nicaraguan Deaf community engaged in to determine a name for the sign language there, and Deuchar (1995) mentions the process through which British Sign Language got its name.

27. Here T-R-I-S-T-E represents a sequence of handshapes from the manual alphabet, not a fingerspelled loan sign. These two are very different. As mentioned in the section titled "The Portuguese Name in the Wider Context," in the former, each manual letter is distinctly articulated, often without any sort of movement. That is, the hand is held relatively steady, and only the fingers move. Differently from this, in a fingerspelled loan sign, the individual manual letters that would appear in a spelling of the Portuguese word are merged into a smooth flow that often entails one of three types of movement of the entire hand: flexion, rotation, or translation (linear path).

28. Note that, with respect to the issue of the autonomy of the sign language from the spoken language, word order within the phrase differs, with the general term initial in Portuguese but final in LSB.

29. The rental application of a deaf woman who had asked me to assist her with an apartment search was refused by a real estate agent who insisted that deafness made her incompetent under the law to enter into a legal contract. Misinformation and prejudice of this sort may contribute to the clustering of deaf people around deaf schools, where the neighbors may be better informed about deaf people's ability and reliability.

30. I take this term from Lucas and Valli (1992) who conducted an in-depth analysis of the language contact situation between ASL and English in the United States.

31. These systems combine ASL signs and English grammar. The expectation was that the combination would facilitate the learning of English by deaf children and simplify the learning of a visual mode of communication for their hearing families and teachers. The results, so far, have been disappointing.

32. A few forms with origins in this language contact situation are gaining currency among some deaf people, particularly those who are younger. These forms are introduced to them by hearing adults (parents, teachers, speech therapists, and the like) who have learned them from deaf people using the "foreigner talk variant." For a humorous and thought-provoking view of a similar situation in the United States, see Ben Bahan's story *A Night of Living Terror* (1989a), a satirical prediction of the impact of English calques on communication within the American Deaf community.

33. Although fingerspelling is sometimes used between deaf and hearing people to render the words of a spoken language, a loan sign has undergone phonological changes that make it quite different from the transliteration that provided its source. As mentioned in the section titled "The Portuguese Name in the Wider Context" and endnote 27, production and interpretation depend much more heavily on the movement of the sign than on the sequence of handshapes that transliterates the spoken word.

34. See Klima and Bellugi (1979) for an analysis of ASL verb modulation, Padden (1990) for an analysis of ASL spatial grammar, and Supalla (1982) for an analysis of ASL classifiers. The general processes reported in these studies are also found in LSB, although particulars will differ between the two languages.

35. This project owes a debt to Tanya A. Felipe, Brazilian linguist, LSB researcher, and advocate for the deaf, who worked with Nelson and Myrna S. Monteiro to produce a set of LSB lessons organized around the presentation of LSB grammar (Felipe et al. 1994). Tanya has continued to develop a grammar-based curriculum, in part, to meet the demands of deaf people who see the formal explication of sign language grammar as impor-

tant to reversing negative judgments of the uninformed as to LSB's linguistic status; see this chapter's section titled "A Brief History of the Brazilian Deaf Community."

36.   There is no orthography in widespread use for any sign language, with the possible exception of SignWriting, developed by the Deaf Action Committee, which is used to write several sign languages, most notably Nicaraguan Sign Language.

37.   Some societies differentiated between deaf people who could speak and those who could not. The former were accepted as co-equals but the latter were denied civil rights such as inheritance and the holding of public office.

38.   The work of Helen Neville, formerly of University of California at San Diego and presently at the University of Oregon, on evoked potentials shows that areas of the brain normally allocated to audition are reallocated to vision in the brains of deaf people who are native signers.

References

Bahan, Ben. 1989a. A night of living terror. In *American deaf culture*, ed. Sherman Wilcox, 17–20. Burtonsville, Md.: Linstok Press.

———. 1989b. Notes from a "seeing" person. In *American deaf culture*, ed. Sherman Wilcox, 29–32. Burtonsville, Md.: Linstok Press.

Berenz, Norine. 1996. Person deixis in Brazilian Sign Language. Ph.D. diss., University of California, Berkeley.

———. 1998. The case for Brazilian Sign Language: A deaf community finds its voice. In *Language legislation and linguistic rights*, ed. Douglas A. Kibbee, 269–87. Amsterdam and Philadelphia: Benjamins.

Blom, Jan-Petter, and John J. Gumperz. 1972. Social meaning in linguistic structures: Code-switching in Norway. In *Directions in sociolinguistics*, ed. John J. Gumperz and Dell H. Hymes, 407–34. New York: Basil Blackwell.

Commissão de Levantamento Histórico de INES. 1990.

Deuchar, Margaret. 1995. Where are they now? *Signpost* 8 (2):61.

Felipe, Tanya A., Nelson Pimenta de Castro, Myrna S. Monteiro, Emeli Marques C. Leite, and Norine Berenz. 1994. *Curso de LIBRAS, Nível 1* (LIBRAS Course, Level 1). Rio de Janeiro: FENEIS.

Gannon, Jack R. 1981. *Deaf heritage: A narrative history of deaf America*. Silver Spring, Md.: National Association of the Deaf.

Gumperz, John J., ed. 1982. *Language and social identity*. New York: Cambridge University Press.

Gumperz, John J., and Norine Berenz. 1993. Transcribing conversational exchanges. In *Talking data: Transcription and coding in discourse research*, ed. Jane A. Edwards and Martin D. Lampert, 91–121. Hillsdale, N.J.: Erlbaum.

Hoemann, Harry, Eugênio Oates, and Shirley Hoemann. [1981] 1984. *The Sign Language of Brazil*. Reprint, New York: Mill Neck Foundation. Originally published as *Linguagem de Sinais do Brasil* (Porto Alegre, RS, Brazil: n.p.).

Kakumasu, James. 1968. Urubú Sign Language. *International Journal of American Linguistics* 34(4): 275–81.

Kakumasu, James Y., and Kiyoko Kakumasu. 1988. *Dicionário por tópicos urubu-kaapor—português*. Brasília: Fundação Nacional do Indio and Summer Institute of Linguistics.

Kegl, Judy, Ann Senghas, and Maria Coppola. 1999. Creation through contact: Sign language emergence and sign language change in Nicaragua. In *Language creation and language change*, ed. Michel DeGraff, 179–238. Cambridge, Mass.: MIT Press.

Klima, Edward S., and Ursula Bellugi. 1979. *The signs of language*. Cambridge, Mass.: Harvard University Press.

Lucas, Ceil, and Clayton Valli. 1992. *Language contact in the American deaf community*. San Diego, Calif.: Academic Press.

Oates, Eugênio. 1983. *Linguagem das mãos*. Aparecida, SP, Brazil: Editora Santuário.

Padden, Carol A. 1990. The relation between space and grammar: ASL verb morphology. In *Sign language research: Theoretical issues*, ed. Ceil Lucas, 118–32. Washington, D.C.: Gallaudet University Press.

———. 1991. The acquisition of fingerspelling by deaf children. In *Theoretical issues in sign language research*, Vol. 2, ed. Patricia Siple and Susan Fischer, 191–210. Chicago: University of Chicago Press.

Padden, Carol, and Tom Humphries. 1988. *Deaf in America: Voices from a culture*. Cambridge, Mass.: Harvard University Press.

Pimenta de Castro, Nelson, Emeli Marques C. Leite, João Carlos Alves Carreira, and Norine Berenz. 1994a. *Curso de língua de sinais: Classficadores e alfabeto manual*. Rio de Janeiro: FENEIS.

———. 1994b. *Curso de língua de sinais para ouvintes*. Rio de Janeiro: FENEIS.

Senghas, Ann. 1995. Children's contribution to the birth of Nicaraguan Sign Language. Cambridge, Mass.: Ph.D. diss., Massachusetts Institute of Technology.

Smith, Cheri, Ella Mae Lentz, and Ken Mikos. 1988. *Signing naturally: Level 1*. San Diego, Calif.: DawnSign Press.

Smith Stark, Thomas C. 1990. Una comparaición de las lenguas manuales de México y de Brasil. Paper presented at the IX Congreso Internacional de la Asociación de Lingüística y Filología de América Latina, Campinas, Brasil.

Stokoe, William C., Dorothy C. Casterline, and Carl G. Croneberg. 1976. *A dictionary of American Sign Language on linguistic principles*. Silver Spring, Md.: Linstok Press.

Supalla, Ted. 1982. Structure and acquisition of verbs of motion and location in American Sign Language. Ph.D. diss., University of California, San Diego.

Thiong'o, Ngugi wa. 1986. *Decolonising the mind: The politics of language in African literature*. Harare, Zimbabwe: Zimbabwe Publishing House.

10 | ## South African Sign Language: Changing Policies and Practice

Debra Aarons and Louise Reynolds

In April 1994, South Africa held its first democratic elections, and as a result of the election of the new government, the policy of apartheid that had governed every aspect of the lives of all South Africans was officially abolished. Needless to say, the simple abolition of apartheid did little to affect the many years of profound damage; the heritage of apartheid will be with us for many years to come. The consequences of the policy of apartheid can clearly be seen in the way that education is carried out in South Africa. Deaf people in South Africa have been affected by the policies of apartheid and by its educational and linguistic consequences in a profound and comprehensive way.

We focus on the Western Cape Province where we both live and work. Both authors are hearing and have been involved in Deaf community affairs for about ten years. The first author is a sign language linguist, and the second author is a language therapist. This chapter was written as an initial step to investigate the issue of variation in the signed language that is used in South Africa.[1]

The Historical Context

Background of the Education System

Under the apartheid regime in South Africa, separate departments of education were set up for each racial group, each with its own directorate, staff, budget, syllabi, curriculum, and standards. From 1910 to 1994, there were four provinces in South Africa.[2] Each of the four provinces had a separate department of education for white scholars. Further, the country had one national department of education for black scholars, another national department of education for so-called colored (or mixed race) scholars, and yet another for scholars of Indian origin.[3] Additionally, the country established a national department of special education for whites and a separate department of special education for each of the other three "race" groups. These departments were by no means equally funded or supported; the funding was based entirely on the relative color ranking in the country. Further, national policy determined what education and training were necessary for each of the population groups, thereby ensuring disparate knowledge and skills bases. The national government also made decisions relating to language policy for each of the communities in question. The education services that were provided were directly related to the pigmentation of the various groups.

Since 1994, South Africa has radically reenvisioned its education structures. Now, the country has one national ministry of education and, in principle, equality of educational opportunity for all. The practice still lags behind the principle; other than some desegregation of white schools in mostly urban areas, schools remain very much the same for the majority of the population because most teachers are undertrained and the distribution of resources is unequal. Thus, although the law has now changed, the reality of the situation remains largely untouched.

A new Constitution of the Republic of South Africa, arguably one of the most democratic and fair in the world today, was drawn up and accepted in 1996. Current educational practices that relate to Deaf people are undoubtedly unconstitutional. However, they will have to be challenged in the Constitutional Court to be changed. This will be lengthy and costly, and will involve major commitment and involvement by the parties most oppressed by this system. Because South Africa is a country in which much must still be challenged and many new institutions are yet to be developed, the lot of Deaf people is not currently perceived as a high national priority. Many of the issues and conflicts surrounding language and education in South Africa can be seen clearly at their extremes by examining the situation of Deaf people in South Africa today, as has been suggested previously by Ogilvy-Foreman, Penn, and Reagan (1994).

Divisions within the Deaf community accurately reflect the divisions in the wider society (Ogilvy-Foreman, Penn, and Reagan 1994). As a consequence of apartheid, there are social strata based on color and racial privilege within the Deaf community. Deaf schools have always been segregated, first, on the basis of color. In apartheid South Africa, and to a large measure, still today, white Deaf students, colored (mixed race) Deaf students, Indian Deaf students, and black Deaf students each attended separate schools. Additionally, the schools for white and colored Deaf children always have been further divided into schools for the Afrikaans-"speaking" Deaf and schools for the English-"speaking" Deaf. The rationale for this division is that the pupils are considered to be either English or Afrikaans "speaking." This is a consequence of oralist teaching strategies and, more recently, of the perception that a signed language is a manual form of a particular spoken language. Furthermore, apartheid education legislation also stipulated that the medium of instruction in the colored schools would be either English or Afrikaans; in the Indian schools, English; and in the black schools, where pupils came from approximately nine different spoken-language backgrounds, (officially) English.

The post-apartheid South African Schools Act of 1996 stipulates that, in schools for the Deaf in South Africa, South African Sign Language should be the medium of instruction. However, as of 1999, not a single school for the Deaf in South Africa had put this provision into practice. The reasons for this are manifold, but crucially, there are at most, only four teachers of the Deaf throughout South Africa who could even conform to the stipulations of this act.

Since the policy of apartheid has officially been abolished, it is interesting to note that—apart from a small number of black and colored pupils who now attend formerly white schools for the Deaf—almost no change has come about in the demographics of schools for the Deaf. Astonishingly, despite the fact that, officially, segregation on the basis of color is no longer practiced and despite the well-established fact that the signed language of a community is not related to the spoken language of the wider community, Deaf schools in South Africa are still segregated on the basis of color and on the basis of the (former) official spoken languages (English and Afrikaans) that were designated by the apartheid education policy.

The previously white schools have good resources, a small pupil-teacher ratio, and some specialized facilities. The schools previously set aside for colored pupils are less well-equipped, with a much larger pupil-teacher ratio and fewer facilities. The schools previously intended for black Deaf pupils have very few resources, a high pupil-teacher ratio, and almost no specialized facilities. In addition, because education for Deaf children was not compulsory under the previous regime, many Deaf children never attended school at all, which is particularly true for black children from poor and uneducated families. Needless to say, then, Deaf people in South Africa are just as oppressed as Deaf people anywhere else in the world, but for some Deaf people, the oppression is multiple, perhaps even exponential.

A Brief History of South Africa

Dutch settlers arrived in 1652; the British, in 1795. Up until 1910, what is now South Africa was under the rule of the British or the Dutch, depending on the various European wars that were being fought and the treaties that were being made. The second Anglo-Boer War ended in 1901 after which the British ruled until 1910. At that point, the Union of South Africa was declared to be a self-governing member of the British Commonwealth. In 1948, the Nationalist government came to power, formally entrenching the policy of apartheid, or separate development. Essentially, this policy meant that services provided by the government were separate and unequal and were determined on the basis of color.

By 1955, only white people in South Africa could vote, and although white people made up less than 20% of the population, they owned 87% of the land. The country had two official languages, English and Afrikaans (the language based on primarily Dutch and some indigenous and slave languages that had developed in South Africa). White South Africans spoke either English or Afrikaans as their first language, and black (African) South Africans spoke one or several Bantu languages, among them, isiZulu, seSotho, seTswana, isiNdebele, sePedi, siSwati, isiXhosa, Xitsonga, and TshiVenda. Additionally, some black South Africans spoke Khoi-San languages. Colored (mixed race) South Africans used English or Afrikaans, or a mixture of both. A significant sector of the community spoke Indian languages such as Hindu, Gujirati, Tamil, and Telugu.

In 1961, South Africa became a republic, and the policies of apartheid became even more deeply entrenched. A student uprising occurred in 1976, starting in

Soweto, one of the black townships, against gutter education for black people. This protest started a new wave of political resistance and consequent repression. From the beginning of Nationalist Party rule until the early 1990s, most of the opposing voices were silenced through torture, banning, and imprisonment. In 1994, after hundreds of years of oppression and minority rule, South Africa had its first democratic election.

DEAF EDUCATION

Little is known about the history of Deaf people in South Africa before colonization (Heap 2001). After colonization and the beginning of publicly provided education, the state authorities took little or no responsibility for establishing schools for the Deaf, leaving that responsibility almost entirely to the different churches. During the course of the 20th century, once schools had been established and were functioning, they were eligible for some state aid. But not until the new constitution was accepted in 1996 did the government declare that education was compulsory for Deaf children. It should be noted that, before 1994, the majority of Deaf children in South Africa had never been to school, so, by 1994, Deaf people who had never been to school outnumbered Deaf people who had attended a school.

The history of sign language in South Africa is, of course, deeply intertwined with the history of apartheid schooling and its complicated language policies. For this reason, we present some of the details of the history of schools for the Deaf in South Africa with particular reference to the role of different churches as well as to apartheid racial and ethnic classifications. Additionally, we highlight the different communication practices that were prescribed or that emerged in the different schools for the Deaf.

To help the reader through a mass of details, we provide a guiding generalization. In general, speaking was perceived by the authorities as the prestigious form of language. Hence, schools for white Deaf students insisted on oralism whereas schools for the other races allowed some measure of manualism (in most cases, not a natural signed language but a mixture of speech and some signs).

In 1863, Irish sisters from the Dominican Order established a school for the Deaf, St. Mary's, in Cape Town, in the Western Cape Province. From the early 20th century, St. Mary's catered to all race groups, using signed language as a medium of instruction. The written language that was taught was English.

By 1904, two other schools for the Deaf had been established in South Africa. These schools served only white Deaf children. Approximately 80 kilometers from Cape Town, the Worcester School for the Deaf and Blind was established in 1881 by the Dutch Reformed Church for the children of the Dutch settlers. Only "European" children were permitted to attend this school.[4] The 1904 census report states that combined oral and manual methods were used in the school. The folklore is that Jan de la Bat, a Dutch Reformed Church missionary, taught his Deaf brother by means of signs and that his use of signs heralded the beginning of the signed language that is used in Worcester, which is claimed by this community to be indigenous.

In 1884, German Dominican nuns established a school at Kingwilliamstown in the Eastern Cape. This, too, was a school for the "European" Deaf and followed a policy of strict oralism, presumably because of the overwhelming influence of oralism in Germany. The German Dominican School later moved to Johannesburg where it became St. Vincent's School for the Deaf, admitting only white Deaf children. In 1933, the Dutch Reformed Church set up another school for the "colored" Deaf known as Nuwe Hoop. The language policy was the same as that at the Worcester school for the white Deaf: spoken Afrikaans and some manualism.

The Grimley Institute for the Deaf in Cape Town remained racially integrated and, in the 1920s, segregated the children on the basis of whether they were to use manualism or oralism. This grouping occurred after one of the sisters visited the German Dominican School in Kingwilliamstown and instituted a policy that all but the most "backward" children would be taught using the oral method. In 1937, the Irish Dominicans opened a separate school for the "non-European" Deaf in Cape Town at Wittebome. Both "colored" and African Deaf children were admitted to the school. However, by 1953, once the Nationalist government refined the policy of apartheid even further, the Dominican Grimley School at Wittebome was declared a school for colored Deaf only.

In the 1960s, the white Dominican Grimley School for the Deaf moved to Hout Bay and adopted a policy of strict oralism that it has continued to this day. Pupils are expected to maintain strict separation from any signers, and absolutely no signing is permitted on school premises.

In 1962, apparently because African pupils were still trying to attend the Wittebome school for the colored Deaf, the Irish Dominican nuns from the Wittebome School set up a separate school for African Deaf children in Hammanskraal (then in the Transvaal Province, about 1,600 kilometers away from Wittebome). Note that no school for African Deaf children existed in the Western Cape, and no attempt was made to set one up until 1986, which was in accord with the Nationalist government's policy of influx control (in terms of which no African children actually officially belonged in the Western Cape). Only after influx control had been officially scrapped in 1986 did the Dutch Reformed Church set up a school for African Deaf children, Noluthando School, in Khayelitsha (an area set aside for black people) on the outskirts of Cape Town.

The first school for black Deaf children, Khutlwanong, was opened in 1941, near Roodepoort in the Transvaal province. Started originally by the Johannesburg Deaf and Dumb Society, it was taken over by Dutch Reformed Church trustees in 1954. At this school, a British system of signs, known as the Paget-Gorman system, was introduced. Teachers and pupils were to speak and simultaneously use the Paget-Gorman signs. This system would eventually spread to other schools for black Deaf pupils. The Paget-Gorman system, however, is not a language but a set of invented signs based on unnatural handshape permutations and lacks a grammar at any level.

As a result of the homelands policy,[5] several additional schools for African Deaf students were established in the rest of the country, divided according to the spoken language of each ethnic group and in line with the Bantustan separate development policy.[6] Students in the schools for African Deaf children had little access to hearing aids and speech therapists. Although the official policy emphasized oralism, sign language thrived among the pupils in these schools. Most of the schools for the African Deaf were vastly under-resourced, underfunded, and understaffed (Penn, Reagan, and Ogilvy 1991). In these schools, children were not forbidden to sign, and a very small number of the teachers picked up some sign language from the children. Less school time was wasted teaching children to speak, and although these Deaf children received an atrocious general education, an unexpected benefit of the neglect was the development of strong centers of natural signed language use.

Educational levels and opportunities varied markedly in the different Deaf schools, depending on the color of the students and the attitudes of the churches involved (Reynolds 1995). The government never took a strong position on Deaf issues and essentially allowed religious and educational groups to make policy decisions of their own accord—as long as these did not conflict with the overarching apartheid legislation. The majority of the funding for the schools for the Deaf came from church groups, and these schools were partly subsidized by the government. It is probably worth noting that Deaf people could not have been regarded as even potentially threatening to any aspect of the apartheid state because most institutions in South African life were entirely controlled and monitored by the government to ensure that they could never pose a challenge. As we have already mentioned, schooling for Deaf children (of any race classification) was not made compulsory until after the 1994 elections.

DEAF COMMUNITIES

Deaf communities evolved largely out of school contacts, and because the schools were racially divided, as were all communities in South Africa, the adult Deaf communities tended to be almost exclusively racially divided, too. As a result of sharing the same school for the first half of the century, there is still some colored-white interaction among the older Dominican-educated Deaf people in the Western Cape.

In 1929, a national council was set up to address the needs of the "poor white" Deaf community. This council was called The South African National Council *for* the Deaf (SANCD).[7] Until very recently, this organization was staffed entirely by hearing social and welfare workers. Apart from its obviously paternalistic and noninclusive nature, it also did not cater to the needs of all population groups, focusing largely on the white Deaf community. The SANCD took no stand as far as language policy was concerned. Few, if any, of the workers on the SANCD could sign. The SANCD did not, as a matter of course, consult the Deaf community on any policy issues.

At about the same time that changes in government were beginning in South Africa (the early 1990s), changes were also being forced to take place in Deaf organizations, largely through external pressure. The SANCD approached the World Federation for the Deaf and was advised that it would not be considered for membership because the organization was dominated by hearing people and its constitution was not acceptable. As a result, the SANCD made changes. Now, the professionals in the organization consist of both Deaf and hearing people, and various changes have been made to the constitution. The name of the organization was changed to DEAFSA, the Deaf Federation of South Africa.

By 1994, it had been clear for some time that the many different Deaf communities in South Africa, particularly those who were not white, were not served by the national organization. Various grassroots organizations of Deaf people surfaced that, previously, had been entirely unfunded or supported minimally as nongovernmental organizations, and these groups affiliated themselves with DEAFSA. These organizations are localized racially as well as geographically. However, DEAFSA's national office is still essentially white, and DEAFSA is still perceived by many black and colored Deaf people as a primarily white organization.

Communication among the different Deaf communities had been very poor over the apartheid years. Only since 1994 have television programs (*Sign Hear*, and then later, *Signature*) been produced for Deaf people, programs that use sign language as well as captioning and voice. Very few Deaf people have access to TTYs or to the use of fax machines and e-mail. In fact, it is probably true to say that the majority of South Africa's Deaf does not have access to electricity and that literacy among Deaf people is inordinately low. DEAFSA statistics from 1994 show that 70% of Deaf South Africans are functionally illiterate and 65% are unemployed. We can reasonably assume that most of the illiterate and unemployed Deaf are black or colored.

As we have said, Deaf communities have tended to form from relationships made in school. Even those Deaf people who did not attend school tend to cluster where there are organizations of other Deaf people. South Africa is a large country and travel is expensive. As a result, the majority of people in poor Deaf communities have had little opportunity to make contact with other Deaf communities. Few Deaf people have had the advantage of secondary education, and a handful of these individuals have gone abroad to study further, where they have remained, enjoying the obvious benefits to educated Deaf people that are provided in the United States and Europe rather than enduring the difficulties of life as a Deaf person in South Africa.

ATTITUDES TOWARD DEAF PEOPLE

The prevailing attitude of the general hearing community in South Africa toward Deafness is one of ignorance. Some awareness of minority rights is taking place in South Africa in the current climate of democracy. Essentially, however, Deaf people are seen neither as a minority group nor as members of another cultural or linguistic community. This lack of identity occurs because, to a large extent, their language is neither recognized nor acknowledged.

Deaf people, however, are recognized by medical practitioners and educators as having specialized needs. The reasons for this recognition are obvious, as are the consequences. Hearing people make decisions for Deaf people: Deafness is regarded as a medical problem. The people considered to be most qualified to make decisions about the lives of Deaf people are medical practitioners and special educators, all of whom make their livelihoods through the medicalization of Deafness. Even the bulk of the research that has been done on communication and Deaf people focuses on Deaf-hearing interchange rather than on the language of Deaf people themselves (see Penn, Reagan, and Ogilvy 1991). The medical profession in South Africa (including Ear, Nose, and Throat medical specialists, audiologists, speech and language therapists) favor oralism and take a purely medical view of Deafness. A language therapy model (remediating impaired spoken language) is typically adopted in the language planning that is done for Deaf children, and even though sign language is sometimes considered, the acquisition of a sign language is not considered to be normal language acquisition.

Because the general public has had little exposure to the issues of Deafness and the use of signed language, the media tends to focus on miracle cures such as cochlear implants and on the best ways in which Deaf children can be taught to speak. Lobbying by Deaf people has not made much difference in changing the general public's perception of Deafness as a medical problem that is properly to be dealt with by experts in audiological and acoustic matters.

THE CURRENT SITUATION IN EDUCATION AND LANGUAGE USE

The South African Schools Act of 1996, the law concerning the medium of instruction in schools for Deaf students, is clear. The act stipulates that South African Sign Language (SASL) is to be the medium of instruction in schools for the Deaf.[8] Regrettably, this legislation has not changed the practice in the majority of schools for the Deaf. There are only three qualified Deaf teachers in the entire country. Most of the teachers in schools for the Deaf do not sign at all nor do they believe that they should have to do so. The majority of parents would like to see their children learning to speak.

The adult Deaf community has, in the main, not spoken out in a unified way in favor of SASL as the primary medium of instruction. DEAFSA has overseen the development of curricula for SASL as a subject, in line with the new requirements for outcomes-based education. However, no official way exists either to get these curricula into the schools or to persuade the teachers to use them. Local Deaf organizations have exerted a certain amount of pressure on the schools to appoint Deaf adults as assistants to the hearing teachers so pupils will have access to the content of classes and so the teachers can begin to learn how to sign. In addition, proposals have been made to start sign language classes for all teachers in schools for the Deaf. However, these proposals are finding no backing from school authorities, education departments, or teachers themselves. Thus, the act notwithstanding, very little is changing in schools for the Deaf.

In several parts of the country, a very small number of teachers in schools for the Deaf have tried to adopt a language policy that is in line with the wishes of the adult Deaf community, that is, to use signed language as a medium of instruction. In the Western Cape, there is still enormous confusion among educators of the Deaf. Some still maintain a rigidly oralist policy. Others confuse signed language with sign-supported speech, simultaneous communication, and manually coded spoken language. Very rarely, if ever, are Deaf people consulted.

Language policy is determined entirely by hearing people who consider themselves in the best position to do so. As a matter of fact, hardly any educators of the Deaf in South Africa are in any position to determine whether or not the signed language used by the community is a natural language nor are any decisions about medium of instruction based on established research about access to language in education. The decisions are made by hearing educators purely on the basis of belief about the superiority of spoken over signed languages. These decisions also display ignorance of research showing that the acquisition of literacy in a second language (for example, English) is possible once the first language (a signed language) is in place (Strong 1988; Johnson, Liddell, and Erting 1989).

Language Used in the Adult Deaf Community

Apartheid and Variation

Deaf South African adults who consider themselves to be members of a Deaf community sign among themselves and consider the fact that they sign to be the distinctive feature of their Deafness and membership in a Deaf community. As has been discussed earlier, a number of historically distinct Deaf communities have developed in South Africa. Their distinctness is, in general, school related. The separation of the schools is due to apartheid policies and spoken language apartheid as well as geographical distance.

One could logically and reasonably hypothesize that, as a result of apartheid and the historical distinctness of the communities, the language used by each of the communities would be different, as suggested by Penn and Reagan (1990); Penn, Reagan, and Ogilvy (1991); and Penn (1992a, 1992b, 1993–1994). Despite the historical differences among Deaf communities, however, Deaf people from different communities in South Africa seem to understand one another reasonably well, much more than Zulu- and English-speaking South Africans do.

Currently, local and national Deaf events of a sporting, cultural, and educational nature are frequent. Initiatives have been launched for the Deaf people within provinces to hold regular forums; in the last few years, national Deaf *indaba* (a Zulu term meaning a "big meeting of great importance") have been held. At these meetings, Deaf South Africans seem perfectly able to communicate easily with one another, although it is revealing that many Deaf people believe different sign language varieties exist in South Africa.

For the past few years, the Deaf Forum has held regular meetings in the Western Cape. This practice is a huge departure from the past. The Deaf Forum is a gathering of Deaf people from white (English and Afrikaans), colored, and black Deaf communities that is held on a rotating basis in different localities in the Western Cape and hosted by different communities. In the past, it was most unusual for these communities to meet. Now, they meet and discuss matters of mutual interest to Deaf people.

The proceedings are run entirely by Deaf people and are open to everyone. Often, participants express dissension, and occasionally, they make accusations of racism, but essentially, the forum meetings are a major development in the forging of a united Deaf community. Different grassroots communities are represented at the forum, and the group makes policy decisions that affect, among other things, the public profile of the Deaf community. This effort has been a remarkable exercise in communication among the different Deaf communities and has certainly shown Deaf people that they can communicate more easily with Deaf people of other colors and cultures than with hearing people of their own original cultures. The language itself is not a barrier to communication, and people are learning, through exposure, to accommodate other people's varieties.

A fascinating feature of these meetings is that the Deaf people from the different communities all manage to communicate with one another quite effectively but that interpreting is required by the hearing people present. In addition, when interpreters sign, Deaf people do not experience the same common understanding that they do when they sign to one another. For example, if an Afrikaans Deaf person signs, then the hearing people demand that he or she must be voiced by an Afrikaans interpreter. However, when the interpreter signs for an Afrikaans-speaking hearing person, the other (non-Afrikaans) Deaf people cannot understand the interpreter and, consequently, the interpreters who serve each community need to interpret the spoken Afrikaans into signed language for their community. This phenomenon seems to be the case in these settings for any interpretation that is made from spoken language into signed language.

Obviously, the problem does not lie with Deaf-Deaf communication, but with the hearing-Deaf communication. We must assume that the interpreters are sticking very closely to signed Afrikaans or signed English or signed Xhosa, which is indeed the case. This practice explains why Deaf people who do not know the structure of Afrikaans will not understand the interpreter who is interpreting from spoken Afrikaans into signed Afrikaans. The interpreter is not interpreting into signed language but is putting Afrikaans on his or her hands and mouth. The problem created by this form of signing is not a sign language variation problem. It is, instead, a fine example of how hearing people who are involved with Deaf people often believe that signed language is merely spoken language on the hands.

Finally, Deaf people have very recently started training other Deaf people to teach signed language. As a result of this training, Deaf people are exposed to other varieties without being required to change their own. Since the elections in 1994, signed language programs have been regularly broadcast on television. These kinds of contacts are also beginning to harmonize the different varieties.

Variation and the SASL Dictionary

Clearly, signed language has not been nurtured or encouraged in schools for the Deaf in South Africa. Needless to say, however, many Deaf people use signed language among themselves. As we have shown above, the various Deaf communities have not mixed much over the years, and as a result, the signed languages used show some lexical variation, a variation perpetuated by apartheid divisions (Penn and Reagan 1990; Penn 1992a, 1992b, 1993–1994; Ogilvy-Foreman, Penn, and Reagan 1994; Penn and Reagan 1994). This effect of apartheid is one of the reasons why many people, both Deaf and hearing, refer to an Afrikaans sign language or an English sign language or a Xhosa sign language; past practices have kept the communities separate for so long. The other reason, of course, is that many people still believe there is a direct relationship between the spoken and signed languages of a particular ethnic community.

In the mid-1980s, the Human Sciences Research Council advertised for a researcher to work on the standardization of South African Sign Language. The *Dictionary of Southern African Signs* (Penn 1992b, 1993–1994) was the final outcome of the work commissioned by that research council. It was developed at much cost over seven years and focused on lexical differences, attempting to correlate different lexical items with the spoken language communities from which the Deaf users came (see Penn 1992a; Penn and Reagan 1994). To this end, the project team documented signs from 11 different racial and geographical communities in South Africa. Researchers used English words and phrases to elicit the signs from representatives of each community. These signs were videorecorded and presented in the dictionary as the signs for the particular English word or phrase used by the different communities. Thus, each page of the dictionary listed an English item and then showed 11 or so different signs that informants claimed were the ways in which this English word was used in their language.

This process is quite analogous to what happened to the indigenous spoken languages under apartheid. State language boards were set up, usually comprising nonnative speakers of a language, for example, Xhosa. Then, the standard Xhosa to be taught in schools was decided on. Native speakers of Xhosa found that the language they actually used was often deemed to be faulty as a consequence of the decrees of the language board (see Nyamende 1994).

It should be also noted that the dictionary had a stated pedagogical purpose (Penn 1992a; Penn and Reagan 1994). Thus, its purpose was not only to describe the different varieties used by the different communities but also to use them for teaching one or another signed language. The question of signed language syntax is not addressed in the dictionary itself, and the pedagogical purpose seems to be to teach some vocabulary in the context of an English sentence. We believe that the pedaogogical approach set forward in the dictionary is fraught with many dangers.

A close examination of some of the signs that are listed in the dictionary as translations into different varieties for the same English word reveals that some of these signs differ only in one or another inflectional aspect or perhaps a handshape alternation and should not be considered as different signs but as different inflections of the same sign. Thus, we use as an example the entry for the English word *look* (see figure 10.1). The dictionary entry is accompanied by photographs, but their quality is not adequate for reproduction here.

The dictionary presents only one possible sign for a given lexical item in a variety. We believe the way that the dictionary is presented leads to the false impression that only one sign per variety is suitable, even given a restricted context of use, and ignores how SASL, just like other languages, has different registers for formal and less formal occasions with polite and less-polite signs, slang, fast signing, in-group signing, and all the other variations that other languages boast, depending on the context of their use. The elicitation and presentation of items for the dictionary does not take these factors into account.

It seems clear that Deaf people in South Africa understand one another but that the problem arises when hearing people declare that they understand only Afrikaans or English sign language (meaning signed English or signed Afrikaans). The standardization issue is one that seems geared to accommodating hearing people who cannot really claim knowledge of signed language (so-called interpreters, many of whom have had no training whatsoever, and others, including teachers of the Deaf and speech pathologists) at the expense of unity among the Deaf of South Africa. Our observation and that of other researchers such as Penn and Reagan (1994) is that, when Deaf people gather from different communities, they all seem to communicate rather well with one another. We have seen that, as soon as hearing people are involved, a tower of Babel is erected, involving up to six interpreters, all of whom use different spoken languages and different sign systems.

In fact, not enough research has actually been conducted on the sign language (or perhaps signed languages) used in South Africa to make the claim one way or another that there is one sign language. Our intuition tells us that some lexical

LOOK

Grammatical category: verb.

Level: preschool.

Theme: Sight-act.

Translations: *Kyk* (Afrikaans), *Buka* (Zulu), *Sheba, tadima* (Sotho).

Synonyms: See/watch.

Example of usage: Look at the beautiful bird with the red beak.

Kyk vir daardie pragtige voel (Afrikaans).

Variation 1: One-handed sign in which G-hand, palm left, hand up, moves outwards and downwards from eye level. Used by Northern Transvaal Tswana and Zulu Natal.

Variation 2: One-handed sign in which B-hand, palm left, hand up, moves diagonally outwards and downwards from eye. Used by Transvaal Indian.

Variation 3: One-handed sign in which V-hand, palm left, hand up, moves outwards and downwards from eye. Used by Natal English and taught in the Department of Education and Training Schools (i.e., the black schools).

Variation 4: One-handed sign in which V-hand, palm down, hand away, moves outwards and downwards from bridge of nose. Used by Cape English.

Variation 5: One-handed sign in which V-hand, palm towards, hand up, moves outward and downward from eyes. Used by Soweto Sotho, Zulu Natal, Cape Afrikaans, Transvaal Afrikaans.

GENERAL: Transparent sign. All versions involve movement from eye level.

FIGURE 10.1. Entry for "look" in the *Dictionary of Southern African Signs for Communicating with the Deaf* (Penn 1992b, 356, italics added)

variation exists in the choices of the signs that are used but that SASL can be considered to be one language, generally understood by signing Deaf people. However, we believe it would be hasty to make the claim without sufficient linguistic research. Several of the authors of the dictionary claim that a syntactic unity exists in the signed language used in South Africa (Ogilvy-Foreman, Penn, and Reagan 1994; Penn and Reagan 1994).

Much more linguistic research needs to be done, using a considerably wider sample of the Deaf population, a sentiment shared by the makers of the dictionary (see Penn and Reagan 1996). Further, this process of investigation essentially must involve Deaf people being trained to do linguistic research, research that feeds back into the Deaf community and is of some use to that community by empowering Deaf people to be the experts on their language (Aarons 1994; 1996). Aarons and Morgan (1998) have been researching the structure of the signed language used in different communities in the Western Cape Province and Gauteng Province.

In any event, continued debate on what variety of signed language should be the standard seems misplaced. Far more important is for Deaf and hearing people to recognize that signed language is not merely a manual coding of spoken language. Much energy is still required to convince the broader public—especially speech pathologists, educators, legislators, and those in the medical profession—who wield enormous power over the lives of Deaf people that signed languages are natural languages and that Deaf people should have the right to use the language of their choice.

Interpreting

There are only limited opportunities to train to be an interpreter in South Africa. The University of the Free State has offered several short courses for potential interpreters, but these have merely identified likely candidates and presented the essentials of the language. As of 1999, both the University of the Witwatersrand and the University of the Free State have initiated interpreter training diploma courses. There are currently very few skilled interpreters providing services in South Africa, and none of them has been trained in the country.

No professionalization of interpreting has occurred. Interpreters are very seldom paid, no code of professional ethics has been created, and no certifying or controlling body governs interpreting practices. In addition, no legislation requires interpretation to be provided for Deaf people. In the courtroom, interpreting services are provided on an ad hoc basis by hard of hearing people who have no training in interpreting at all and who often have not attained as much as a tenth grade educational level. In South Africa, any person can claim to be able to interpret for the Deaf. In addition, Deaf people do not yet consider themselves to be clients or consumers who are entitled to fully professional interpretation because they are not yet mobilized to the point where they demand full access to everything that is available to the rest of the society.

The constitutional rights of Deaf people are a crucial feature in the future development of sign language in South Africa and in the establishment of interpreter training programs. Full access for Deaf people will necessitate highly trained, available interpreters. These, in turn, will have to be trained by Deaf and hearing people who are fluent in and conscious of the natural signed language used by a wide variety of Deaf people in the country. Additionally, interpreters must be trained by people highly skilled in interpreting theory and practice, irrespective of language or modality. The issue of variation should be acknowledged, but given that Deaf people in South Africa understand one another, it should be accorded no more attention than, for instance, that given to different regional dialects of English used on the BBC shows.

The South African Constitution and the Bill of Rights

Deaf consciousness in South Africa does exist but is still very young. As a result of lobbying by Deaf activists, SASL was put on the agenda to be included in the constitution as one of the official languages of South Africa. The battle for official language status was lost, but in fact, the protection and development of SASL has a particular mention in the constitution, and the constitution has been written in such a way that the rights of Deaf people are protected. Much of current practice will have to be challenged in the Constitutional Court, and these challenges will be time-consuming and costly, but the mechanisms are in place.

One relevant extract from the Constitution of the Republic of South Africa, as adopted on May 8, 1996, follows:

Languages

6. (5) The Pan South African Language Board must—

    a. promote and create conditions for the development and use of

        i. all official languages;

        ii. the Khoi, Nama and San languages; and

        iii. sign language (Constitution 1996).

Note that, although sign language does not enjoy the status of an official language, the fact that it has a clause of its own may, in fact, give it a different and special status. In reality, the eleven official languages (isiZulu, isiXhosa, seven other Bantu languages, English, and Afrikaans) are equal only in an official sense. In practice, English is the language of the parliament, although the majority of its members are not native speakers of English. Afrikaans still enjoys widespread usage, particularly in officialdom. Historical inequality will continue to last for a long time. People will have a right to education through the other official languages only if it is practicable to do so in the area in which they live. In general, this reality will serve the majority of South Africans' language needs, and the official languages will be given parity of esteem. The Pan South African Language Board has a constitutional brief to create conditions for the development and use of sign language. Seven years down the line, these conditions have not yet been determined.

As far as education is concerned, the constitution makes provision only for education in official languages.

Education

29. (2) Everyone has the right to receive education in the official language or languages of their choice in public educational institutions where that education is reasonably practicable. To ensure the effective access to, and implementation of, this right, the state must consider all reasonable educational alternatives, including single medium institutions, taking into account—

    a. equity;

    b. practicability; and

    c. the need to redress the results of past racially discriminatory law and practice. (Constitution 1996)

It is clear from the spirit of the clause above that, if the majority of stakeholders in a school for the Deaf demanded sign language as the medium of instruction, this demand would be their constitutional right. What the constitution does not enforce, however, is that sign language actually should be the medium of instruction in schools for the Deaf. As discussed above, the South African Schools Act of 1996 has made this law, but it has not been enforced. The Pan South African Language Board has, however, been made aware of the problems of providing instruction only through the medium of official languages for Deaf people and the impracticability of so doing. Its brief is, among other things, to monitor unfair language practices, and it has declared itself willing to entertain alternative proposals for the elimination of discrimination on the basis of language. Thus, it seems that the door may open in the future for an appeal to be made to the Constitutional Court to declare that the way in which Deaf children are educated in South Africa is unconstitutional.

Furthermore, should Deaf people be able to make the case that they are a linguistic and cultural community, they are entitled to protection through the Commission for the Promotion and Protection of the Rights of Cultural, Religious, and Linguistic Communities. Should Deaf people feel that their human rights are being violated, they are also entitled to request the aid of this committee.

Thus, although the constitution does not provide explicitly for sign language as a medium of instruction in schools for the Deaf, it does provide, in principle, a means by which Deaf people can ensure that they have equal access. The South African Schools Act should be considered as law, and schools for the Deaf are thus in contravention of the law. However, for the provisions of the constitution to be explicitly articulated, Deaf people will have to mobilize themselves and challenge existing educational and language practices. As a result of the legacy of the past, there are myriad ways in which Deaf people are oppressed on the basis of language. None of these will change unless they are challenged by Deaf people.

IMPLICATIONS OF MULTILINGUAL LANGUAGE POLICIES FOR THE USE AND STATUS OF SIGN LANGUAGE

As has been outlined above, the education that Deaf people receive is inadequate and inferior, further aggravated by the deep racial inequalities still at work in South Africa and the fact that the relevant ministries consider Deafness to be a disability equivalent in some ways to mental retardation. Information collected by DEAFSA in 1997 indicates that only three Deaf teachers are employed in South Africa and that no more than 15 Deaf university graduates live in the country. The educational level in schools for the Deaf is inferior to that in schools for the hearing, and Deaf students are deeply disadvantaged by inadequate access to the medium of instruction. As is common worldwide, many Deaf people do not acquire literacy at all while some are just barely literate. It is also true that, given the inadequate resources in large parts of the country, more Deaf black children are most likely out of school than are in school. Many Deaf children find themselves in schools for the multiply handicapped, sharing classes with mentally retarded, physically handicapped, and blind pupils, all of whom have different educational and language needs. This situation is not going to change despite the new constitution and the new educational dispensation unless it is challenged by Deaf people who unite on the basis of a common language and who understand that they are entitled to all the rights that others in the country have.

As long as Deaf people are not trained and employed as teachers, Deaf children will be taught by hearing people who, often, are unable to sign well enough to function effectively. Until there are Deaf researchers and Deaf linguists, hearing people will make official decisions about signed language. Until interpreters are trained and professionalized, Deaf people will not have their voices heard in the hearing world. Up to now, resources and an infrastructure to train interpreters in South Africa have not been made available, and this situation is not yet perceived by the majority as an urgent priority to break the cycle of Deaf needs going unheard and unmet.

Thus, as must by now be obvious, the Deaf community in South Africa is largely untouched by the change of government and the development of a new constitution. However, the empowerment of Deaf people is now possible. The Deaf community has the rather formidable task of organizing and mobilizing itself to determine the course of its future. For the first time, the law does not stand in its path. As a community united through linguistic oppression, it now has to transform the ignorance and accepted wisdom of the wider society of which it is a part.

NOTES

1. Subsequent to the presentation of the chapter, a research project to investigate the linguistic structure of the signed language used in two provinces (the Western Cape Province and Gauteng) has been initiated by Aarons and Morgan, "An Investigation into the Linguistic Structure of the Signed Language/s Used by the Deaf Communities in the Western Cape Province and Gauteng," Research Grant Number 15/1/3/16/0125 from the Centre for Science Development of the Human Sciences Research Council, South Africa; Principal Investigator, Debra Aarons. A more detailed discussion of the signed language used throughout South Africa may be found in Aarons and Akach (1998, forthcoming).

2. These provinces were the Transvaal, the Cape, the Orange Free State, and Natal.

3. The terminology related to color in South Africa is very complex and was developed according to apartheid divisions. Some of the terminology has now been reclaimed. Thus, nowadays, some white South Africans might refer to themselves as "Africans," and mixed-race South Africans may refer to themselves as "black." To make the apartheid distinctions clear for the purpose of this chapter, however, we refer to negroid South Africans as either "African" or as "black," and for the purposes of discussing apartheid and its aftermath, we use apartheid terminology, although we regret that this use is necessary here.

4. This label was one more of the many racial classifications used during the apartheid years. "Europeans" referred to whites, and "non-Europeans" referred to everyone else.

5. This policy was the apartheid policy of separate development in which the idea was to separate white South Africa from black South Africa and then further divide black South Africans into a number of ethnic groups, each with its own "homeland." Black people were then considered "citizens" of their designated homeland and not South Africans.

6. The different homelands were also known as Bantustans.

7. The italics are ours.

8. However, the same act makes provision for the medium of instruction to be decided by the governing body and the community. It does seem that schools for the Deaf are a special case, but this situation will eventually be decided by further legislation and possible litigation.

References

Aarons, Debra. 1994. Aspects of the syntax of American Sign Language. Ph.D. diss., Boston University.

———. 1996. Signed languages and professional responsibility. *Stellenbosch Papers in Linguistics* 30: 285–311.

Aarons, Debra, and Philemon Akach. 1998. One language or many? A sociolinguistic question. *Stellenbosch Papers in Linguistics* 31:1–28.

———. Forthcoming. South African Sign Language—one language or many? In *Language and social history: Studies in South African sociolinguistics*, ed. Rajend Mesthrie. 2d ed. Cambridge, Mass.: Cambridge University Press.

Aarons, Debra, and Ruth Morgan. 1998. The structure of South African Sign Language after apartheid. Paper presented at the Sixth Conference of Theoretical Issues in Sign Language Research, November, at Gallaudet University, Washington, D.C.

Constitution of the Republic of South Africa. 1996. Available on the Internet: <http://www.polity.org.za/html/govdocs/constitution/saconst.html> (accessed in Jauary 2003).

Heap, Marion. 2001. An anthropological perspective of the deaf people in Cape Town. University of Stellenbosch, Department of Anthropology. Typescript.

Johnson, Robert E., Scott K. Liddell, and Carol J. Erting. 1989. *Unlocking the curriculum: Principles of achieving access in deaf education.* Gallaudet Research Institute Working Paper 89–3. Washington, D.C.: Gallaudet University Press.

Nyamende, Abner. 1994. Regional variation in Xhosa. *Stellenbosch Papers in Linguistics* 26:202–17.

Ogilvy-Foreman, Dale, Claire Penn, and Timothy Reagan. 1994. Selected syntactic features of South African Sign Language: A preliminary analysis. *South African Journal of Linguistics* 12 (4):118–23.

Penn, Claire. 1992a. The sociolinguistics of South African Sign Language. In *Language and society in Africa*, ed. Robert K. Herbert, 277–84. Johannesburg: Witwatersrand University Press.

Penn, Claire, ed. 1992b. *Dictionary of Southern African signs for communicating with the deaf.* Vol. 1. Pretoria: Human Sciences Research Council.

———. 1993–1994. *Dictionary of Southern African signs for communicating with the deaf.* Vols. 2–5. Pretoria: Human Sciences Research Council.

Penn, Claire, and Timothy Reagan. 1990. How do you sign "apartheid"? The politics of South African Sign Language. *Language Problems and Language Planning* 14 (2):91–103.

———. 1994. The properties of South African Sign Language: Lexical diversity and syntactic unity. *Sign Language Studies* 84:319–27.

———. 1996. Language policy, South African Sign Language, and the deaf: Social and educational implications. Typescript.

Penn, Claire, Timothy Reagan, and Dale Ogilvy. 1991. Deaf-hearing interchange in South Africa. *Sign Language Studies* 71:131–42.

Reynolds, Louise. 1995. Philosophies and practices in deaf education in the Western Cape, South Africa. *Signpost* 8 (2):66–71.

Strong, Michael. 1988. A bilingual approach to the education of young deaf children: ASL and English. In *Language learning and deafness*, ed. Michael Strong, 113–29. Cambridge: Cambridge University Press.

11 | U-Turns, Deaf Shock, and
the Hard of Hearing:
Japanese Deaf Identities at
the Borderlands

Karen Nakamura

A growing body of anthropological and sociolinguistic research (Lane 1976, 1984; Kegl 1994; Senghas and Kegl 1994; Parasnis 1996) has confirmed what Deaf people in the United States have known all along—that schools for the deaf are the birthplace of Deaf communities, Deaf identities, and signed languages. Japan is no different in this respect, although two factors add a particular variation to deaf identities there. The first factor is the relatively late introduction (for an industrialized nation) of widespread educational opportunities for deaf people. Although the first school for the deaf opened in the late 19th century, compulsory education for deaf students was introduced only after the end of World War II. The second factor is the combination of a drastically falling birth rate, improved medical care, and a trend toward mainstreaming during the past three decades that has led to a decimation of ranks within schools for the deaf.

The two pivotal historical moments in this ethnography of Japanese deaf communities are 1948 and 1970: 1948 being the date of the introduction of compulsory education for the deaf after World War II and 1970 signifying the beginning of a rapid increase in the practice of mainstreaming deaf children into hearing schools. These events segment deaf identities in Japan into age-demarcated categories because a deaf person's date of birth will profoundly influence the types of educational opportunities he or she may have had, his or her peer group, the type of signed language he or she used, and his or her general political and cultural outlook. This chapter analyzes how the histories of Japanese deaf communities affect the proliferation of deaf identities in contemporary Japan.

A metaphor in current use within the anthropology of identities is that of nations and nation building, mainly inspired by Benedict Anderson's (1983) key text, *Imagined Communities: Reflections on the Origin and Spread of Nationalism*. Within this frame, this chapter discusses the emergence of deaf identities in Japan from a process-oriented, anthropological standpoint; that is, the same historical and cultural processes that we typically attribute to nation building can also be used to understand how identities and institutions come together and disperse. Whether one identifies as "Japanese" or "Deaf" or "American," a person relies on processes of "imagined" similarities with others in the same category and differences with those categorized as other. The processes that make us identify as Japanese, Deaf, or American also blur history, so we tend to imagine that these identities have always existed—which is the nature of identities.

In reality, processes of identifications are never quite so simple and have become more fragmented in recent times. There are no natural identities, whether being culturally Deaf or ethnically Japanese; rather, identifications in themselves all result from processes of historical and political machinations on the macro scale and from active psychological construction within individuals.[1] The reader may have noticed that I have not used the "big-D" *Deaf* term when referring to deaf people in Japan—a common practice in American Deaf studies when referring to cultural Deafness, a position that situates itself in opposition to hearing culture or "audism" (Wilcox 1989; Lane 1992). In many ways, the goal of this chapter is to challenge and denaturalize (a) the notion of a singular Deaf culture, whether in other cultures or in Japan, and (b) artificial, rigid boundaries between hearing and deaf cultures.

Methodology

This chapter is based on 16 months of participant-observation research among deaf groups in Japan. Most of the research time was centered in the Tokyo-Kanto area, although I also attended numerous deaf events and functions across Japan from the northern island of Hokkaido to the southern island of Kyushu. The mainstay of my research was a period of eight months as a research intern within the Japanese Federation of the Deaf (JFD), the oldest and largest of the deaf groups in Japan. My primary job responsibility was to translate JFD public relations material and correspondence with and between the World Federation of the Deaf (WFD) and WFD member organizations. I also attended many JFD meetings at all levels as an observer and, occasionally, as a staff helper. Supplementing this ethnographic research was archival work conducted at the JFD and the National Library in Tokyo and interviews with leadership, activists, and members of the JFD within Tokyo and other prefectures.

I am hearing and fluent in both spoken and written forms of English and Japanese, and I have spent almost equal thirds of my life growing up in Australia, Japan, and the United States. I studied American Sign Language (ASL) during a summer at Gallaudet University and at the American School for the Deaf for a year and a half before my fieldwork in Japan. I learned Japanese Sign Language (JSL) through private tutoring and through a process of immersion while in Japan.

During the fieldwork period, my JSL signing abilities, though not spectacular, were sufficient to conduct interviews and conversations without the use of an interpreter, once we got past the initial question of dialectal differences in Japanese signed language forms. By the latter part of my research, most deaf informants thought I was deaf myself or, at least, hard of hearing. They may have made this assumption because of the ASL "accent" on my signing, for example, the use of ASL grammatical forms (such as the use of classifiers, facial and non-gestural grammatical markers, not mouthing or vocalizing words, not following the spoken Japanese word ordering, and so forth) and my anomalous role as participant-observer, one who was neither an interpreter nor a member of a deaf organization. My gender certainly played a role in being identified as deaf or hard of hearing as did my being seen as partly American or Americanized.[2]

Defining Deafness

In Japan, one finds no single, hegemonic definition of what it means to be "Deaf." No group has yet managed to gain control of the discourses surrounding deafness or levels of hearing impairment. Various factors have caused new deaf identities to emerge and proliferate, mainly along age-demarcated lines. In particular, although pre–World War II and immediate postwar deaf groups tend to retain an encompassing and singular notion of deafness that includes all those with hearing disabilities, younger deaf activists have fragmented along the fault lines of cultural Deafness and hard of hearing assimilation, thus creating new identities at the borderlands. Just like the contemporary reconstitution of nationhood and national identity in the Baltic region, new deaf groups in Japan are re-creating and synthesizing new concepts of deafness along often radical lines while older groups reformulate themselves in a more fragmented world.

In Japan, deaf people differ greatly in the types of signed language that they use and in what they define as "Deaf culture"(*rou bunka/defu karucha*) and deaf "identity" (*aidentiti*). One way we can see these differences is in the proliferation of terms used to identify being "deaf." For example, in written and spoken Japanese, there are at least five major ways of identifying as deaf:

- *Rou/roua/rouasha/rousha*—Deaf /Deaf-mute (from classical Chinese)

- *Tsunbo*—Deaf (derogatory; archaic; classical Japanese)

- *Defu/D*—Deaf (from English)

- *Choukakushougaisha*—Hearing disabled (literal)

- *Nanchousha*—Hard of hearing (literal)

- *Mimigakikoenai-hito*—Person whose ears do not hear (literal)

Compounded against these written and verbal systems are also at least six ways of signing "deaf," "hearing disabled," or "hard of hearing." Voicing and mouthing are important parts of Japanese Sign Language, so the voicing and mouthing options add further complexity (see figures 11.1, 11.2, and 11.3).

One is tempted to see in this array of identities the same forms that are found in the American academic discourse on deafness. We could easily map *roua* to indicate big-D Deaf and *nanchousha* to indicate hard of hearing (HOH; in America, those people who have some degree of hearing loss but who use primarily oral forms of communication such as speaking and speechreading). But this mapping would be problematic as we shall soon see. Deaf groups in Japan that have the name "hearing disabled" in their titles, for example, the *Tokyo Chokakushougaisha*

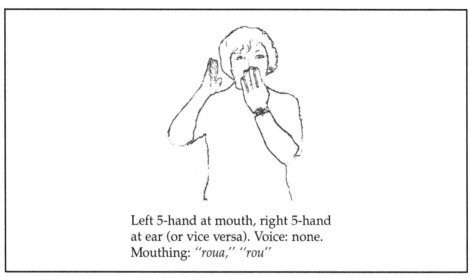

Left 5-hand at mouth, right 5-hand
at ear (or vice versa). Voice: none.
Mouthing: *"roua," "rou"*

FIGURE 11.1 Classical Japanese sign for "deaf mute"

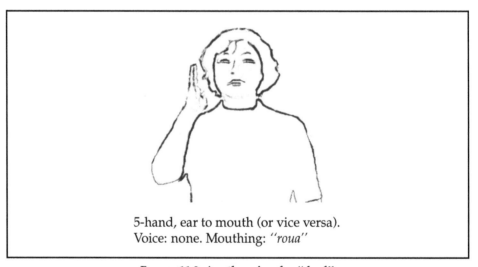

5-hand, ear to mouth (or vice versa).
Voice: none. Mouthing: *"roua"*

FIGURE 11.2 Another sign for "deaf"

Renmei (the Tokyo Association of the Hearing Disabled), seem like anachronisms from the perspective of those in the field of American Deaf Studies. They strike one as being dinosaurs that will inevitably follow the modernization path toward removing such "discriminatory" language from their titles. We would expect them to soon change their names. American Deaf Studies avoids discussion of the physical aspect of deafness while focusing on the cultural and linguistic aspects. This approach follows the general trend in American identity politics of deemphasizing the material and physical while privileging the cultural, for example, the shift from *negro* and *black* to *Black* or *African American* and the shift from *homosexual* or *homophile* to *Gay* and *Lesbian*.

However, when trying to map the American model onto Japan, reading it as

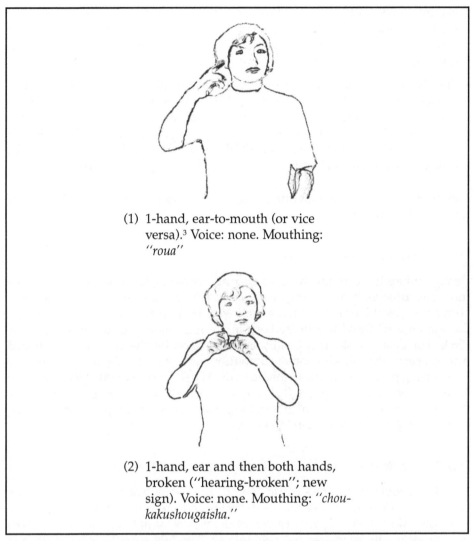

(1) 1-hand, ear-to-mouth (or vice versa).[3] Voice: none. Mouthing: *"roua"*

(2) 1-hand, ear and then both hands, broken ("hearing-broken"; new sign). Voice: none. Mouthing: *"chou-kakushougaisha."*

FIGURE 11.3 Two additional signs for "deaf" using one hand and mouthing

protomodern in its identity constructions, we run into phenomena that do not match the American case. For example, consider the following three situations:

- During the national meetings of the Japanese Federation of the Deaf, most of the board of directors—deaf men ages 45 and above—used simultaneous voicing while signing. The audience was ostensibly almost all deaf (except for myself), so the voicing was not for hearing people's sake. Why would the leaders of the largest and most politically active deaf group in Japan be so far away from the Deaf cultural model (i.e., only signing)?

- Apparently, predominantly young people identify as hard of hearing or hearing impaired, and rarely do people who are middle-aged or older use the term. Many young "hearing impaired" people in Japan seem to prefer the HOH or hearing impaired label over "deaf" and do not join deaf groups. Most of the local and regional organizations of the deaf in Japan are having a very difficult time recruiting younger deaf members. Why are younger deaf avoiding the traditional deaf organizations?

• The Tokyo Association of the Hearing-Impaired used to be called the Tokyo Association of the Deaf (Tokyo Roua Renmei), but they changed their name from "deaf" to "hearing impaired" in the last decade. Many of the local associations of the deaf also are switching their names, and the Japanese Federation of the Deaf has also contemplated a similar name switch. Why would they be changing to a name that emphasizes the disability aspect of deafness?

The following discussion will attempt to understand the dynamics behind Japanese trends such as these.

Demographics and Identity

Demographically, deaf and hard of hearing people in Japan fall into much the same categories as their hearing peers. That is, they comprise (a) those who were born before World War II, (b) those who were born in the baby boom soon after the war, and (c) those who were born in the fully modernized period after the 1960s. For deaf people, this history is demarcated by the two aforementioned pivotal events: the introduction of compulsory education for the deaf in 1948 and the growing practice of mainstreaming in the 1970s. These two pivotal events have created three main groupings that map onto the three groups above. They are the pre-compulsory-education group, the postcompulsory and premainstreaming group, and the postmainstreaming group.

Pre–World War II, Pre-Compulsory-Education Deaf People

The deaf people in the pre–World War II, pre-compulsory-education category were born sometime during the 1900s–1930s and are now between 70 and 100 years old. Most deaf people born before the war were not able to attend school because deaf education was not compulsory. The first school for the deaf (and blind) opened its doors in 1878 in Kyoto, and a similar school opened a few years later in Tokyo. This development was part of a trend led by the Meiji government to modernize and Westernize, and this government realized that universal education, especially for those who were handicapped, was the hallmark of leading European nations. Thus, deaf education became a concomitant part of the same nationalistic political movement that would later embrace colonization and lead Japan into World War II.[4]

Not many children attended these early schools for the deaf, which were funded by a combination of state, city, and private money.[5] Even when tuition was free, the cost of room, board, and school supplies together with the potential loss of household labor kept many families from sending their deaf children to school. Not until education was universal and mandatory did deaf children started attending school in droves.

Because the great majority of those deaf people born before mandatory education had no formal schooling, they are often illiterate—an unusual thing in a Japanese society with its much vaunted 98% literacy rate. The pre–World War II generation's sign language consists in large part of local or home signs with very little use of the spoken Japanese grammatical structure that marks contemporary JSL. Many were kept at home by their families and not allowed to go to school or associate with other deaf individuals. There is little evidence that Japanese Sign Language as such existed as a uniform sign language system before the Meiji Restoration (1868).

Deaf children growing up during this period were exposed to local sign systems (if they were exposed to any signs at all), and only in later adulthood were they exposed to a larger number of deaf adults. The post–World War II period brought deaf people together through the JFD, but their childhoods were spent separated from other deaf peers. As a result, most of these older deaf people sign in an idiosyncratic style. Even deaf adults in their same area have difficulty understanding what they are signing while hearing interpreters throw up their hands in frustration.[6] Because hearing people in authority (doctors, welfare officers) have trouble understanding them, they often do not receive proper medical attention and social welfare services.

Many deaf women were forcibly sterilized when they were young to prevent them from having offspring—a sad result of Japan's own meddling in eugenics, a common worldwide trend during the early 20th centuries (including not only countries influenced by Nazi propaganda but also the United States). Other deaf women whom I interviewed were not allowed to marry by choice and were forced into marriages with hearing spouses.

One example of this generation was an elderly deaf woman I met in the northern Hokkaido region. She had been sterilized when her parents took her to a doctor for menstrual cramps. Her parents kept her in the house for most of her early life, and she was later forcibly married to a hearing man. Only after her husband died did her life start to open up. She converted to Nichiren Buddhism and started to meet other people (mostly hearing) through her religious activities. When I was introduced to her, she was the only deaf person in an independent-living nursing home facility for the elderly.

This population of elderly Deaf is difficult to reach because most of them are socially isolated, and the poorer health care they receive because of communication problems means that they have a much shorter life expectancy than the average hearing Japanese person. As Japan becomes more aware of its rapidly aging populace (the *koreikashakai* problem) and as the baby-boomer deaf adults enter the age of retirement, more attention has been paid to this older age group, but communication and socialization problems remain a major issue.

WORLD WAR II AND POST–WORLD WAR II BABY BOOMERS

The deaf people born during and after World War II (who were born during the 1940s and 1950s and who are now in their 50s and 60s) are the largest demographic segment of the deaf community—the baby boomers. The increase in births in the immediate postwar period combined with the difficult economic times, crowded cities, corresponding increase in prenatal and postnatal diseases, and the introduction of streptomycin and other new antibiotics and immunization drugs all led to a large number of babies with hearing disabilities in the 1940s and 1950s.

On April 1, 1948, compulsory education for the deaf began, and large numbers of these children began attending schools for the deaf, which were being constructed all across the country. This effort was part of the postwar modernization project started by General MacArthur and his General Headquarters (GHQ).

Because transportation systems were still not developed in rural areas, many of these schools were residential. The educational methodology was oral (speech-reading and speech skills), but it was hampered by the lack of effective and economical hearing aids. Many of the children were what we would now call hard of hearing or late-deafened (many were deafened between the ages of 6 and 8 when they received inoculations or streptomycin shots), but they were lumped into the schools for the deaf without being identified according to hearing ability.

Japanese society places a strong emphasis on literacy, and the deaf community has not been isolated from this social valuation. Both in the schools for the deaf and in organizations of the deaf that developed out of these schools, high "verbal" skills (as in written and spoken Japanese) were valued rather than signing skills. Deaf culture and sign language were being formed in the playgrounds and dorms of these schools, but the history of the schools is so much shallower than those in Europe or America. We find no "golden age" of deaf education in Japan.[7] From the beginning, deaf education was very much embedded in the value systems of the dominant hearing culture.

Thus, children who were late-deafened or merely hard of hearing tended to rise within the school system. They became the class leaders as well as the liaisons between the teachers and other students, and they went on to become leaders in the deaf community. An American Deaf person visiting a JFD national meeting would be astonished to find that most of the meeting would be conducted in manually signed Japanese, with voicing taking precedence over signing. Part of this communication style is the result of the different regional dialects of JSL that make spoken Japanese the lingua franca (common language). Another factor is that, although the JFD is an organization *of* deaf people, they do not engage in identity politics per se, so the leaders of the organization do not necessarily seem to epitomize deafness the same way we demand minority leaders in the United States to be representative in every sense of the word. One aspect of Japanese deaf people's approach to communication is pragmatic (and not a little indicative of a lack of faith in interpreters). The deaf leaders who can speak and speechread the clearest are also seen as the most able to work most easily with the bureaucrats in the governments to secure social services for the rest of the group.

This age group of baby boomers defines themselves as *roua* (Deaf)—as in the Zen-nihon-roua-renmei (Japanese Federation of the Deaf)—and sees themselves as relatively homogenous. Little differentiation is made on the basis of hearing ability or signing skills within the community itself. The base criterion is that one cannot hear; no statements are made concerning cultural or linguistic outlook. In many ways, the "imagined" homogeneity of this age group reflects the same type of social unification without bounds in the "imagined nation" approach to the rebuilding of Japan in the World War II and postwar period.

The JFD is both a political organization and a social services provider. Politically, they lobby for deaf civil rights and welfare benefits, but they also are the nonprofit organization that receives government-outsourced contracts related to social services for deaf people (interpreter training and dispatch, video captioning). This material and legal perspective toward deaf organizing characterizes deaf people within this middle group. They are old enough to remember the period of rampant discrimination and the political changes that brought about the current, relatively benevolent present. And, although they do not see themselves as particularly disabled, they are fluent in the disability (*shougaisha*) discourse and have been able to use it to gain key political ground. Entwining themselves into the welfare bureaucracy has enabled members of the JFD to leverage Japan's increasing investment in social services.

One example of a member of this generation, Susumu Ohya, one of the founders of the first nursing home designed especially for the deaf, falls within this age category. He attended high school in the mid-1960s and was an active participant in the famous Student Strike at the Kyoto School for the Deaf in 1965—Japan's own version of the Gallaudet Deaf President Now movement—where the students boycotted the school for the poor education it provided to its students. He remembers his high school days as a time full of talk about social movements, political protests, and the like. He was active in organizing the community to create funds to build the first nursing home for the deaf in Japan then managed to secure prefectural and local social welfare grants to continue to fund its existence.

Not coincidentally, the period during the 1960s and 1970s when this age group was most politically active (then in their twenties and thirties) was also a time of huge upheaval for Japan as a whole. The GHQ government led by General MacArthur of the United States withdrew, and Japan found itself, once again, a sovereign nation. The joint Japan–United States security treaty questioned the meaning of this sovereignty. Communism and socialist activities threatened to tear the nation apart. In Osaka and Kyoto, former Burakumin (outcaste groups) became political. In Japan, the key concept of the turbulent 1960s and 1970s was *kenri*—civil and human rights—and the deaf young adults of the time emerged within this environment.

The JFD and its regional affiliates have traditionally been political action groups with cultural and social activities a secondary sideline. The JFD made *kenri* a central part of their political efforts and, as a result, were able to effect changes in a great number of welfare and labor laws. The 1980s and 1990s have been JFD's most powerful and active period. Sweeping political changes that have been enacted include the introduction of a volunteer interpreting system, driver's licenses for the deaf, a national welfare pension plan, and Japanese Sign Language textbooks. The JFD has also fostered widespread understanding of deaf issues.

The one area in Japan that has been totally unaffected by outside political turbulence has been the educational system. The Ministry of Education (Monbusho) is perhaps the most powerful ministry in the government in terms of its ability to act independently of any external influence. The JFD along with other social reformers and political activists have been unable to change the Japanese educational system despite much effort. Japanese is the only language recognized within Japanese schools, which means no approved curricula can be developed using signed languages. This educational policy toward teaching speech and speechreading skills as well as adhering to the same curricula as hearing schools has remained the same from 1948 until the present. Signed languages are "permitted" to be used, but only at the middle and high school levels and only as an aid to Japanese-language materials. The strong adherence to Japanese as the primary language base has influenced JSL strongly, with many of the students using JSL signs in Japanese word order and grammatical forms.

A good number of students stayed in the schools for the deaf after graduation in the 1960s and 1970s. They took positions as adjunct teachers, and their presence played an important role in ensuring continuity within the school system (and also making sure their hearing coworkers learned at least a few signs)—even though their placement was often limited to teaching woodwork, beautician skills, sewing, physical education, or other noncore courses. These deaf teachers played a critical role in stabilizing the community and ensuring a more uniform sign language system both within the schools and in Japan itself.

NEW GENERATION POST-BOOMERS

The deaf people born during the period of 1960–1980, the new generation post-boomers, are now in their twenties, thirties, and forties. In the 1970s, two major changes occurred that would later prove to have significant effects on Japanese deaf communities and, in particular, this age group. The first was the start of a rapidly plummeting birth rate and the second was a strong shift toward main-streaming within schools for the deaf. The conjunction of these two forces has meant that enrollment in schools for the deaf has also correspondingly plummeted. School enrollment for all schools for the deaf in Japan was at its peak in 1960 at 20,723 students. By 1995, enrollment had dropped to 7,537 students, approximately 36% of the earlier figure (Japanese Federation of the Deaf 1996, 71). The number of "hearing impaired" children, as classified by the government, was 26,000 in 1965; 26 years later, by 1991, this number had dropped by 57% to 11,200 (Ministry of Health and Welfare 1998).

The significance of this shift cannot be underestimated. Many of the schools for the deaf that I visited during 1997–1998 had significantly lower enrollments than at any other time in their history. Classrooms that used to hold 40 or more students now held an entire grade in one classroom of three to four students. At some schools, entire grade years were missing. The general atmosphere at these schools was a bit like a ghost town. Students, teachers, and parents recognized that the best educational (and thus, social) opportunities existed for the students who could be mainstreamed outside of the schools for the deaf.

This generation of students began graduating about ten years ago and are currently in their twenties, thirties, and forties. Those who were mainstreamed after kindergarten or primary schools often identify themselves as hard of hearing (*nanchousha*) or as hearing-disabled (*choukakushougaisha*), but not as deaf (*rouasha/defu*), despite having the same level of hearing loss as their peers in the schools for the deaf. Many of these young deaf adults do not know any sign language or learned it only after graduating from high school. Many of these people see themselves as simply not hearing very well, and they avoid deaf groups and asso-ciating with the deaf community.

In one family in Tokyo with two girls who were hearing impaired, only the older sister identified herself as Deaf (either *rou* or *defu*). She went to a school for the deaf and signs fluently. The younger sister identifies herself as "not-deaf," goes to a hearing school, and does not sign, even though she has the same amount of residual hearing as her *defu* sister. This pattern is one that I have also seen in other families. Note that, in many cases, the students themselves (and not necessarily the parents) are the ones who want to mainstream and who want to be just like any other (hearing) child. One teacher of the deaf in Osaka, deaf himself, explained: "In the past, a whole class of us would join the local deaf association when we graduated from [a high] school [for the deaf], but now, kids go to mainstream schools and might never meet a deaf person."

The brighter students with strong academic records are usually encouraged to mainstream. Looking at deaf school records for children, one sees a huge drop in the number of students continuing from the kindergarten to the first grade at the school and then some slow attrition in the higher grades.[8] The culling of the top layer of students for mainstreaming has the significant effect of removing any potential leaders of the deaf community and reinforcing the image that schools for the deaf are for the nonacademically minded.

The children who have remained in the schools for the deaf are often painfully aware that they are considered slow in comparison to their mainstreamed or hearing peers, and we see demoralization in this age group. Most of the graduates from schools for the deaf are unable to attend college because no interpreters are provided at colleges, and even the single technical college for the deaf has unsigned and uninterpreted lectures. Only students with extremely strong oral skills and a dedicated academic attitude can make it into an undergraduate program. The great majority of the graduates of schools for the deaf enter the job market directly, aided by the Employment Promotion Law for Disabled Persons that stipulates a 1.6% quota of disabled employees in large companies.[9]

On the whole, students from this most recent generation who have graduated from schools for the deaf or who have been mainstreamed are not political. They also lack ties to the older deaf population. Most of the high school students I have talked to are only dimly aware of the Japanese Federation of the Deaf, their own local organizations of the deaf, or the various services and offices for the deaf that are available.

The Challenge of the New "Hard of Hearing" Generation

The growing number of younger people who identify themselves as either hard of hearing (*nanchousha*), hearing disabled (*chokakushougaisha*), or not-deaf (*roudewa nai*) has caused much concern to the Japanese Federation of the Deaf and its affiliated organizations. In fact, the aforementioned change of name from the Tokyo Association of the Deaf to the Tokyo Association of the Hearing Disabled was designed to attract the younger generation who do not identify as deaf.

Roua (deaf) is seen as a passé term by the younger generation. It is not a common term and often carries negative connotations, especially for hearing Japanese who think it is outdated or discriminatory. The word *roua* is a close homonym to *rou* (elderly).[10] Well-meaning hearing people in Japan often correct *roua* with *mimigakikoenai* (a person whose ears cannot hear; a Japanese term) or *choukakushougaisha* (hearing disabled; a Chinese-based term).

"U-Turn Deaf"

New trends are developing in this rather bleak picture of contemporary deaf education. The first is the "U-Turn Deaf." The term *U-Turn Deaf* refers to students who were mainstreamed but who then "U-turned" back into schools for the deaf. From the oralist perspective, these kids failed out of mainstream schools. Indeed, some children did return to the schools for the deaf because of educational difficulties, but during my school visits, I also met some children who returned out of choice. "Why did you return to a deaf school?," I asked a high school student who attended hearing school at the primary and middle school levels. She replied, "I was doing OK in the hearing school, but I decided to come back because this is where my friends are."

It is difficult to ascertain the real reasons why the children return. School becomes much more difficult at the middle school level, and in Japan, students are advanced into the next year even if they do not finish a previous year. This practice means that students who are having problems are left even further behind. Many middle and high schools have entrance exams, and most of high school is preparation for "exam hell" for colleges, so U-turning at those junctures makes sense.

However, despite the educational system's negative opinion of these children, I also see reflections of pride in the choice to come back. Returning to a school for the deaf is not easy, but the transition is supported by the small class sizes. Many of the U-Turn Deaf do not know sign language because they were mainstreamed just after kindergarten. Others know only how to sign using a Rochester-like method of fingerspelling each word. Reentering schools for the deaf, these students need to learn or relearn sign language and reassimilate into a deaf environment. But for many, the school for the deaf is a welcome change from the demanding and often lonesome existence as a mainstreamed deaf child in a hearing school system.

Unfortunately, a large majority of the deaf teachers of the deaf described above are now in their late fifties and early sixties and are retiring. Not many new young deaf teachers are available to fill their ranks—mostly because of recent Ministry of Education requirements that make it more difficult for deaf people to become teachers. But some young new teachers, both hearing and deaf, are bringing in a cultural deaf perspective and bilingual educational models, so there is some hope for the future. The increasing numbers of Japanese who are returning to the country and of foreign children as well as the growing pressure from resident Koreans has also helped to liberalize the mindset within Japanese educational circles.

Perhaps the most promising development is that some schools for the deaf such as the Nara Prefectural School are adopting a much more lenient approach to sign language and deaf education. Rather than force speechreading and speech training on their kindergartners (which is the emphasis at most other schools), the Nara School emphasizes the fun nature of learning and group skill-building exercises. The school is also unique in that it has the only deaf kindergarten teacher in Japan.[11] This school does not experience the massive flight of students into mainstream primary schools from the kindergarten level; its kindergartners think that learning is fun and that the school for the deaf is an exciting place to be. They enjoy being with their deaf peers and decide to stay. Speech training comes later, academic quality is better than the other schools, and the school positively bustles with kids. Other schools are very slowly looking at the Nara School for inspiration, but it is still seen as a radical, experimental approach, and the long-term effects on the deaf community and deaf education are still to be seen.

"Deaf Shock"

One other new trend involves mainstreamed students who are discovering their Deaf identities as they become adults—usually when they enter college or when they hit the internal glass ceilings at their places of employment. The typical pattern is that they are invited into or simply join sign language circles (groups of people who get together to learn JSL), and there, they meet other deaf, hard of hearing, or "hearing impaired" people and gradually start to form an idea of themselves as Deaf. Concomitant to this practice has been the importation of American Deaf identities. These younger Deaf students and adults are most keen to learn about how U.S. Deaf identity is organized along the lines of identity politics or cultural Deafness.

"Deaf Shock" is the name of a new organization in the Osaka area. One of the members told me that its name comes from the feeling of shock one gets when one realizes that he or she is a cultural and linguistic minority and not merely disabled. The Japanese for "Deaf Shock" is a combination of the loan words *defu shokku*. The new groups are notable in their use of American loan words and ASL loan signs. In their writings, they often use the roman character *D* to denote cultural Deafness and a culturally Deaf person. They identify as *defu* and reject both *roua* and *choukakushougaisha* as labels.

One of the interesting aspects of the members of these "D-groups" or "*Defu*-groups" as they are known, is that they are not only much younger than the JFD members but also have very little intergenerational and intergroup contact with the older groups. Very few members of D-Pro (the principle group in Tokyo) are active members of the JFD or Tokyo Association of the Deaf and vice-versa. The separation is most striking when attending D-Pro sponsored events because most of the audience is below the age of 40 whereas the opposite is usually the case for JFD meetings.

The D-Pro group has been active in inviting prominent Deaf activists from the United States to Japan. Deaf cultural activist MJ Bienvenu has been their guest in the past, and in 1998, they invited Deaf poet, linguist, and activist Clayton Valli. The age gap and lack of intergenerational ties was most apparent when Valli arrived because he (in his late forties) was easily the oldest person there, and most of his audience was a full generation younger.

D-Pro and the other D-groups have been able to attract a growing number of younger deaf people in the metropolitan areas. In taking an overtly American perspective, they also erect the same definitional boundaries between deaf and hard of hearing that we find in the United States and the same definition of Deaf-born-Deaf at the core of Deaf society. I have been calling the process one of "imagined community" building within deaf communities in Japan. Cultures erect their own language and identity barriers to define themselves against others. Within the D-groups, signing is done without voicing or mouthing. This method was not the version of signing used by the D-Pro members when they were still students in high school, so they undergo a process of language learning or alteration when they join the D-group. I often heard laments from teachers of former deaf students. One teacher's comment typified these laments: "She had such a beautiful voice before she joined D-Pro." The tone of the teacher's comment almost made it seem like she thought D-Pro was a cult, at least, that was how many of the (hearing) teachers viewed it. Older deaf people also view D-Pro warily.

The D-groups, especially D-Pro, have come under some harsh criticism, mostly from older deaf people and from hearing people related to the deaf community. The D-group's thinking is too "American" and they simply "copy American Deaf ways," or they are "too radical, too right wing," or "too exclusionary." They are criticized for centering on only the culturally Deaf within the Deaf community, marginalizing the hard of hearing, and rejecting hearing people. D-Pro leaders have been known to refer to leaders as, not deaf, but hard of hearing because they do not use true Japanese Sign Language but, instead, use SimCom (Simultaneous Communication).

I found the comment that D-Pro was "right wing" (made by a principal of a school for the deaf) to be the most interesting. It makes sense within a political frame of nationalism because what D-Pro is trying to do is erect a new national Deaf movement. The criticism that D-Pro marginalizes the hard of hearing is true, but it is important to note that the hard of hearing problem is one that is almost uniquely specific to D-Pro's generation.[12]

D-Pro's generation has had to contend with the emerging multiple new identities and the lack of identity that many younger deaf people feel. Ironically, much of this struggle has been prompted by a greater acceptance of deaf people and a drop in discrimination against those who are deaf, victories that were achieved because of JFD activities over the past half century. But like all new identity-based movements, others are likely to view it as being too fervent, and the process to build a history while building a new movement at the same time is difficult. D-Pro members struggle with constructing themselves both as Deaf and as different from the older generation. For example, when D-Pro lectures about "Deaf history," it talks mainly about Deaf history in America and Europe, rarely about the history of deaf people in Japan, and it talks especially seldom about any of the political activities of the JFD in the post–World War II period.

LANGUAGE DIFFERENCES AND LANGUAGE WARS

The different groups mentioned in this chapter all complain that they find the other groups difficult to understand. Although the following categories were not determined through rigorous linguistic analysis, I believe they summarize the primary linguistic differences:

- Prewar deaf: JSL and home signs; JSL grammar; no fingerspelling; no voicing
- Postwar deaf: JSL signs; mixed JSL and Japanese grammar; voicing
- New generation—
    - Hard of hearing: JSL and new signs; Japanese grammar; fingerspelling; full voicing
    - D-Groups: JSL and new signs; new JSL grammar; no voicing

Adding to this mix of communication styles and problems is the fact that JSL is not standard across Japan, and even basic vocabulary terms differ. Any descriptive grammar of JSL would set artificial bounds on what to include and exclude as JSL. While a form of fingerspelling was used in the first school for the deaf in Japan (1878), a new standardized form was introduced after the war (1948). Similarly, the numerical system was not standardized until this period. As a result, the JFD board meetings that I described at the beginning of the chapter use spoken Japanese partially out of necessity as a lingua franca. Overhead captioning is almost always used at meetings, ensuring that those who do not understand the signing form used can catch up with the captions.

A large part of the problem is that there has been no single center where JSL can develop and promulgate. The schools for the deaf cannot serve in this role for many reasons: they are oral, they are too small, the schools have little contact with each other, the teachers are all hearing and rotate out of the schools every seven to ten years, the Ministry of Education recognizes only Japanese as the language of education in Japan, the students commute to rather than reside at the school, the students have little contact with the Deaf community, and worst of all, the students experience little intergenerational contact.[13]

The Japanese Federation of the Deaf does have a JSL committee that is developing new signs and publishing them in dictionaries, but the spread of these new signs is limited because the JFD's reach as an organization is limited, especially among the younger age groups. The situation is comically sad for interpreters. They go to their sign language courses and learn one set of signs. They watch the *Sign Language News* on the national public television station and learn other signs. Their dictionary has yet another set of signs. And when they interpret, the audience members often stop and correct them as they interpret.

CONCLUSION

Because the main focus of this chapter was intended to be ethnographic rather than theoretical, I will only very briefly touch on the three key theoretical lenses through which I am analyzing deaf communities in Japan. The theoretical aspects are developed further in my Ph.D. dissertation (Nakamura 2001).

The first lens is that of the shift from the JFD to the new D-groups, which can be examined analytically as a shift from a "classical social movement" to a "new social movement" (NSM), a concept developed in the works by Alberto Melucci (1980) and Aldon Morris and Carol McClurg Mueller (1992). Classical social movements, such as communism and other political philosophies, emphasize group identity and participation. In contrast, NSMs emphasize individual identity and individual identity politics. Examples of these NSMs would be the feminism, environmentalism, and the gay and lesbian movement. In NSMs, the concept that the "personal is political" is more important than the participation in any group membership.

The second analytical lens explores deaf identity in Japan in relation to the growing literature on postcolonial studies, identity as narrative, and postmodern critical thought, drawn from the recent works of Homi Bhabha (1993), Jean and John Comaroff (1993), Etienne Balibar and Immanuel Wallerstein (1991), and Arjun Appadurai and Carol Breckenridge (1988). The deaf community in Japan in many ways can be compared with the situation in Algiers during and immediately after the French occupation. The process of mainstreaming and the culling of the brightest students into mainstream schools can be historically compared to similar colonial practices. We find analogous groups to the U-Turn Deaf and Deaf Shock in the Algerian nationalism movement, and yet, the problem of uniting a new nation seems comparatively easier because a nation has a delineated geography and a visible colonial presence.

Building on this body of literature is literature related to a growing interest in identity within Japan studies itself. Texts within this frame include Marilyn Ivy's (1995) *Discourses of the Vanishing*, Michael Weiner's (1997) *Japan's Minorities: The Illusion of Homogeneity*, William Kelly's (1986, 1990, 1993) various articles on identity and process in Japan, and Dorinne Kondo's (1990) work on Japanese identity as constructed within a frame of gender and power. All index the mechanisms by which one's identity as Japanese is narrated as homogenous, yet the actual workings of identity carefully interact with systems such as power, age, and gender.

Postscript

The Japanese Deaf community has a relatively short history compared to the United States or Europe. Although my ASL tutor in Connecticut can point out with pride that she is a sixth-generation Deaf person (with a daughter who is also Deaf), even second-generation Deaf-of-Deaf are rare in Japan, and those who have passed JSL down as an inheritance are even fewer. Consequently, the deaf community in Japan is only three or four generations deep, and the political and social changes of the 20th century have fragmented the community along age lines. In a way, Deaf communities in Japan are not only young, having a still thin lineage, but also very old, having weathered the profound effect that mainstreaming has had over the past 20 years.

Acknowledgments

This chapter is based on my dissertation field research on Japanese deaf identities (Nakamura 2001). The author would like to thank the organizations that made her research possible: the Wenner Gren Foundation for Anthropological Studies, Small Grant (#6144); a dissertation research fellowship from the Yale Council on East Asian Studies; the Social Science Research Council; and a research internship at the Japanese Federation of the Deaf. She also greatly appreciates the kind support and encouragement from the Japanese Federation of the Deaf and all of its members and staff, especially the executive board and the Tokyo office of the JFD. Finally, she would like to thank the many informants who have contributed to this research project.

Notes

1.   This view is, of course, a postmodern perspective on identity strongly associated with the works of Michel Foucault (1973, 1979, 1990) and Judith Butler (1990). This chapter will not deal explicitly with the notion of power in the creation of deaf and hearing identi-

ties. For an excellent example of how race (another category we often consider natural) has been constructed within anthropology, popular understanding, and the law, see Braman (1999).

2.   My name, Karen, is both a Japanese and American name; but I was alternately seen as either Japanese or American. My informants and I both emphasized either my Japanese or my American aspect, depending on the situation, and this behavior often created a struggle for me to negotiate my cultural identity.

3.   The 1-hand-ear-to-mouth is signed the same way as in ASL and several other European sign languages. I would hazard a guess that this sign and the variant, 5-hand-ear-to-mouth, are the result of adoption of ASL and other forms into the deaf community. This analysis is reinforced by the observation that older (>70-year-old) Japanese deaf people do not use the ASL-like ear-to-mouth form, rather, sign *roua* by bringing both hands to the ear and mouth simultaneously (see figure 11.1).

4.   As a historical side note, when the Japanese colonized Taiwan (1895–1945) and Korea (1910–1945) in the early part of the last century, one of the many changes was the establishment of Japanese-style schools. The regular schools taught the students Japanese whereas Japanese Sign Language was evidently used in the schools for the deaf. Even now, many older, hearing Koreans and Taiwanese can still speak Japanese while the signed languages used in Korea and Taiwan remain heavily influenced by JSL, enough so that they are still mutually intelligible.

5.   In addition to the private schools, historical evidence indicates *teragoya* or temple schools in the Meiji period that taught deaf and blind students. Not much is known about the existence of these schools (e.g., number of schools, pupils, teaching methods).

6.   Interpreters in Japan are not usually taught what is called "traditional sign language" (*dentoutekishuwa*) but only how to sign while simultaneously mouthing the sentences, what we would call SimCom, Manually Signed English, or pidgin sign in the United States. Thus, they have difficulty understanding the older generation of signers.

7.   The teachers are caught in a conundrum. Clearly, a student from a deaf high school in Japan would have an extremely difficult time successfully getting into a good college. The high schools for the deaf are often two to three years behind the hearing schools, and they do not do exam preparation. Japanese colleges do not have any sort of affirmative action for students. They judge them by only their written and oral test scores. And Japanese schools are not required by law to provide interpreters. Although, clearly, an overhaul of the educational system is needed (for many more reasons than just the deaf students), the best advice would be to encourage students to make the decisions that lead to the best opportunities, even if those decisions are not necessarily best for the larger picture of deaf cultural development or deaf political activism. This situation appears similar to the situation facing resident Korean students in Japan (Ryang 1997).

8.   Other factors behind the push to mainstreaming are that, after kindergarten, children have picked up some degree of speech skills, they want (or their parents pressure them) to attend a primary school that is closer to their own homes where their neighborhood friends are. Also, many children do not have a positive impression of schools for the deaf (especially if speech skills are forcibly taught at a young age), and they want to leave as soon as they can. The Nara School (see later text), which does not teach speech skills until the primary school level, does not have this attrition problem.

9.   The law does not stipulate what positions these employees must be in or what their working conditions must be. It also does not concern itself with the type of disability. Many companies bypass the quotas by hiring many disabled part-timers or by employing them in only low-level clerical jobs. The fines for not meeting the quota are so low that many companies simply opt to pay the fine rather than deal with hiring disabled employees. Japan has no equivalent of the Americans with Disabilities Act, which mandates an equalization of job opportunities regardless of disability status.

10.   The homonym can be confusing: an elderly deaf person is a *rou-rou-jin*. In English, a similar confusion occurs around "death" and "deaf."

11.   One major component of the exam for kindergarten teachers is the ability to sing and play the piano.

12.   In contrast, D-Pro accuses the JFD of being left-wing communists (which may be closer to the mark than JFD leaders want to acknowledge).

13.   For example, a hearing teacher at a school for the deaf in Tokyo has noted that, although a residential facility for deaf children used to have its own particular name sign of arbitrary origins, younger students are starting to use a new name sign based on the kanji spelling of the facility. The origin of the new name sign appears to be the hearing teachers themselves.

REFERENCES

Anderson, Benedict. 1983. *Imagined communities: Reflections on the origin and spread of nationalism.* London: Verso.

Appadurai, Arjun, and Carol A. Breckenridge. 1988. Why public culture? *Public Culture* 1 (1):5–10.

Balibar, Etienne, and Immanuel Wallerstein. 1991. *Race, nation, class: Ambiguous identities.* London: Verso.

Bhabha, Homi K. 1993. *The location of culture.* London: Routledge.

Braman, Donald. 1999. Of race and immutability. *UCLA Law Review* 45 (5):1375–463.

Butler, Judith, ed. 1990. *Gender trouble: Feminism and the subversion of identity.* New York: Routledge.

Comaroff, Jean, and John Comaroff, eds. 1993. *Modernity and its malcontents: Ritual and power in postcolonial Africa.* Chicago: University of Chicago Press.

Foucault, Michel. 1973. *The birth of the clinic: An archaeology of medical perception.* Translated by A. M. Sheridan Smith. New York: Vintage Books.

———. 1979. *Discipline and punish: The birth of the prison.* Translated by Alan Sheridan. New York: Vintage Books.

———. 1990. *The history of sexuality.* Vol. 1, *An introduction.* Translated by Robert Hurley. New York: Vintage Books.

Ivy, Marilyn. 1995. *Discourses of the vanishing: Modernity, phantasm, Japan.* Chicago: University of Chicago Press.

Japanese Federation of the Deaf. 1996. *Kaigi shiryoushuu I* (Conference resource material, Vol. I). Prepared for the 44th Annual All-Japan Deaf Meeting and 45th Annual Board Members Meeting, June 13–16, Matsuyama City, Aichi Prefecture. Tokyo: Japanese Federation of the Deaf.

Kegl, Judy. 1994. The Nicaraguan Sign Language project: An overview. *Signpost* 7 (1):24–31.

Kelly, William W. 1986. Rationalization and nostalgia: Cultural dynamics of new middle-class Japan. *American Ethnologist* 13 (4):603–18.

———. 1990. Japanese No-Noh: The crosstalk of public culture in a rural festival. *Public Culture* 2 (2):65–81.

———. 1993. Finding a place in metropolitan Japan: Ideologies, institutions, and everyday life. In *Postwar Japan as history,* ed. Andrew Gordon, 189–217. Berkeley: University of California Press.

Kondo, Dorinne K. 1990. *Crafting selves: Power, gender, and discourses of identity in a Japanese workplace.* Chicago: University of Chicago Press.

Lane, Harlan. 1992. *The mask of benevolence: Disabling the deaf community.* New York: Knopf.

Lane, Harlan, ed. 1976. *The deaf experience: Classics in language and education.* Cambridge, Mass.: Harvard University Press.

———. 1984. *When the mind hears: A history of the deaf.* New York: Random House.

Melucci, Alberto. 1980. The new social movements: A theoretical approach. *Social Science Information* 19 (2):199–226.

Ministry of Health and Welfare, Disability Insurance and Welfare Group. 1998. *Heisei 10-nen shintaishougaiji jittaichousa oyobi shintaishougaisha jittaichousa no gaiyou ni tsuite* (1998 Report on the status of disabled children and adults). White paper dated July 2. Tokyo: Ministry of Health and Welfare.

Morris, Aldon D., and Carol McClurg Mueller, eds. 1992. *Frontiers in social movement theory.* New Haven, Conn.: Yale University Press.

Nakamura Karen. 2001. Deaf identities, sign languages, and minority social movement politics in modern Japan (1868–2000). Ph.D. diss., Yale University.

Parasnis, Ila, ed. 1996. *Cultural and language diversity and the deaf experience.* New York: Cambridge University Press.

Ryang, Sonia. 1997. *North Koreans in Japan: Language, ideology, and identity.* Boulder, Colo.: Westview.

Senghas, Richard J., and Judy Kegl. 1994. Social considerations in the emergence of Idioma de Signos Nicaraguense (Nicaraguan Sign Language). *Signpost* 7 (1):40–46.

Weiner, Michael, ed. 1997. *Japan's minorities: The illusion of homogeneity.* New York: Routledge.

Wilcox, Sherman. 1989. *American deaf culture: An anthology.* Silver Spring, Md.: Linstok Press.

12 The Chiying School of Taiwan: A Foreigner's Perspective

Jean Ann

My route to studying sign language in Taiwan was roundabout. I began learning American Sign Language (ASL) in 1977. In the mid-1980s, I spent a year in Beijing, China, teaching English as a foreign language. As a graduate student in linguistics several years later, I decided to write my doctoral dissertation on the phonology and phonetics of signed language in use in Beijing. But by 1989, the People's Republic of China was in political turmoil. The Tian An Men Square massacre made a return to China difficult. Searching for an alternative field site, I recalled the unique history of a school for the deaf in Kaohsiung, Taiwan.[1] The Chiying School, founded by Chiang Ssu Nung, a deaf man originally from mainland China, had used the Chinese Sign Language (CSL) as a medium of instruction for many years while Taiwan's other schools for the deaf used Taiwan Sign Language (TSL) (Yau 1977, 7; Chao, Chu and Liu 1988, 9–10; Smith 1989, 1–2). Circumstances seemed to have conspired to create a living archive of CSL in Taiwan.

Taiwan is an island that lies off the southeastern coast of mainland China. For the last 500 years, it has been populated by Chinese immigrants and by a long-standing local population. Taiwan was occupied by Japan from 1895 to 1945, returning to Chinese control after the Sino-Japanese War. Chinese Nationalist Party leaders and followers fled to Taiwan in 1949 when the Communists took over mainland China. Ever since, the island has been estranged from the mainland.

Kaohsiung is Taiwan's third largest city and is situated on its southwestern coast. It is the industrial center of Taiwan and, throughout the 1990s, had supported one of Taiwan's largest economies. In the Tsoying area of Kaohsiung is the Chiying Private Elementary School for the Deaf. Like many schools for the deaf, the Chiying School occupies a position of great importance in the history of the deaf community in Taiwan. To my delight, the Chiying School agreed that I could visit for nearly five months to gather Chinese Sign Language data. A dissertation grant from the American Council of Learned Societies financed the project.

During the course of gathering data for my work in linguistics at the Chiying

School, I enjoyed sustained contact with deaf children who boarded there and with deaf staff members. In addition, I came into frequent contact with the deaf and hearing friends, acquaintances, and family members of these people. My observations from this time form the basis of this chapter. Though some of what follows is based on actions or conversations caught on videotape, most of it is based on the notes I took as I came to know, sometimes through formal interviews and sometimes through more casual conversation, the people who were part of the Chiying School in the early 1990s. The period of time that I spent at the Chiying School might be described as a temporary fusion of individuals from disparate worlds: deaf people who had long been deeply connected to the Chiying School, to Kaohsiung, and to Taiwan and a curious stranger who was neither Taiwanese nor deaf.

THE CHIYING SCHOOL IN THE EARLY 1990S

THE PHYSICAL APPEARANCE OF THE CHIYING SCHOOL

The two-story school was constructed largely of cement. It was roughly U-shaped, with classrooms, dining area, and dormitory space on two wings and the administrative offices on the other. There were a few air conditioners and fans in various locations, and an old automatic washer. Some of the classrooms were carpeted, and the teachers and students entered those classrooms without their "slippers"—plastic or rubber sandal-like footwear. Most of the classrooms had prominently placed televisions and VCRs. The school owned a computer, which one or two teachers used regularly.

The school had a well-worn appearance that bespoke a proud but difficult history. The privately controlled and funded Chiying School was indeed struggling, and this struggle was not the first financial challenge it had faced (Smith 1999). Its current travails, I learned, contrasted the situations of the better-funded government-run schools for the deaf in the other Taiwanese cities of Taipei, Tainan, and Taichung. The Chiying School somehow continued its work in the face of difficulties. The school was apparently known for accepting and attempting to educate some of the most unfortunate of Taiwan's children.

THE SETUP OF THE CLASSES

The Chiying School began as a school for the deaf, but over the years, enrollment of deaf students had declined, necessitating that the school also accept developmentally disabled students. Everyone in the school—members of the administration, staff members, and students themselves—perceived the deaf students as having very different educational needs from the developmentally disabled students, who, thus, were taught in separate classrooms and on separate floors. The deaf students were often scandalized by some of the behavior of the developmentally disabled children and were blunt about their disapproval. However, the deaf children seemed to take the view that the developmentally disabled children were not as responsible for their behavior as they themselves would have been.

Smith (1999) reports that about 100 students per year enrolled at Chiying in the 1970s. The school that I saw in the early 1990s greatly resembled his description of the school in the 1970s, except for the fact that, by the 1990s, enrollment had gone down to about 65–75. The Chiying School offered classes for deaf children and developmentally disabled children from first to sixth grade. Occasionally, students who were much older than the appropriate age for the grade appeared in the classrooms. Several of the deaf staff people told me about friends and acquaintances who had, for example, begun school at age 13 and graduated from sixth grade at age 19. Ten to 15 students boarded at the school during the time that I was there; perhaps another 55 to 60 children from the Kaohsiung area commuted to the Chiying School daily. Some students took a bus sent out by the school, and others arrived at the school by means of public buses and alternate means of transportation. Many of the people in the Tsoying area, such as shop owners, were familiar with the school, partially because over the years, the school had maintained a bakery that supplied baked goods to eating establishments in the area.

When I was at the Chiying School, both deaf and hearing teachers worked there, which, I was told, had been the case since the school's inception. In fact, the descriptions of the faculty compositions at not only the Chiying School but also the other schools that Chiang Ssu Nung established suggest that this situation was typical (Smith 1999).[2] The Chiying School apparently took care of its own, hiring some graduates for positions such as teachers and bakers. Over the weeks, as I met the people at the school, I observed that all of them had a conscious appreciation for Chiang Ssu Nung's contribution to deaf life with the establishment of the Chiying School. Although they did not see him regularly or often, they seemed to feel respect and fondness for him.

LANGUAGE AT THE CHIYING SCHOOL

A visitor to the Chiying School is struck immediately by the fact that signing is the preferred mode of communication there. Closer inspection also reveals linguistic diversity.

LANGUAGE USE DURING THE CHIYING SCHOOL'S DISTANT PAST

The Japanese are believed to be the first Asians to formally educate their deaf citizens (Hodgson 1953, 267). The 50-year Japanese occupation of Taiwan from 1895 to 1945 is important to deaf history in Taiwan because, during this time, the two schools for the deaf were established in Tainan and Taipei. The Tainan school was set up in 1915 and was staffed with teachers from Tokyo. The Taipei school, set up in 1917, was staffed with teachers from Osaka. The teachers from Japan "used their respective dialects of Japanese Sign Language in their classrooms" (Chao, Chu, and Liu 1988, 9; Smith 1989, 1). That language, which originated in Japan and which took hold in Taiwan through the schools for the deaf in Tainan and Taipei, is today known as TSL.

Chiang Ssu Nung left mainland China in 1949 (Smith 1999) when the communists took over and, like many refugees, he settled in Taiwan. When he arrived in Taiwan, he established a school for the deaf in Keelung, Taiwan, that lasted less than a year.[3] Chiang then moved south to Kaohsiung and established the Chiying School (Chao, Chu, and Liu 1988, 9; Smith 1999).

TSL was entrenched in the schools for the deaf by the time Chiang Ssu Nung arrived in Taiwan. But Chiang, who was late-deafened and had learned to sign in the Shanghai area (Smith 1999), neither knew nor cared to know TSL.[4] He preferred to use the Chinese signs as a medium of instruction in his schools.[5] Deaf children in Tainan and Taipei learned TSL throughout their schooling, but the children who attended the Chiying School used only CSL during their elementary school years. When they graduated, some went on to middle school in Tainan and learned TSL (Chao, Chu, and Liu 1988, 7). I met some of these former students at the Chiying School during the early 1990s. To my knowledge, they always produced TSL, but they continued to understand CSL.[6] I also met signers who did not attend middle school and, so, did not have to learn TSL in school. Some of them still sign CSL, and some learned TSL on their own.

In Taiwan, a high school education was the highest level to which most deaf people could aspire; higher education has always eluded deaf Taiwanese. A discussion I had with a consultant revealed her genuine shock that I had a Deaf American professor on my dissertation committee.

LANGUAGE USE DURING THE CHIYING SCHOOL'S RECENT PAST

The tradition of using CSL as a medium of instruction remained in place at the Chiying School until sometime in the late 1970s or early 1980s when the school changed over to TSL. In a conversation I had with Wayne Smith in 1999, he recalled seeing teachers from the Chiying School use CSL at a conference in Taipei in 1980. Neither Chiang Ssu Nung nor Jennifer, his daughter, elaborated on the reasons for the change with me. I sensed that the change was not a particularly welcome one. Although the Chiying School was private, in 1991, Smith surmised that the school changed from CSL to TSL "under pressure from the provincial government."

By the time I arrived in Kaohsiung in the early 1990s, Chiang Ssu Nung had essentially retired and was living most of the time in Taipei. Although all the Chiying deaf people whom I met had learned CSL at the school when they were young, the changing times and evolving deaf community in Kaohsiung and Tainan had dislodged CSL, and, in the 1990s, it was a somewhat distantly remembered part of their linguistic lives. Few of the people I knew used it exclusively or even mostly, but it was remembered somewhat affectionately.

Although I had come to Taiwan in search of CSL, these circumstances suggested that I would need to change my research focus to TSL. In principle, the CSL signers at Chiying were willing to help me locate other CSL signers, but they conceded that the endeavor would be difficult. They told me that the few CSL signers in close proximity were older deaf people or people unaccustomed to and uninterested in the idea that they could serve as linguistic consultants for research on their language. Some of the Chiying CSL signers were willing in spirit but, for various reasons, not able to serve as consultants for my research themselves. In the end, I did not push my original agenda of finding CSL signers, which seemed to be a great relief to the Chiying CSL signers. In contrast, the Chiying TSL signers were noticeably interested in and, perhaps, a bit bemused by the idea that I would ask them to serve as linguistic consultants.

Taiwan's Linguistic Variation

Given the long tradition, indeed historical bias, of geographic region named as a major marker of linguistic variation (Wardhaugh 1998), it is not surprising that the literature reports two dialects of TSL, one centered around the school in Taipei and one centered around the school in Tainan. The literature contains little direct evidence to support this claim; the differences between the two dialects are reported to be lexical (Smith 1989, 1; Chao, Chu, and Liu 1988, 9–10). However, given the historical facts, we might expect to find morphological and syntactic differences between Chiying TSL and Taipei/Tainan TSL. In fact, there is some evidence that this is the case.

Smith's work on TSL is based on data he gathered largely from Taipei signers, with a few from Tainan (Wayne Smith, 1991, personal communication). My work is based on data I gathered at the Chiying School. I can report two pieces of evidence that suggest that Chiying signers use a slightly different system than the Taipei/Tainan signers Smith describes. First, Smith explains that the Taipei/Tainan signers have agreement verbs that mark gender of subject or object and number of subject or object (1989, 1990). Consider the following examples. In figure 12.1, the extended pinky on the weak hand serves as the object of the verb TELL. TELL is articulated with the strong hand. Figure 12.2 shows how the idea "tell the two of them" would be expressed. In figure 12.2, the weak hand assumes the handshape for the number two, while the strong hand articulates the verb TELL.

The Chiying signers mark the gender of subject and object on verbs the same way that other TSL signers do, so the sign in figure 12.1 was acceptable to them. However, the Chiying signers rejected expressions like that in figure 12.2. Though other TSL signers can inflect the weak hand's handshape for number, the Chiying signers cannot. For them, the way to express the idea "tell the two of them" is for the strong hand to articulate the verb twice while the weak hand maintains a handshape not marked for number.

Second, TSL has been analyzed as having three auxiliaries called Aux 1, Aux 2 and Aux 11 (Smith 1989, Smith 1990). Aux 1, the most frequent, looks like a point from location x to location y. Aux 2 looks like the TSL sign KAN (SEE). Aux 11 looks like the TSL sign DUI YU (MEET) (Smith 1989, Smith 1990).[7] Although the

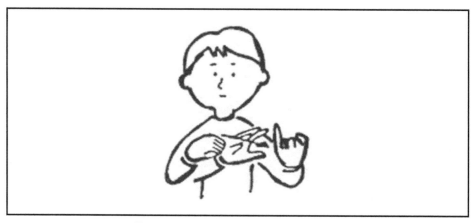

Figure 12.1 TELL HER **(Smith 1989, 175)**

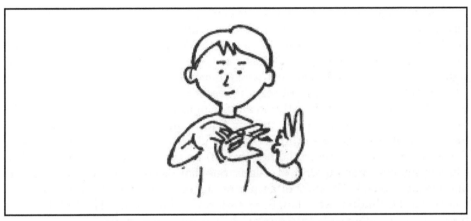

FIGURE 12.2 TELL THE TWO OF THEM **(Smith 1989, 194)**

Chiying signers regularly used Aux 2 and Aux 11, I did not observe nor could I elicit Aux 1. When I asked directly if Aux 1 was possible, all of the Chiying TSL signers were certain that it was not (Ann 1998). Clearly many questions remain about TSL dialects.

ATTITUDES TOWARD LANGUAGE: WRITTEN CHINESE, SIGNED MANDARIN, AND TSL

As a signer of ASL as a second language, I had a sense of what communicating in a visual language is like, how my hearing interferes with aspects of learning a sign language, and how I might best learn a new sign language. Armed with this knowledge, I was a ready student of TSL. But the Chiying deaf people, who hold the Chinese language in high esteem, seemed convinced that I had come to the school to interact in some way with the hearing people there, for example, as an English teacher. My real purpose was not understood until later and was always regarded, I sensed, to be a bit absurd. After all, as the Chiying deaf people asked me point blank, who would come halfway around the world to learn TSL and interact with them? In the beginning, then, as I would try to engage the Chiying deaf adults and children in TSL conversation, they would try to help me with my written Chinese characters. For example, if I asked about a particular sign, people seemed to think I was asking them to show me the Chinese characters for the word. But I showed little interest and less promise in practicing my characters, and day by day, I was learning to articulate my thoughts more clearly in signs, so the Chiying deaf people eventually gave up using written characters with me.

Although linguistic and cultural issues occupy a central place in the lives of many Deaf Americans, the same could not be said about the situation among Taiwanese deaf people, according to what I saw at the Chiying School. The Chiying deaf people considered the views and preferences of the hearing world to be important and certainly dominant. Despite this view, the tacit understanding was that deaf people also had their own needs and concerns. These needs would simply not be addressed by society, but that issue seemed to be an entirely different matter to them.

The notion of Signed Mandarin was expressed in TSL by a one-handed sign that could be roughly described as placing Chinese characters in space one by one from top to bottom. Because of the way the Chiying deaf people defined the sign for me, I eventually glossed it as SIGNING-THE-CHARACTERS-IN-ORDER. TSL signers sometimes rolled their eyes when they mentioned SIGNING-THE-CHARAC-TERS-IN-ORDER, but they did not seem to resent it. SIGNING-THE-CHARACTERS-IN-ORDER was not positive or negative in an ideological sense. Rather, people's slight impatience with it had to do with it being "slow" and "tiring." I rarely saw more than stock phrases expressed in Signed Mandarin among the Chiying signers. The Mandarin phrase "return home" (huì jiā) was one of these expressions. The Chiying signers signed it with two signs: one that meant "return" and a second that meant "home." The only other use of Signed Mandarin that I encountered was when the children were taught to perform a signed song. The Chiying deaf people never used SIGNING-THE-CHARACTERS-IN-ORDER with me.

As would be expected, the Chiying deaf people had no understanding of the ASL fingerspelled expression T-S-L. They referred to their way of signing with one another using two different ways. One was a two-handed sign that I glossed as SIGNING-THE-CHARACTERS-OUT-OF-ORDER, based on the way they explained the meaning of the sign to me. I glossed the other as CONDENSE. They considered SIGNING-THE-CHARACTERS-OUT-OF-ORDER to be clear and fast from the standpoint of both production and perception. They did not seem particularly enamored of their language or loyal to it in a philosophical sense. Rather, SIGNING-THE-CHAR-ACTERS-OUT-OF-ORDER was simply the most economical way to communicate and was the agreed-on way in the community.

One might question how much agreement exists with respect to sign use. The Chiying signers could often come up with as many as four to seven signs for the same referent without trouble. In fact, deaf people from both Kaohsiung and Tai-pei told me that an abundance of synonymous signs was in use.[8] Smith (1976, revised 1988) discusses the same phenomenon. The Ministry of Education in Tai-wan is aware of the proliferation of local signs throughout Taiwan, and through the years, the government has attempted to standardize TSL. The Chiying deaf people seemed to feel a need for standardization and wanted, at least in principle, to cooperate with the government's attempts. On several occasions, I observed deaf teachers advise the students to use a sign in one of the sign language manu-als compiled by the government rather than a sign the child picked up from one of the teachers.

Perhaps in some deaf communities, hearing people and foreigners would be looked at with some suspicion. I did not perceive this to be the case at the Chiying School. In fact, my circumstances were certainly a language learner's paradise, although the challenge of communicating with a well-intentioned but foreign guest did affect the conversations that the Chiying deaf people had with me. At some point during my stay there, they began to consider me an actual participant in some conversations, despite my obvious inability to be completely independent in my signed discourse. And often, they seemed to feel a responsibility to include me as much as I wanted to be included. They checked to see whether or not I had understood and were often willing to rephrase what was said in ways they knew I would understand better. Fast and fluent conversation sometimes slowed appre-ciably on my behalf.

Many deaf people at the school were adept at more than one language and were observant about linguistic matters. For example, after seeing several ASL name signs, including mine, the Chiying deaf signers decided that name signs in ASL often involved the fingerspelled letter that represented the initial. Then, they explained to me that name signs in TSL often referred to physical characteristics of a person such as "eyes that wander" or "tall woman" or "scar on the head" (see Yau and He, 1989, for similar observations about name signs in a school for the deaf in southern China).

And although the Chiying deaf people acknowledged that SIGNING-THE-CHARACTERS-IN-ORDER and SIGNING-THE-CHARACTERS-OUT-OF-ORDER were two very different ways of signing, they sometimes would claim they were using Signed Mandarin when they were actually using TSL but signing slowly. Similarly, fast signing was labeled as TSL even if it was Signed Mandarin. The Chiying deaf people sometimes claimed that Signed Mandarin and TSL were distributed according to geography. They might assert, for example, that signers from Tainan "signed the characters in order" whereas Kaohsiung signers "signed the characters out of order." Out of all Taiwan's signers, I was once told, Taipei signers were the best at "signing the characters out of order." They also shared other similar theories. These statements were rarely consistent and reflected fleeting impressions rather than reasoned generalizations that were based on data analysis. However, as research continues on TSL, we might find truths about regional variation beyond Smith's (1989) claims.

THE PEOPLE AT THE CHIYING SCHOOL

This section describes both the children and the adults I came to know the best. To protect the privacy of the people I write about, each person's name has been rendered as a single letter followed by a long dash, and some identifying characteristics have been changed.

THE CHIYING STUDENTS

The children, mostly boys, except one girl who was developmentally disabled, ranged in age from about 7 to 16. The older deaf boys were the clear leaders whereas the younger deaf boys and all the developmentally disabled children were the followers. A few of the students had a deaf parent, but most were the only deaf member of hearing families. During the time that I was there, one deaf boy's hearing father removed him from the school for 30 days in an attempt to cure his deafness with Chinese medicine. When the boy returned to school, he was still deaf. A few students had strong hearing or deaf families who cared deeply for them. But a significant number came to attend the Chiying School through circumstances that seemed reflective of relations between deaf and hearing people in general, ranging from benign neglect to abuse. Some had been dropped off years before by unstable families who rarely, if ever, visited. Others were found abandoned and brought to the Chiying School.

All of the children had energy to spare, and almost all were boisterous. Their lives, from my perspective, revolved around playing. Playing involved forming a group of eight to ten, a great deal of physical contact among those in the group, and the constant movement of the group around school premises. Although the boys tickled one another mercilessly, tackled one another to the floor on a regular basis, and seemed to infuriate one another often, they rarely hurt one another intentionally. A hard of hearing child who wore a hearing aid, was not a fluent signer, and had negative attitudes toward signing was more of a target than any of the deaf boys. The deaf boys called the hard of hearing child by the sign TING REN (hearing person).[9]

THE CHIYING STAFF

Both deaf and hearing teachers and staff members worked at the Chiying School. A hearing woman called "*obasan*" (aunt) prepared breakfast and dinner for the boarders as well as lunch for all the children. She also laundered the boarders' clothes. Her title was one of the many signs of Japanese influence in Taiwan; *obasan* is a Japanese word used to refer to a housekeeper. Obasan clearly cared about the deaf students, and her conversation with them was sparsely peppered with signs.

T———'s precise job at the school was unclear to me, but he seemed to serve as an all-around caretaker and administrator. He became deaf at age 7 and began first grade at the Chiying School at age 14. After graduation, he continued to work for the school and had worked there ever since. When I met him, he was in his early 50s, animated, and fun. His life up till then had spanned a number of hard years in Taiwan. As a child, he had known poverty, and when I met him, he talked of younger people (who had grown up in a richer, more modern Taiwan) not understanding his struggles to survive back then as a poor man and as a deaf man. The toil of his young adulthood yielded better times. He eventually became reasonably financially secure, married, and had children.

T———'s linguistic repertoire included both sign and spoken languages. He subscribed to the belief that CSL was preferable to TSL. He seemed to be a fluent signer of CSL, and though he understood TSL, he did not produce it. The TSL signers and T——— conversed often. A frequent observer of these interactions, I thought that TSL signers produced TSL and understood CSL, and that T——— produced CSL and understood TSL. All of the Chiying deaf people said this method was exactly how T——— and the TSL signers communicated. (Things were a bit different when the Chiying TSL signers saw Chiang Ssu Nung. Despite the fact that CSL had essentially fallen into disuse in the community at large, the Chiying TSL signers said they either had to remember their CSL signs or simply not communicate with Chiang.)

In addition, before T——— became deaf, he was a speaker of Taiwanese and also knew some Japanese. I saw him use both languages in a few circumstances, for example, with hearing people who could not sign, when he had not established eye contact with a hearing person, or when he believed a hearing person would not understand his signing. Several times, after sessions with me lasting more than an hour, he spoke with Jennifer in Taiwanese. A patient and excellent communicator, he seemed determined to establish a channel of communication with whomever he pleased regardless of any differences in linguistic backgrounds. When his interlocutor was less energetic or creative than he was, he took on the burden of the extra work enthusiastically—freely making use of mime, gesture, CSL, some TSL, and his spoken languages. The consequence was that nonsigners and signers who were not fluent understood what he was saying almost in spite of themselves. Though T—— was the first deaf person to spend a significant amount of time with me, I saw him regularly only at the beginning of my stay at the school. When his responsibilities beckoned him elsewhere, I turned toward other members of the Chiying School's deaf community.

When I met him, F—— was a teacher at the school in his early 30s. He had been born deaf into a family with only one other deaf relative. He had been educated at the Chiying School and then attended middle school and high school in Tainan, so he had learned CSL first and then TSL. He said that both languages were part of him but that he regularly used TSL and not CSL because not many people understood CSL. By all accounts, he read and wrote Chinese well. He seemed to be a successful student of languages; he had learned some written Japanese in childhood, which he used when the occasion called for it.[10] F—— seemed endlessly interested when I used a fingerspelled word or a sign from ASL. On these occasions, he often learned the sign and signed it back to me in other contexts, assuming I would be amused. I never heard F—— speak a word of any language.

Though I was able to chat one on one with the deaf people around the school, it was difficult or impossible to participate in discussions in which people were signing but not directly to me. However, I wanted to take advantage of every chance to learn as much TSL as possible, so when I lost the thread of the conversation, I would get someone's attention and ask for help. In so doing, I routinely tried to focus my questions on a specific sign rather than a general topic. Further, I decided not to depend on one person all the time. I intuited from my experience at the school that doing so might suggest that I was more confident in a particular person than in the community at large and that this would not be acceptable. Apparently I was wrong; most of the deaf people seemed to feel that it took special talents to deal with me. For weeks, everyone I questioned would hesitate a moment before beginning to answer and then suddenly turn to or summon F——. "She doesn't understand GONG (public)," they'd say. "Explain to her." F—— was able, effortlessly it seemed, to construct the perfect canonical scenario to make the meaning of the sign obvious to me. So it came to be that for most of my stay at Chiying, F—— was considered the person who could get through to me, no matter what.

F—— radiated a confidence in himself as a deaf person that was unique among the people I met. He never talked of being hearing or what life might be like if he were a hearing person. He seemed not only to accept but also to cherish his deafness, to have the sense that it was not a bit regrettable to be deaf. He appeared to attach no great importance to the fact that, as a deaf person, he was a member of a minority. F—— talked of opportunities as though he had access to them and not at all as though they were unattainable. I had the sense that, although F—— knew perfectly well what the world would offer him as a deaf man, in small ways each day, he simply refused to accept it. F——'s attitudes were neither motivated nor reinforced by a politically active deaf community around him. They seemed simply to be a part of his nature. And, in fact, he was relatively successful in gaining some of society's advantages.

As a linguistic consultant, F—— was superior. He had intuitions about TSL that he discussed easily with me. More than any other person I worked with, he seemed after a short time to know what I wanted when I asked him "linguist" questions. When he taught, the children were rapt. They asked questions and participated fully in their lessons. F——— seemed well suited for the job of teacher because he understood what his students (including me) knew and pushed them forward from there.

W——— was a baker at the school. Intelligent, reserved and hard working, he did not bring too much attention to himself. He had learned CSL at the Chiying School as a child and then had acquired TSL as a middle school student in Tainan. If at first W——— was somewhat hesitant to deal with me, he quickly became both an expert at that task and one of the people who greatly supported my work while I was at Chiying. For example, when other deaf people would want a chance to sign on videotape but were not sure how to do so, W——— would patiently explain what I wanted and stay around long enough to make sure the person truly understood and got off to a good start.

The community I came to know at the Chiying School was larger. However, these descriptions introduce some of the people with whom I interacted at the Chiying School and provide a sense of the key people who contributed to my research.

Social Constructions of Deafness and Hearing

In many societies, "disabilities" such as deafness are hidden from view because they are not the norm and are, therefore, negative (see Tsuchiya 1994, 65). In Taiwanese society, young deaf adults (and people with other "disabilities") who have never been to school are still sometimes discovered.[11] At worst, hearing society in Taiwan seems to view deaf people as lawless and uneducable; at best, pitiful and incompetent. Certainly, I sensed that nearly every Taiwanese person believed on some significant level that deafness is at least a somewhat negative attribute. In this section, I focus on how the deaf and hearing people in the Chiying School saw deafness and hearing.

Deaf People's Attitudes about Deafness

Although deafness often "creates unique social groupings and identities," the mere fact that deaf people have a particular audiological status does not necessarily cause them to cohere into a social unit (Johnson 1994, 102). Although many sorts of relationships could be found among the Chiying deaf people, they did not seem to primarily help or socialize with other deaf people. Hearing family members were often involved with supporting deaf people. Deaf people probably socialized as much with hearing people as with other deaf people.

Although the Chiying deaf people were not explicit about this, they believe that to be born deaf is less desirable than to be born hearing and become deaf later. Certainly, someone who was born deaf would prefer to marry a hearing person, a hard of hearing person, or a deaf person who had been born hearing. This preference was related to the fear that deafness might be passed on to one's children if one were born deaf. Most of the deaf people I met described themselves as "born hearing and became deaf in childhood because of a fever."

Despite the oppressive treatment of society, the Chiying deaf people seem to regard their deafness more as an inconvenience that could be dealt with than as a tragedy. But I sensed that the views of deaf children and deaf adults were different. If asked directly whether deafness was a positive or negative thing, the children's faces registered surprise—apparently, at the question. "Of course it's bad!" they signed. Although the children permitted me, with great enthusiasm, to videotape them playing, they unequivocally refused my requests to videotape them signing. I wondered why they did not want to appear on videotape answering my off-camera questions or even having signed conversations with each other.

I asked one of the teachers whether the children would consider their signing on videotape to be a display of a disability and, therefore, an embarrassment. The teacher laughed off this suggestion and offered another explanation. Taiwanese children are not used to being experts, he said. For them, adults are experts. The idea that I might ask them something that they might not know how to answer would involve a great loss of face. Even assuming that I left them to talk with one another while taping them, knowing what to talk about presented problems, particularly if I were to ask them about something they said. It was safer for them to avoid the whole issue by not getting involved at all.

The adults had somewhat contradictory attitudes about their deafness. A few deaf people said they deeply regretted not being able to speak. One man, visibly moved, told me that only some students, those who had residual hearing, had opportunities for speech training in childhood. He had not been among them. Throughout his whole education, no one had attempted at any time to teach him to speak; he had signed from the beginning at the Chiying School. But most deaf people seemed to have no particular interest in hearing or speech. Its utility as a means of communication notwithstanding, it simply had nothing to do with their lives. It had long been recognized and accepted that, for some deaf people, speech training served no practical purpose; it was simply too much effort for scanty results. According to a conversation I had with Yau Shun Chiu in 1991, this view is also prevalent in mainland China.

With the onus of learning to speak lifted from the shoulders of deaf students, one might imagine that the Chiying School, if not the educational system, would have actually fostered a cohesive and strong deaf community, intended or not. That community, we might imagine, might have great pride in its own natural sign language and even, perhaps, not much regard for what was going on in the hearing world. In fact, I did not observe this. The educational system, set up for hearing children and merely adapted to the needs of deaf children, and the constant contact with hearing families ensure that hearing people and their concerns are always a factor in deaf life in Taiwan. In general, deaf people seemed to defer their own communicative needs to the needs or perceived needs of the hearing people around them.

One of the deaf people with whom I shared a collegial and friendly relationship invited me to visit his hearing family. At their home, his nonsigning family members and I communicated in a mixture of spoken English and spoken Mandarin. I felt the need to try to sign at least the gist of what I was saying so I would not exclude my deaf consultant. He seemed content enough to read my signs and know approximately what was being said. However, with my unequal abilities in English, Mandarin, and TSL, he knew that the communicative burden quickly became too much for me. I thought he might then begin to communicate with me in TSL and leave his family to fend for themselves. But he seemed to want me to talk with his family rather than with him. He readily walked away or looked away, clearly indicating that he was content not to be included.

The deaf people and I were invited out one evening by some hearing people who were closely involved with the school. Some of them could sign. We sat at a large round table, intermixed, deaf and hearing. All were Taiwanese but me. The hearing people spoke Taiwanese, and those of us who could not were quickly left in the dark. I felt uncomfortable eating in silence while people were speaking around me, and I looked for ways to be part of a conversation.

I began to sign with the deaf man across the table, and we held a brief and tenuous conversation. When it ended, I turned to the deaf woman seated beside me. Although we began what turned out to be a long interchange, when I compared her signing style and demeanor in this instance to that of conversations we had had in other settings, she seemed restrained and self-conscious. I concluded that something about this setting made them feel awkward to sign.

When I later asked some deaf and hearing people about my impressions of the evening, all said it was perfectly acceptable—even normal—for the deaf people to sit silently, whether seated together or apart, in mixed social groups with hearing people while spoken conversation buzzed around them. I had the impression from both deaf and hearing people around the school that mixed gatherings were not infrequent and that the deaf people were not excluded in that sense when "everyone" went out to dinner. Still, signing at the table in mixed groups seemed marked. However, I could detect no discomfort among the deaf or hearing people with respect to this arrangement.

One Chiying deaf person whose linguistic prowess was clear once remarked, "It's hard to be deaf because I can't talk easily to you." This remark reflects her assumption that it is her responsibility to bridge the gap in our linguistic abilities and that I had no responsibility for our successful communication. I did not clearly understand how my status as a foreigner and as a hearing person might have interacted to produce this result.

One might assume that the deaf Taiwanese, by constantly deferring their communicative needs, bore a great burden of oppression without being aware of it or angered by it, but I do not think that assumption explains the whole picture. Although I never heard a deaf person raise concern about any of the communicative matters, deaf people openly revealed among themselves and, many times, in my presence profound dissatisfaction with their economic situation. They believe that their lives have been harder because they are deaf. They believe that the government should do something to help them, and indeed, in recent years, policies have been put in place to ensure that deaf (and other "disabled") people are charged a lower fee for amenities such as public transportation and admission to parks. Deaf people do not mind paying less because, I was told, they are acutely aware of the fact that they routinely work with hearing people who are paid higher salaries for the same work. Apparently, this pay differential goes without saying in Taiwanese society. Deaf people will work for less, and so they are paid less, which puts them at a distinct disadvantage given Taiwan's rather high cost of living.

Many deaf people consider themselves to be loyal and hardworking, less because they are endeared to their employers than because they have few choices in employment. Even a job at which they are exploited is better than no job. People or organizations that are perceived as culprits in wronging deaf people are said to be "in cahoots with each other." To express this idea, they use the sign GUAN XI (relationship), inflected to indicate a group of them. And all the deaf adults said that, in their lifetimes, things for deaf people had greatly improved in Taiwan.

One day during a long and spirited conversation, one Chiying deaf person asked me whether I was aware that deaf people often engaged in socially deviant behavior. I nodded. "People say deaf people steal, and that is sometimes true," he went on. "I myself stole when I was younger. But do you know why they steal?"

I had a few ideas. I responded that, during my stay in Kaohsiung, I had noticed many negative attitudes about deafness in conversations with deaf and hearing people alike. I suggested that, as children, deaf people learn to have low self-esteem. In addition, cultural and linguistic barriers are placed in the way of their success. They experience enormous frustrations associated with being deaf in an unfriendly society. Why shouldn't they steal?

"That is only part of it," the man said. "They steal because they work for little money. If they don't steal, they go hungry."

DEAF PEOPLE'S ATTITUDES ABOUT HEARING PEOPLE

If deafness is an inconvenience, then the ability to hear is a profound convenience and a great gift. In the minds of Chiying deaf people, being hearing was related to literacy, perhaps to intelligence, and ultimately to success in life. They seemed to feel that their only impediment to success is their deafness and that hearing people's success in their society is entirely because of their hearing. I found out soon after my arrival that the children saw my hearing status as utterly incongruent with the fact that I could not write Chinese characters very well. My obvious racial and cultural differences did not excuse me in any way. To them, it was preposterous that I was not literate in Chinese because I was hearing. Indeed, particularly at the beginning, even the adults seemed surprised that I could not be counted on to read the simplest of sentences written in Chinese characters. Over the months, in casual discussions that mentioned one hearing person or another who found the perfect spouse, wrote a book, or made a lot of money, the unsurprised response was, "Of course. She (or he) is hearing."

Although the deaf people seemed to envy and admire the ease with which a hearing life may be lived, they were a little "afraid of" or put off by hearing people. On an outing one day, two of the children and I attracted a great deal of attention from hearing people who saw us walking and signing together. Five or six people began to gather and stare. They seemed to be talking about us, but they spoke in Taiwanese, so neither the children nor I understood what they were saying. I was extremely uncomfortable with the attention; it was a great shock after being inside the gates of the Chiying School where signing was not only accepted but also expected and was certainly nothing special. In my annoyance, I realized that, outside the school, signing was fair game for this sort of attention, as are many behaviors that the local community thought of as odd in some way. I tried to ignore the attention, as did the children—or so it seemed. But after we had managed to catch a bus and leave the interested crowd, one of the children told me, "I'm glad to be out of there. I'm afraid of hearing people."

No one I knew admitted to disliking or liking hearing people simply because they were hearing. Most of the deaf people I talked with seemed to hold hearing people in general in high regard; some said they had a number of tolerant hearing friends. Some deaf people thought deaf people were kinder and easier to get to know whereas hearing people were stiffer and harder to talk with. Others seemed to want to have hearing friends but did not know quite where to begin to cultivate any. Other deaf people did not much care whether their friends were deaf or hearing as long as they had some of the same beliefs and attitudes. In a memorable conversation, one deaf man said, "If a hearing person's heart and my heart are going the same way, fine, but otherwise, I'm not interested in hearing people."

Hearing People's Attitudes about Deafness and Deaf People

In many parts of the world, a signed language seems to hold a certain attraction for hearing people, and Taiwan is no exception. These days, ample evidence indicates that hearing Taiwanese are attracted to and interested in TSL. According to a conversation with Smith in 1991, sign language classes available in Taipei in the 1970s were full as soon as they were offered (Chao 1994, 347). Interpreters appear in boxes on Taiwanese television, and Taiwanese airlines feature interpreted safety announcements. Many hearing people accept the abstract idea that deaf people are valuable citizens and should be treated and thought of well, all things being equal. However, some hearing people harbor a deep disdain for deaf people, including some hearing people who are intimately tied to deaf people.

A hearing child of deaf parents told me a painful story of eating in a restaurant with his parents as a young child. The waiters made fun of his parents' signing, and he retaliated by throwing food on the floor. During his later childhood years, children from hearing families teased him because of his deaf parents. Classmates treated him in this manner until he reached college age. Deaf parents reported again and again that their hearing children wanted little to do with them. Deafness flags possible social problems, and few would want to marry someone whose parents do not have advantages of money and position needed in Taiwanese society.

Whether or not deaf people deserve the judgment, hearing people do not necessarily consider deaf people to be competent workers or desirable colleagues. One Chiying deaf man described a setting in which he worked with hearing people. He felt his hearing coworkers looked down on him, and he resolved to change their opinions of him. He made it a point to sit down and talk with each one about the job and his qualifications for it. He told me that they respected him after that.

Perhaps nowhere is the disdain for deaf people more evident than in the lack of services for them. It is probably not surprising that interpreting services for hearing people wanting to talk with deaf people or deaf people wanting to talk with hearing people did not seem available with any certainty in Kaohsiung in the early 1990s. As far as I knew, none of the Chiying staff members, deaf or hearing, knew of any service like that, although arrangements might be made among individuals for particular events to be interpreted.

A hearing person deeply involved with the deaf community once explained to me that an interpreter was someone who "explained for the deaf people at the police station." When I asked whether interpreters served other functions, he seemed surprised and said that that was the usual task. Although he was admittedly untrained and not confident as an interpreter, he nevertheless functioned as one from time to time. He refused payment for his services, saying deaf people would be angry with him if he accepted payment. Hearing people who sometimes functioned as interpreters and knew personal details of deaf people's lives routinely revealed them to me. The mere fact that someone was the interpreter for an event was not necessarily enough to prevent that person from assuming other roles. For example, at a large, formal event, the interpreter on stage stopped functioning as interpreter to help someone with a mobility impairment up the stairs as the spoken parts of the event continued. The interpreter resumed the task of interpreting once the mobility-impaired woman reached her destination, and many minutes of interpretation were lost.

A deaf woman from a hearing family came to the Chiying School one day looking for an interpreter. Although she had engaged in antisocial behavior as a young girl, she had finally married. But her deaf husband committed petty crimes to provide for them and wound up in jail. Now, she wanted to see a lawyer about a divorce. An interpreter I knew refused to interpret for the deaf woman because the interpreter disapproved of the woman's desire to divorce her jailed husband.

In the most jarring of interpreting-related experiences I had, I observed a court hearing at which an interpreter was present. The proceedings dealt with a deaf person accused of an extremely serious crime. The accused deaf person and spouse would begin to sign as if to question the interpreter (not the lawyers), and the interpreter would sign (not interpret) DENG, DENG ("wait, wait") and convince them to stay silent while the tense court proceedings continued. To my knowledge, the accused person was found guilty and received the harshest of sentences.

SUMMARY AND CONCLUSIONS

The Chiying School in Kaohsiung, Taiwan, has existed for nearly 50 years. The description of the school in this chapter suggests that there were always "many ways to be deaf" at Chiying. Linguistic diversity has always been a feature of deaf life at Chiying, with both spoken and signed languages as part of the environment. Spoken and written Japanese and Chinese have been and still are significant in aspects of deaf life there. The Chinese language continues to be held in very high esteem by deaf Taiwanese. Signed languages have occupied an important place in life at Chiying: for many years, CSL was Chiying's medium of instruction, and now, TSL serves that role. TSL conversation outside of classes is abundant while remnants of CSL remain in everyday life for many people. TSL was not viewed as superior to Signed Mandarin by the Chiying deaf community. However, most people seemed to consider it much more efficient than Signed Mandarin. ASL signs were a curiosity to the Chiying signers, and without exception, they admired ASL fingerspelling.

Apart from linguistic issues, the Chiying deaf people have a range of opinions and attitudes where deafness is concerned. Most of the people with whom I came in frequent contact had very early ties to a signed language. A majority of them learned CSL first at the Chiying School, and when they went off to middle school in Tainan, they learned TSL, which had long been the medium of instruction in the public schools for the deaf in Taiwan. Their early contact with a signed language notwithstanding, many of the Chiying deaf group hold hearing people and their values as an ever present concern. A statement made to me by Chiang Ssu Nung captured this idea. I had heard that Chiang believed that CSL was a better language than JSL, and I was anxious to hear him articulate this position. But my question seemed to bore him. "The best sign language," he said, "is the sign language which hearing people can easily understand."

In contrast, many deaf people are indignant about some of the social and economic issues they face. Indeed, some of the Chiying deaf people seem to have developed a secure sense of themselves as human beings with every right to inhabit the largely hearing world around them and to be beneficiaries of all it has to offer.

Acknowledgments

This chapter was developed from a paper presented at the International Sixth Conference of Theoretical Issues in Sign Language Research at Gallaudet University in Washington, D.C., November, 1998. I could not have written it alone. I gratefully acknowledge the assistance of the following people. Leila Monaghan encouraged me to write this chapter and gave me anthropological guidance in the form of many patient and helpful comments throughout the process. Long Peng's comments on the very underpinnings of the chapter changed it for the better. Without a doubt, much of what we know about TSL and deaf life in Taiwan, we know from Wayne Smith's treasure trove of published and unpublished work. He has shared all of his resources with me throughout the years. The illustrations for the figures in this chapter are from Smith's work and are used by permission. Grants from the American Council of Learned Societies, the American Association of University Women, and the University of Arizona financed my work in Taiwan. With a great deal of help from Jane Tsay, Jennifer Chiang, and Chiang Ssu Nung, I was able to arrange to live at the Chiying School. Finally, the contributions that the deaf adults and children in the Chiying School community of the early 1990s made to my work and to my life are incalculable. I, alone, am responsible for any inaccuracies within this chapter.

Notes

1.   The common orthographic convention, especially in the United States, is to use uppercase *D* and lowercase *d* to signify different worldviews and attitudes of people with a particular audiological status. The usefulness of the terms *deaf* and *Deaf* for describing communities in American society seems clear; Padden and Humphries (1988, 2) remark on the terms' complexity and interrelatedness. However, it seems inappropriate to assume that the Taiwan deaf community need necessarily fit this model. In fact, as far as I can tell, Taiwanese deaf people possess both deaf and Deaf characteristics, as well, perhaps, as others that do not fall neatly into either category. Because neither the orthographic convention nor the philosophical positions that the words are meant to express were familiar to my consultants, I refer to Taiwan deaf people as "deaf." When I discuss the American Deaf community, I use "Deaf."

Also, throughout this chapter, I use the word *community* to signify that the people I refer to live in a particular geographic area and share some experiences as well as some political and social conditions. One cannot necessarily assume that they see themselves as a cultural or linguistic community.

2. In mainland China, Chiang had worked in several schools for the deaf. In fact, he himself founded one in the Shanghai area, "but before the school ever got on its feet, Chiang was forced to flee Shanghai" (Smith 1999). Later, in Taiwan, Chiang founded a school in Keelung before he established the Chiying School (Smith 1999). In all of these schools, at least some of the teachers were deaf.

3. On this point, sources disagree. Chao, Chu, and Liu (1988, 9) claim that Chiang Ssu Nung worked with another man, Lu Chun-ou and that, together, they established the school in Keelung.

4. In my contacts with Chiang during the early 1990s, he regularly used either speech or what would be called "sign supported speech" (Johnson, Liddell, and Erting 1989) to communicate with me and with the people around him. He spoke Shanghainese and signed the Chinese signs.

5. On this point, Chiang never expressed any reason for his preference when I met him in the early 1990s. Chao Chien-Min expresses his preference for CSL by saying, "Japanese Sign Language is not suited for the thoughts, concepts and characters of our country" (Chao, Chu, and Liu 1988, 9–10).

6. I showed some of the deaf staff members one authoritative work titled *Long Ya Ren Shou Yu Tu* (Deaf-Mute People's Sign Language Manual) published in Shanghai, China. Each volume has illustrations of the signs of mainland China and written explanations of how to form each sign. The Chiying deaf people said they had never seen the manual before, but they were immediately familiar with 80%–95% of what they saw. As they examined the book, some confirmed with smiles that they had indeed learned particular signs in the book but had not used or thought of them in a long time.

7. In this chapter, I follow the orthographic convention of using small capital letters to write the glosses for signs. In the case of TSL signs, I provide a Mandarin gloss and an English translation in parentheses. Where possible, I refer to the Mandarin gloss in Smith and Ting (1979, 1984). However, because Smith and Ting (1979, 1984) do not use Roman letters to provide a gloss, I gloss signs in Mandarin using Chinese pinyin, a romanization system not much used in Taiwan but standardly used in the linguistic literature on Mandarin.

8. I became aware of these multiple signs because I would often point to an object or perform an action and ask for the sign. I once commented that my inquiries must be tiresome for my consultants, but they brushed off my concern, saying that my effort was similar in kind, if not in quantity, to that of Taiwanese deaf people from different parts of Taiwan, who often used this strategy to learn the local signs.

9. Reilly (1995) finds the same pattern in a Thai school for the deaf.

10. Once, I wanted F——— to use the sign RI BEN (Japan). To that end, I showed him a written Japanese ad I had found in a magazine. Though I recognized one or two kanji, I had no idea what the ad said in total; for me, it was only an example of Japanese writing. I asked F——— where the writing was from, assuming his response would be RI BEN and that would start us off. But F———'s answer was more than just the sign RI BEN, and he launched into a discussion I had not predicted. I quickly got lost. It turned out that he had read the ad and made a comment about its content. When he realized that his assumption that I could read Japanese was incorrect, he explained meticulously what each character meant and also deconstructed his comment about it.

11. Indeed, to be kept isolated at home is part of many deaf Taiwanese young people's lives, even if they are educated. Sometimes as a punishment for misbehavior, they are

kept home by their parents. In such cases, their friends sadly say that so-and-so is "at home."

REFERENCES

Ann, Jean. 1998. Variation in Taiwan Sign Language: Evidence from morphology, syntax and the lexicon. Paper presented at the Sixth Conference of Theoretical Issues in Sign Language Research, November, at Gallaudet University, Washington, D.C.

Chao, Chien-Min James. 1994. Taiwan Natural Sign Language research work. In *The Deaf Way: Perspectives from the international conference on Deaf culture*, ed. C. J. Erting, R. C. Johnson, D. L. Smith, and B. D. Snider, 347–49. Washington, D.C.: Gallaudet University Press.

Chao, Chien-Min, Hsi-hsiung Chu, and Chao-Chung Liu. 1988. *Taiwan Ziran ShouYu* (Taiwan Natural Sign Language). Taipei, Taiwan: Deaf Sign Language Research Association.

China Deaf and Blind Association. 1981. *Long Ya Ren Tong Yang Shou Yu Tu* (Deaf Persons Common Sign Language Manual). Shanghai: China Deaf and Blind Association.

Hodgson, Walter Kenneth. 1953. *The deaf and their problems: A study in special education*. London: Watts.

Johnson, Robert. 1994. Sign language and the concept of deafness in a traditional Yucatec Mayan Village. In *The Deaf Way: Perspectives from the international conference on Deaf culture*, ed. C. J. Erting, R. C. Johnson, D. L. Smith, and B. D. Snider, 102–9. Washington, D.C.: Gallaudet University Press.

Johnson, Robert, Scott Liddell, and Carol Erting. 1989. *Unlocking the curriculum: Principles for achieving success in deaf education*. Working Paper 89. Washington, D.C.: Gallaudet Research Institute.

Padden, Carol, and Tom Humphries. 1988. *Deaf in America: Voices from a culture*. Cambridge, Mass.: Harvard University Press.

Reilly, Charles. 1995. A deaf way of education: Interaction among children in a Thai boarding school. Ph.D. diss., University of Maryland.

Smith, Wayne. 1976. Taiwan Sign Language. Revised 1988. Typescript.

———. 1989. The morphological characteristics of verbs in Taiwan Sign Language. Ph.D. diss., Indiana University.

———. 1990. Evidence for auxiliaries in Taiwan Sign Language. In *Theoretical issues in sign language research*, ed. Susan D. Fischer and Patricia Siple, Vol. 1, 211–28. Chicago: University of Chicago Press.

———. 1999. A history of the development of education of the deaf in the Republic of China. Typescript.

Smith, Wayne, and Li-fen Ting. 1979. *Shou neng sheng chyau* (Your hands can become a bridge). Vol. 1. Taipei: Deaf Sign Language Research Association of the Republic of China.

———. 1984. *Shou neng sheng chyau* (Your hands can become a bridge). Vol. 2. Taipei: Deaf Sign Language Research Association of the Republic of China.

Tsuchiya, Michiko. 1994. The deaf Japanese and their self-identity. In *The Deaf Way: Perspectives from the international conference on Deaf culture*, ed. C. J. Erting, R. C. Johnson, D. L. Smith, and B. D. Snider, 65–68. Washington, D.C.: Gallaudet University Press.

Wardhaugh, Ronald. 1998. *Introduction to sociolinguistics*. 3d ed. New York: Basil Blackwell.

Yau, Shun Chiu. 1977. *The Chinese signs: Lexicon of the standard sign language for the deaf in China*. Kowloon and Hong Kong: Chiu Ming Publishers.

Yau, Shun Chiu, and Jingxian He. 1989. How deaf children in a Chinese school get their name signs. *Sign Language Studies* 65:305–22.

13 The Changing World of the Russian Deaf Community

Michael Pursglove and Anna Komarova

On September 7, 1995, Igor Abramov, chairman of the Moscow branch of VOG, the All-Russian Federation of the Deaf, was shot dead by a contract killer outside his flat in the Strogino suburb of Moscow. The often violent world of hearing Moscow had impinged on that of the Moscow deaf community. One of Abramov's last acts was to chair a committee that produced a modest little booklet titled *Zhesty* (Signs), published only a few days before his death. At the time, the booklet did not attract much attention but, in hindsight, it marks an important stage in the development of the Russian deaf community in the post-Communist era.

Zhesty is probably best described as a phrase book and contains what are claimed to be the 472 most used signs in Russian Sign Language (RSL), the first language of many profoundly deaf people in Russia. It makes no claim to being academic but, instead, is offered as an "elementary teaching aid." Although some deaf people in Moscow are rather critical of the book, claiming that some of the signs are wrong, it does have its uses, and it is extremely user-friendly, a rare virtue in a country not noted for its user-friendliness. For example, one of the two double sections, each containing 40 signs, is given over to the numbers that any user of any language, sign or otherwise, needs from a very early stage.

What is most important about this booklet, however, is not its contents nor its format, but the circumstances of its publication. It was published by the organization that Abramov had headed, MOSGORVOG, the Moscow branch of the All-Russian Federation of the Deaf. Its parent organization, VOG, is virtually the sole organization for deaf people in Russia. Founded in 1926, it has branches—72 in all—in every major city in the Russian Federation and a total membership of approximately 156,000. *Zhesty's* publication marks a striking shift from years of VOG's oralist policies.

The coauthors of this chapter, one English and one Russian, both hearing,

---

This chapter is an edited and updated version of a paper presented at the Sociolinguistics Symposium 11, Cardiff, Wales, September 1996.

have experience working for the central directorate of VOG, which provided insight into the workings of both it and its subordinate branches. We have also been involved from the beginning with the Moscow Bilingual School for the Deaf, set up in 1992 to promote the bilingual approach to deaf education in a country where attitudes toward sign language still range from lukewarm to downright hostile, despite the changes in society begun by Gorbachev in 1985. With the first pupils having graduated in 1998, this time seems to be an opportune occasion to attempt an assessment of the changes that have occurred since 1991 within what we will call the Russian deaf community. As we will show, a generally accepted definition of that term still remains elusive, but sufficient evidence is available to enable us to draw some tentative conclusions.

Gorbachev's Reforms and Their Impact on Russian Deaf People

The reforms initiated by Mikhail Gorbachev from 1985 onward are associated with the concepts of *glasnost* (openness, transparency) and *perestroika* (restructuring), both of which were originally intended to relate only to the workings of the Communist Party and the government. It is beyond the scope of this chapter to discuss the effect of these reforms on Soviet society as a whole, although the generalization could be ventured that, although Gorbachev's attempts at restructuring largely failed, his policy of openness was widely interpreted as a green light for the introduction of freedoms that had been rigorously suppressed in the pre-Gorbachev era—freedoms of speech, association, and travel. For deaf people, the freedom to meet their Western counterparts and the removal of restrictions on travel to Western countries had a dramatic effect. From 1987 onward, contact between Russian deaf people and foreigners grew to an extent that enabled Russia to send a group of more than 50 to the "Deaf Way" conference at Gallaudet in 1989. The fact that users of RSL were able to communicate readily with users of other sign languages came as a revelation to them, as did the fact that, in some countries at least, sign language was accorded the same status as the national spoken language.

The Role of VOG in the Soviet Era

Despite its theoretical status as a nongovernmental organization, VOG was under close party control and was, therefore, inevitably affected by Gorbachev's reforms. Indeed, from the time of its foundation, VOG had had all the features of a typical Soviet organization if not of the Soviet state itself. It had, for example, a pyramidal structure at the top of which was the presidium, chaired by the president of VOG. He—and in true Soviet fashion it always was a "he"—was helped by a number of vice presidents and a large bureaucracy, the central directorate (*tsentral'noe pravlenie*), based in a seven-story building on 1905 Street in Moscow.

In the deaf world, VOG was all-powerful, not least because it held the purse strings. Its income came from 63 "UPPs," Russian initials for "training and production enterprises," that is to say deaf workshops and deaf factories, making all sorts of things, from electronic parts to clothing, from badges to furniture. The money from the UPPs went up to the presidium of VOG, which then redistributed the money downward to the local branches, which in turn distributed money to a host of activities such as deaf clubs, schools, the famous Theater of Mime and Gesture in Moscow, deaf artistic groups (such as the poetry group Kamerton), sports groups, and sanatoria for deaf people.

With money came power. VOG decided everything from sign language policy to the composition of delegations of deaf people who might travel abroad. All the people who mattered in VOG were members of the Communist Party, which was true within any Soviet organization. A particular deaf Soviet dimension was the absence of any profoundly deaf people in positions of power and an attitude toward sign language that ranged from lukewarm to downright hostile. The pyramidal structure of VOG as a whole was replicated in each of the branches (Pursglove and Komarova 1991; Pursglove 1995).

After the Soviet Union ceased to exist on December 31, 1991, VOG and many other Soviet-type organizations had to change or risk extinction. How profound these changes have been and how irreversible they may be are matters of great interest if not great anxiety for anyone interested in the country. Change had actually begun in the Gorbachev era between 1985 and 1991, but after 1991, the most dramatic change in VOG, as in Russia, concerned the so-called "switch to the market," which meant that free enterprise was allowed. For VOG, the first effect of this change was a dramatic loss of income because the UPPs, hit by the loss of regular orders from the state, declined to send their hard-earned profits up the pyramid and, instead, kept some or all of it for themselves.

VOG was forced to fill the gap in its income by renting large parts of its headquarters to commercial interests. Many regional headquarters followed suit. The whole of the central administration of VOG underwent its own version of perestroika, with a "representative" section staffed by deaf people and an "administrative" section staffed by hearing people. There was also a small indication that VOG's attitude toward sign language might be changing insofar as the diehard journal of the national VOG, *V edinom stroiu* (In United Rank), printed a sign language lexicon on the back page of several of its issues. This apparent change proved illusory, and by 1997, the journal was running what almost amounted to an anti–sign language crusade.

The pressure for change was seen at the 15th Congress of VOG, held in St. Petersburg in June 1995. In his preelection address, the incumbent president, Valerii Korablinov, went so far as to say that, in his personal view, the only hearing people who should be allowed to join VOG were those with a knowledge of sign language. Nevertheless, a large number of hearing delegates were elected, especially by provincial branches. Some of these branches were thrown into turmoil by the pressure for a less Soviet and more open modus operandi.

In Vologda, for instance, the local chairperson refused to accept the fact that she had been voted out of office. Yet in another instance, in Murmansk, in Russia's Far North, a young reformist chairperson took office. The Petersburg meeting to choose delegates for the 15th Congress was picketed by deaf people who disapproved of the choices made. These events were reported in *V edinom stroiu* whose newfound relative openness even extended both to expressing the view that most deaf people regarded VOG "skeptically" and to printing, without refutation, a letter from the deaf poet Ivan Isaev, editor of the rival publication *Maiak* (The Beacon), now known as *Mir glukhikh* (Deaf World), in which he said bluntly that VOG was "sick." Some things, however, remained the same. The 11-member VOG presidium elected at the congress was much the same as the previous one, with both Korablinov and his vice president, Mikhail Mamonov, reelected.

Change, then, however reluctantly undertaken, has been in the air since at least 1991. VOG managed to keep open all but one of the branches it had in 1991, that at Naro-Fominsk, a town 44 miles southwest of Moscow. However, the pyramid began to fall apart as soon as the Soviet Union disintegrated. One important symptom of this disintegration was the breakaway movement by the most important of the VOG branches, the Moscow branch. This branch began to oppose VOG on issues of policy, an opposition that it symbolized by calling itself, on the masthead of its newspaper, not "The Moscow Branch of VOG," but "The Moscow Federation of the Deaf." As with so much that has happened in Russia since 1991, this change was, perhaps, more apparent than real.

Abramov's Impact

Abramov became chairman of Moscow VOG in April 1985 at the age of 28, which would be considered young in any country. But in Russia—for years, a gerontocracy under the Soviet regime—such a youthful appointment was unusual. April 1985 was the very beginning of the period of perestroika, and at that time, a person in Abramov's position had to be a member of the Communist Party. Born in 1956, he was deafened in early childhood. Although he mastered sign language, his oral speech remained good. He trained as an engineer at Moscow's Bauman Institute and was also a published writer of short stories. He gained a doctorate and had a long sabbatical in the United States. In 1989, he became the first deaf person to stand for elected political office in the hearing world when he stood, unsuccessfully, for the Congress of People's Deputies in 1989 and for the Moscow City Council in 1990.

Abramov founded the newspaper *Maiak* and saw it through the transition to the post-Soviet era, mainly by astutely removing the slogan "Workers of the world unite" from its masthead and replacing it with the apolitical "The traveler will master the road." Within a month of the demise of the Soviet Union, in a reversal of his previously skeptical attitude toward sign language, he sanctioned an evening titled "Sign language is your native language," consisting of lectures on all aspects of sign language and a competition to find the best signers among the audience.

Most impressive of all, perhaps, he managed to persuade the Moscow City Council and the formidable mayor of Moscow, Yurii Luzhkov, to adopt, on paper at least, a series of measures designed to improve the financial position of deaf people and to improve communications for them. This dynamism did not make Abramov universally popular. Even his own executive criticized in print his prolonged absence in the United States. Among Moscow deaf people, his strictly unofficial sign name was a sharp jab with the elbow. For all his faults, however, his forceful, dynamic personality did pose an obvious threat to the considerably less dynamic presidium of central VOG. It attempted to get him on board by making him a vice president, but he was still seen as a threat to Korablinov.

All sorts of theories have been put forward to explain Abramov's murder in 1995, but there is little doubt that it had something to do with the newly acquired financial power of Moscow VOG. Since 1991, charitable organizations have been granted big tax concessions on imports and exports, which enable them to set themselves up as rivals to other businesses. This granting of tax concessions makes sense only in a country that has large monolithic organizations, a hangover from Soviet days. In today's Russia, wherever one finds money, one also finds corruption and violence. The head of the charitable organization for disabled veterans of the Soviet war in Afghanistan was murdered a few months before Abramov, presumably for the same reason, and in February 1995, the head of a company that had made several lucrative deals with Moscow VOG was also the victim of a contract killing. Moscow VOG had itself set up scores of companies in 1995, a perfectly legal move that may, however, have had an illegitimate side. As the Moscow newspaper *Kommersant* reported,

> Half the staff in these businesses were disabled, which legally exempted the companies from paying duty. But it was not necessary to have disabled people on staff to gain exemptions; fake agreements can be signed and wages paid to non-existent personnel. Legally, profit from businesses owned by public organizations is not liable for tax if it is intended to fund the ostensible activities of these bodies. This makes them an attractive channel for laundering money. (*The Guardian* 1995, 13)

Thus, the murder of Igor Abramov, to nobody's surprise, remains unsolved. It seems to have been a direct result of the nature of the organization that he ran, and the nature of that organization is a product of the tension in contemporary Russian society between the old (in this context, "Soviet"), exemplified by the operation of central VOG, and the new, exemplified by the wheeling-dealing Moscow VOG.

The more cautious approach of central VOG to the new circumstances of post-Communist Russia, however, did not render it immune from the violence that engulfed Abramov. On November 1, 1996, its chairman Valerii Korablinov, chairman of national VOG since 1984 and whose appointment, like that of Abramov's, had come as a result of Gorbachev's reforms, was shot dead outside his country cottage near Moscow. Korablinov was the only figure in the Russian deaf community whose power rivaled that of Abramov's and, like Abramov, he was murdered. No one has yet been charged in either case.

CHANGING TIMES

Although understanding VOG is vital in understanding the situation of Deaf people in Russia, other institutions are also beginning to play important roles. A tentative move away from oralism and toward a wider recognition of sign language was made in December 1990, just one year before the end of the Soviet period, when the Russian Federation passed a draft law on disability, which was finally put on the statute books in late 1995. Members of VOG were on the advisory commission that drew up this legislation, which, in its 14th clause, does contain one brief sentence on sign language: "Sign language is acknowledged as a means of inter-personal communication." This sentence, which survived from the earliest published draft legislation, may seem vague and half-baked, but it was, at least, a start.

In 1992, within a year of the end of the Soviet Union, the Moscow Bilingual School for the Deaf admitted its first pupils. It is still in existence and has become the core of a new Center for Deaf Studies, entirely separate from VOG and from the prestigious but very conservative Institute of Remedial Teaching (formerly the Institute of Defectology). The leading and practically the only researcher on sign language in the whole of Russia, Galina Zaitseva, has left her post at the Institute and is now the driving force behind the Bilingual School. In addition, she was instrumental in organizing the Conference on Bilingual Education of the Deaf, which was held in Moscow in April 1996 and was attended by 140 delegates from 15 countries (Zaitseva, Komarova, and Pursglove 1998). The school has established a bilingual kindergarten, and the bilingual gospel has been spread by the school as far afield as Kursk, Novgorod, and Novosibirsk in Russia; Minsk in Belarus; and Panevezys in Lithuania. Converting to a bilingual approach is a slow process, and opposition is strong. During the 1996 conference, for example, Irina Tsukerman, a deaf senior researcher at the Institute of Remedial Teaching, gave her paper using sign only. Afterwards, she was told by her superior at the Institute that "Sign language demeans deaf people."

Notions of Deaf Community

One reason for the lack of acceptance of Russian Sign Language as a full-fledged language is that, in Russia, there is still no concept of "deaf community" that would be recognizable to a Westerner. There is not even a generally accepted term to express this concept. The word for "community" in Russian is *obshchestvo*; the word, which also means "society," makes up the middle of the three words that constitute VOG. This association makes that word unsuitable for rendering the Western concept of "deaf community." Galina Zaitseva has put a prefix on the word and has come up with *soobshchestvo*, which is the dictionary word for "commonwealth." Taking a different approach, the Orthodox Church, which has put a cathedral at the disposal of deaf people in Moscow and employs at least one signing priest, prefers the cognate word *obshchina* (commune) to describe its organization for deaf people. In a recent article, Zaitseva uses the term *mikrosotsium* (microsocietal unit), but the term is limited to academic discourse and has no general currency. However, Zaitseva uses this term in a passage that comes as close as any commentator has come yet to defining "deaf community" in Russian terms. It will readily be noted that the definition lacks any reference to empowerment, to enabling deaf people to take control of their own affairs:[1]

> With a knowledge of sign language and an understanding of the history and culture of deaf people, they [deaf people] will turn out to be capable of participating fully in the activities of their community, which are directed towards the struggle to realize their civil rights, as well as the right to develop their traditions and their language. (Zaitseva 1995, 6)

Similarly, Russian has no established terms for "deaf culture," "deaf awareness," "deaf identity," "deaf pride," or "deaf heritage." Interpreters have to resort to elaborate periphrases to render them in Russian or RSL. Indeed, even the concepts expressed by these terms probably do not exist in Russia today. It is perhaps symptomatic that one eminent hearing specialist on deafness reacted to the term *deaf pride* with the comment, "What rubbish! What is there to be proud about in that?" Only the term *deaf culture* has a ready translation, *kul'tura glukhikh*, but when the term is used, it almost always refers to deaf actors, deaf poets, or to deaf "cultural" events taking place in premises known as "houses of culture" (*doma kul'tury*). These "cultural" events can include anything from a performance of Chekhov's *Cherry Orchard* by the celebrated Theatre of Mime and Gesture to a hairdressing competition for deaf people. The Russian translation of *deaf culture* is usually used alongside other words with strong Soviet resonances, for example, *kul'trabotnik* (cultural worker), *kul'tuchrezhdenie* (cultural institution), *kul'tmasso-vaia rabota* (mass cultural work), and indeed, *Ministerstvo kul'tury* (Ministry of Culture). In Russia, according to one expert, the term *deaf culture*, in its Western sense, is understood by no more than 20 people.

The difficulty in expressing these concepts is hardly surprising when one considers that not until 1991 did the term for Russian Sign Language (*russkii zhestovyi iazyk*) gain currency by analogy with British Sign Language and American Sign Language as contacts grew between Russian deaf people and their counterparts in the United Kingdom and the United States. Even the originator of the term, Galina Zaitseva, used the term *Conversational Sign Language* in her groundbreaking book on RSL (1991) and in an important article on bilingualism published the following year (1992). A certain degree of confusion was caused by the fact that the Russian word for "conversational" (*razgovornyi*) and the Russian word for "Russian" (*russkii*) begin with the same letter.

The Russian term for Russian Sign Language did not appear in print in Russia until as late as February 1995 (Zaitseva 1995), where a footnote specifically draws attention to the change in terminology. Despite that, however, many Russians, both hearing and deaf, still decode the first letter of the acronym as "conversational." The mistake is more than a linguistic error; it betrays an attitude toward sign language that appears to be widespread in Russia in which few subscribe to the view that sign language is, in the words of Oliver Sacks, "a language equally suitable for making love or speeches, for flirtations or mathematics" (1989, 127). Official pronouncements, the educational system for deaf people, and the deaf press all point to this lack of respect for sign language, and a pilot survey carried out by the authors in Moscow in 1992–1993 seems to show that many deaf people share this view. Among 19 statements put to a sample of 29 deaf people, four were particularly revealing (see table 13.1).

The table shows apparent contradictions: The responses to statements 1 and 4 indicate a negative attitude to sign language whereas the responses to statements 2 and 3 indicate a positive attitude. The explanation for the negative attitude reflected in responses to statement 1 may simply be the product of years of oralist education in Russia while the response to statement 4 may be explained by the fact that deaf Russians, like their hearing counterparts, have suffered for decades at the hands of overweening, corrupt, and inefficient officials with whom communication in any language seems, at times, impossible. Deaf people, furthermore, have had to endure receiving official information on television through sign-supported Russian rather than RSL. Sign-supported Russian, based on the syntax of Russian, is largely incomprehensible to users of RSL.

TABLE 13.1   **Survey Responses by 29 Deaf People**

Survey Statement	Agree	Disagree
1. Sign language is a simplified form of communication.	19	10
2. Sign language is suitable only for everyday communication.	5	24
3. In sign language it is impossible to explain complex concepts.	9	20
4. Sign language is no good for conveying official or complex information.	16	13

The same four statements shown in table 13.1 were put to 17 hearing people about to embark on a course of RSL (see table 13.2).

Although the hearing and deaf responses to statements 2 and 3 are analogous, the hearing responses to statements 1 and 4 differ markedly from the deaf responses and are, in fact, more positive. Results from such small samples are highly tentative, and the very fact that the responses are so mixed seems to indicate a degree of hesitancy, even among deaf people, about the role of sign language in Russian society.

The lexical gaps in spoken and written Russian pertaining to the term *sign language* are confirmed when one consults two recent Russian-English/English-Russian dictionaries that were published in 1993 and 1994 respectively and that both make use of Russian-born native speakers of Russian. Neither gives *zhestovyi iazyk*, the correct term for "sign language." The *Oxford Russian Dictionary* (Howlett 1993), whose compiler has been sent the correct terminology by the present writers, nevertheless persists with the mistakes it made in its first edition: talking about *azbuka glukhonemykh* (alphabet of the deaf and dumb) and confusing sign language and fingerspelling. The 1994 *Collins Russian Dictionary* (Knight 1994) makes the same mistake, although it does manage a phrase for "sign language" that is partially, but not wholly, correct.

The attitude toward sign language in Russia is very different from that in

TABLE 13.2   **Survey Responses by 17 Hearing People**

Survey Statement	Agree	Disagree
1. Sign language is a simplified form of communication.	5	12
2. Sign language is suitable only for everyday communication.	2	15
3. In sign language it is impossible to explain complex concepts.	4	13
4. Sign language is no good for conveying official or complex information.	3	14

Western countries. In Soviet times, despite lip service to the ideas of L. S. Vygotsky, the oral tradition predominated, especially after Stalin appeared to advocate it in 1950 (Zaitseva, Pursglove, and Gregory 1999, 9). In schools, sign language was banished to the playground or beyond, although fingerspelling was used in classroom activities. The first chairman of national VOG, Pavel Savel'ev, whose term of office ran from 1926 to 1948, was an excellent signer who nevertheless felt it appropriate to use speech whenever possible.

An anecdotal example may serve to reinforce this point. In 1993, a sign language course for teachers of the deaf from all over the Russian Federation was mounted in Moscow. Similar courses, which used sign language without any use of voice and were taught by deaf teachers trained at Bristol's Centre for Deaf Studies, had been run since 1991. One teacher from Novgorod reported that, for 15 years, she had used sign language secretly with her pupils. If she had admitted publicly to doing so, she would have risked losing her job.

Russia is probably the only country where the approach to teaching deaf children that was devised and advocated by Emilia Leongard, an approach rooted in oralism, is regarded as successful. Spectacular results are claimed for her method, with some justification in the case of hard of hearing children. Convincing proof has yet to be adduced, however, that the method works with profoundly deaf children, and yet, almost every issue of *V edinom stroiu* gives Leongard considerable space to propound her ideas. Views to the contrary are rarely printed and, when they are, are accompanied by hostile editorial comment. Vygotsky's warnings against pure oralism and treating signing "as an enemy," first published in 1930, were not republished until 1983, and not until the post-Soviet era was a 1992 survey of 15 school-leavers from Moscow's School 101, one of the most prestigious oralist schools in Russia, finally published (Zaitseva 1992). The survey paints a bleak picture of the oral speech skills, speechreading ability, and writing ability of the control group.

Results from the Bilingual School are more hopeful, although the sample (six graduates in 1998 and a further six in 1999) is too small to be statistically viable. The pupils and their parents, both hearing and deaf, have had every encouragement from staff members and from MOSGORVOG through publications such as *Zhesty* to view RSL as a full language.

THE EFFECT OF THESE CHANGES IN ATTITUDE AND LANGUAGE ON THE VOG

For the Russian government, the question What is the deaf community? has always been easily answered: VOG. Official statistics are quoted in support of this view. These claim that the total number of deaf people in the Russian Federation is, in round figures, 171,000, of whom no fewer than 156,000 (91%), are members of VOG. The figures for Moscow are 12,000 out of an estimated deaf population of 20,000. The government and most Russian hearing people also view deaf people as part of a wider, disabled community. Deaf people are often referred to as *invalidy po slukhu* (aurally disabled), and events such as the Day of the Disabled, organized in Moscow in December 1993, include deaf people. Deaf people are classified into one of four disability categories and receive pensions according to the category in which they fall. Little if any evidence indicates that Russian deaf people object to this treatment.

However, rather more evidence is surfacing that suggests deaf people are becoming dissatisfied with VOG as it is currently constituted. Official statistics notwithstanding, there does appear to be a gap between VOG's priorities and those of a growing number of Russian deaf people. VOG attempts to represent people with a wide spectrum of hearing loss and is dominated by hard of hearing people. This situation has led to calls for separate organizations for hard of hearing and profoundly deaf people, as is the case in most Western countries. Profoundly deaf Russian people say that, if one takes "those who regard sign language as their first language" as a working definition of "deaf community," then the gap between national VOG and the emergent "Russian deaf community" becomes more apparent. Increasingly, deaf people appear to be looking to the independence-minded satellite offices of VOG, particularly MOSGORVOG, to take a positive lead in the struggle for recognition of the merits of bilingual education and sign language.

The Way Ahead

Despite continuing resistance to change, the process begun by Abramov continues under his successor Vova Bazoev. Bazoev has recognized, for instance, that deaf Russians need to be aware of their own history, just as hearing Russians have had to reassess and come to terms with the newly revealed and, often, deeply disturbing facts of Soviet history. A seminar on deaf history was organized in September 1996, resulting in a publication by the same deaf-run Zagrei publishing house that put out *Zhesty* (Pichugin 1997). MOSGORVOG organized a Deaf Week in September 1998 at which presentations were given by staff members and pupils from the Bilingual School. Most significant of all, a Center for Deaf Studies and Bilingual Education, independent of government and of VOG, opened its doors in February 1999. The center will coordinate sign language research and its practical application through bilingual education. It has already produced an RSL manual and a videotape of signed fairy tales.

The first graduates of the Moscow Bilingual Deaf School have moved into further education where they have been joined by ten other deaf students who have been taught hitherto by the traditional, largely oral method. In the teeth of political instability and often severe economic hardship, particularly after the collapse of the Russian economy in August 1998, much has been achieved in the years since 1991. The Center for Deaf Studies, the Bilingual School, its thriving kindergarten, and the pedagogical conferences (*pedagogicheskie chteniia*) held in early 1999 at which advocates of bilingualism shared a platform with exponents of more traditional methods all have helped to raise the profile of sign language in Moscow. The message has, as already noted, gone further afield within Russia and the former Soviet Union. One could reasonably assert that the impetus created by the establishment of the Bilingual School in 1992 has been maintained and that, now, Russia holds the nucleus of a confident, independent, dynamic, forward-looking, and outward-looking deaf community.

Notes

1.   My translation, *MP.*

REFERENCES

The Guardian. 1995. September 13.

Howlett, Colin. 1993. *Oxford Russian dictionary.* Oxford: Oxford University Press.

Knight, Lorna S. 1994. *Collins Russian dictionary.* Glasgow and New York: Harper Collins.

Pichugin, Iaroslav B. 1997. *Materialy pervogo moskovskogo simpoziuma po istorii glukhikh.* Moscow: Zagrei.

Pursglove, Michael. 1995. The silent minority: Deaf people in Russia since 1991. In *The new Russia,* ed. Michael Pursglove, 55–63. Oxford: Intellect.

Pursglove, Michael, and Komarova, Anna. 1991. The deaf in Russia: Some current issues. *Rusistika* 4:6–9.

Sacks, Oliver 1989. *Seeing voices.* London: Picador.

Zaitseva, Galina L. 1991. *Daktilologiia: Zhestovaia rech'.* Moscow: Prosveshchenie.

———. 1992. Slovesno-zhestovoe dvuiazychie glukhikh. *Defektologiia* 4:5–11.

———. 1995. Zachem uchit' glukhikh detei zhestovoi rechi? *Defektologiia* 2:3–8.

Zaitseva, Galina L., Anna Komarova, and Michael Pursglove. 1998. *Deaf children and bilingual education.* Moscow: Zagrei.

Zaitseva, Galina L., Michael Pursglove, and Susan Gregory. 1999. Vygotsky, sign language, and the education of deaf pupils. *Journal of Deaf Studies and Deaf Education* 4(1): 9–15.

14 | New Ways to Be Deaf in Nicaragua: Changes in Language, Personhood, and Community

Richard J. Senghas

Annie,
[I] spent an hour and a half today with a 43-year-old Deaf man. . . . It seems he attended a school for 'sordomudos' in the 1960s; the director's name was Berrios. It was oralist pedagogy with finger spelling. . . . The school was on Calle 14 Septiembre, one of Managua's old east-west streets. THE SCHOOL HAD 32 BOYS & 17 GIRLS IN IT. I'm going back to videotape him. . . .

—Richard

EXCERPT OF AN E-MAIL MESSAGE FROM
MANAGUA, NOVEMBER 10, 1995.

When I asked him if he kept in touch with his schoolmates after leaving school, he was very clear that none of them had kept in touch with each other after leaving school. Apparently, even when they were still attending the school, none of them did much with each other after school hours; they all seemed to just go home. And there were no references of any deaf adults. He said that he didn't meet up with any of his old schoolmates until he bumped into them at the ANS-NIC center many [10 or 15] years later. It seems that the best chance so far of finding a pre-existing Deaf community has petered out again.

FROM NOTES OF VIDEOTAPED INTERVIEWS,
NOVEMBER 22 AND 27, 1995.

The book you are reading presents just a few of the many possible ways of being Deaf.[1] Until recently, being deaf in Nicaragua usually offered an existence isolated from other deaf people. Before 1978, there was no established Deaf community in Nicaragua; older deaf people had no ways to pass down the wisdom of deaf experience or to tell stories of the old days. There was no shared sign language.

Today, little more than 20 years later, the new sign language currently used by the growing Nicaraguan Deaf community is drawing the attention of linguists and anthropologists around the world. Accounts of this change have been broadcast on prime-time television in both Great Britain and the United States. Deaf Nicaraguans now have a national association with branches in several cities throughout their country. What happened? And what can this unusual case teach us?

What happened was this: New school programs drew deaf people together, creating an environment where a new sign language could form. In Nicaragua, a Deaf community has grown, and just as a child grows through adolescence into adulthood, this community also has encountered landmark events and developmental stages, many that might have been expected and many that were not. Most children develop where an existing language is readily available to them. And new communities develop where an existing language is already available, too. But 20 years ago, deaf children in Nicaragua were isolated from any existing sign language. Without the ability to hear, young deaf Nicaraguans could not acquire spoken Spanish without great difficulty and effort. In order to satisfy their unmet social needs, these deaf Nicaraguans produced their own new language. There is no record of another case like this anywhere in the world, at any time. This unique case provides clues that help us understand the ways that languages and communities change over time, revealing complex interactions between development at both individual and group levels. Paradoxically, the uniqueness of this case reveals human processes that are normally unnoticed but are possibly universal.

As an anthropologist, I find one development in this case especially compelling. The identification and recognition of the new Nicaraguan sign language, Idioma de Señas de Nicaragua (ISN) as, language has shifted deaf individuals from a category of limited personhood associated with limited cognitive and linguistic potential to one of a linguistic minority—although a particularly problematic one.[2] That is, they are no longer simply relegated to being handicapped dependents but, instead, have the opportunity to be treated as individuals who are capable of acting for themselves and one another. This change, more than any other, demonstrates that ideologies of personhood are significant and operate at many levels simultaneously. The systems of ideas that define what it means to be deaf and what options society allows for such individuals have been challenged and are changing.

Furthermore, Deaf Nicaraguans now use their new language as a central cultural form, as both means and medium of social relations. But when deaf Nicaraguans are acknowledged as having the capacity to acquire language, several more issues then demand attention, including social identification and responsibility; issues of standardized language use; Deaf identities in local, national, and international spheres of interaction; and the still-contested potential for deaf Nicaraguans to achieve "full" personhood attainable by other Nicaraguan adults.

This case shows that descriptions that include the interplay between individual development and other social processes (including group formation) can provide useful explanations of social phenomena. Language change and group identity developments are affected by events that involve individuals as they develop and act within larger social systems. The main point of this chapter is that individuals by themselves should not be seen as the sources of linguistic and social change. Rather, it is the acting and developing of individuals—within a developing social system—that are bringing about new or changing forms at all levels.

I have written elsewhere (Senghas, Kegl, and Senghas 1994; R. J. Senghas 1997) on the history of the Nicaraguan Deaf community and the stages of its development. Here, I present highlights of the interrelatedness of individual development, especially child language acquisition, and the development of the new Nicaraguan sign language as part of more complex social phenomena. Most theories of community development do not account sufficiently for the effects of individual development, and most explanations of individual development do not address issues of community development. Keep in mind that the childhood process of learning a first language is the cultivation of cognitive processes that later become the means by which individuals and communities interact. Thus, categories and structures that make language possible have significant social effects. Similarly, socialization is the cultivation of effective actions and responses of individuals as they interact in their community. For example, teaching children who may say what to whom and how significantly affects the patterns of language use in a community. Clearly, a unified model of social development and change is needed.

IDEOLOGIES OF PERSONHOOD

For this chapter, I focus on one particular set of categories and structures that operates at both individual and social levels. These categories and structures taken together form systems of ideas that allow society to identify and treat individuals as particular types of persons. I refer to these systems as "ideologies of personhood." I choose to focus on them because we see these ideologies in both the structure of language itself and in expressed ideas about language (talk about talk).

The term *ideologies of personhood* is based on an anthropological definition of the term *person*. In conversational American English, seven individuals might be referred to as seven people. But if one of these individuals were a pharaoh who was considered a god-king, two of these individuals were free adults, another a bonded slave, and the remaining three were children, then we could sensibly refer to this collection as having four kinds of persons. Each category could be seen to have significantly different characteristics, including specifically what each is considered responsible for, capable of doing, or allowed to do. This kind of thinking is actually quite common and affects our daily actions. Consider that, in the United States, a person cannot sue a child. However, U.S. law does allow a person to sue the child's parents because parents are considered responsible for their children's actions. Personhood, then, involves the relationship of an individual to other individuals or groups or of an individual to events—real or potential.

These ideologies operate simultaneously at many levels. They range from the levels of linguistic grammar that are normally unconscious to levels of group and community interaction that are frequently political and often quite conscious. These levels are typically studied by different sorts of researchers: linguistic processes are studied by linguists and psycholinguists; social and cultural processes, by sociologists and anthropologists. But an interdisciplinary approach that combines these usually separate perspectives provides a more coherent and complete view. Such an approach is adopted here, allowing for a study of ideologies of personhood that reveals complex interactions often overlooked.

METHODOLOGY

My own ethnographic research is part of a larger, long-term effort to document the emergence of ISN and its linguistic community.[3] Using qualitative and primarily descriptive methods of participant-observation, I build on the quantitative linguistic and psycholinguistic work of others. My field methods include directed interviews, observations of physical environments, and living as a resident in Managua for periods as long as a year. My own trips began in 1993. The longest stay was from early 1995 through early 1996, and my most recent follow-up visit was in June 1999. During these trips, I developed social relations and engaged with local residents in daily activities and special events, including rituals and celebrations. For this chapter, I draw on my field notes and observations of social phenomena among deaf and hearing Nicaraguans as well as the content of interviews (rather than their form). I also consider field experiences, including incidental experiences and experiences reported by fellow researchers of the Nicaraguan sign language resulting from structured interviews as parts of psycholinguistic research. In sum, my method here is to document social processes involving deaf people in Nicaragua and to identify connections between social and linguistic phenomena.

The majority of my fieldwork has been conducted in the greater Managua area, although I made frequent trips to areas outside of this capital city, including visits northwest to León, east to Matagalpa, southeast to Masaya and Granada, and south to several cities and towns in the department of Carazo. In addition, I traveled several times to the Caribbean coast to observe and assist at a pilot educational program for deaf *costeños* (residents of the Caribbean coast) being established in Bluefields. If rates of deafness in Nicaragua are at all similar to those around the world,[4] the deaf population in the greater Managua area probably numbers in the thousands, although official Nicaraguan census figures do not tally deaf residents.[5] Figures provided by the Ministry of Education (MED) do indicate, however, that, in 1995, approximately 500 deaf children were officially enrolled in special education programs throughout Nicaragua.[6] My field observations centered around but were not exclusive to those deaf Nicaraguans who attended special education programs (mostly children) or those beyond school age who were relatively active in the National Association of Deaf People of Nicaragua (Asociación Nacional de Sordos de Nicaragua, ANSNIC). I also studied some families and neighbors of these deaf people and consciously observed other hearing people I encountered in the normal course of living and working in Nicaragua. Although I am a hearing, native English speaker, I learned and used ISN when interacting with Deaf Nicaraguans and used Spanish when dealing with hearing Nicaraguans.

Background History and Social Context

I now would like to focus on the larger sociohistorical context of this case. By the time the Swedish parliament recognized Swedish Sign Language in 1981 as the first and natural language for Swedish Deaf people (Wallin 1994, 318; chapter 4 of this volume), almost halfway around the world, the still unrecognized Nicaraguan sign language was in its early formative stages. This new language emerged during major social and political changes of the Sandinista Revolutionary Period of Nicaraguan history, a time well documented by Hazel Smith (1993). Many of these changes would affect the social environment of most Nicaraguan children, including those who were deaf.

Prior to 1978, public education was not generally available to many Nicaraguans. Special education programs were even more inaccessible and were limited in size; the few that included deaf students were nonresidential day programs based on oralist pedagogy.[7] The earliest deaf education programs date back only to the 1940s, and the largest had only one or two dozen students at a time. Some programs tutored as few as one to three students.[8] When deaf children left these programs, they rarely maintained contact with fellow deaf students. The 43-year-old man mentioned in this chapter's epigraph is one example. According to former students and teachers, some gestures and signs were used in these environments. In the classrooms, certain signs and gestures (including fingerspelling systems) were used to support spoken language as part of an oralist pedagogy. Teachers and parents did not consider these signs and gestures as actual language but, instead, as merely *mimicas* (mime). Outside the classrooms, particularly among the students, some signs and gestures were used in social interaction.

Former students of the Berrios school in Managua, which was founded in 1946 and closed in the 1970s, have shown me signs they used in their childhood. These signs and the signed alphabet used by those students, who are now mostly in their thirties, are noticeably different from those currently used among the Nicaraguan deaf population and seem similar in quality to homesigns used by deaf individuals who are not part of linguistic communities of deaf signers (see Jill Morford 1996 for a review of the literature on homesign systems). The former students had little contact with one another once they left their special education programs, at least until they rediscovered one another as they became involved in the Deaf community during the 1980s and 1990s.

In the late 1970s and early 1980s, the Nicaraguan Ministry of Education and the Social Security and Welfare system (INSSBI) established special education and vocational training programs that brought many deaf students together. The largest of these programs was the Centro de Educación Especial Managua (CEEM), based in Barrio San Judas, Managua. Hope Somoza, wife of then-President Anastasio Somoza Debayle, inaugurated this special education center the year before the Somoza government finally fell to the Sandinista revolutionaries in 1979. Shortly after the overthrow, as part of the general literacy and educational program of the revolutionary Sandinista government, a vocational program for older students (that is, post–sixth grade) was also established in another barrio of

Managua called Villa Libertad.[9] For most of the deaf students brought into the special education system, CEEM was their first experience being together with many other deaf people. Formerly, most deaf Nicaraguan children remained in or near their hearing families' households and, throughout their lives, had only limited contact with other deaf people.[10]

Before the 1980s, most of the social life of deaf Nicaraguans revolved around family and neighborhood relationships, and undoubtedly, they developed home-sign systems to communicate with their families and neighbors. Evidence so far, which includes videotaped conversations made in the mid-1980s and interviews of deaf adults and older special education teachers, suggests that no commonly shared sign language system existed in Managua until recently.

Many researchers I have talked to have been skeptical of the idea that no Deaf community existed in a place as large as the city of Managua. How can we be so sure that a community didn't exist that we have simply overlooked? Weren't all the required factors for Deaf community emergence that Jerome Schein (1992) identified present in Managua?[11] Nevertheless, the social circumstances in Nicaragua seemed to have prevented any such community formation. The stigma associated with having a deaf person in one's family may have caused people to isolate their deaf children from others outside their own family or immediate neighbors (R. J. Senghas 1997; Polich 1998). Another possible obstructing effect on any potentially emerging or even existing Deaf community in Managua may have been the major earthquakes of 1931 and 1972, which both caused considerable casualties and relocation, and disrupted communication and social relations for years.

My own extended fieldwork, combined with the very thorough work of Polich (1998), makes me confident that no coherent Deaf community existed in Nicaragua before the late 1970s. Every time I located older deaf people who grew up before the 1980s, they always indicated that social interaction with other deaf people had been a very rare event. Only after generally available special programs for deaf students were developed and only after significant numbers of deaf students attended these programs (as many as 180 at one time in the central school in Managua in the mid-1980s and early 1990s) did an identifiable Deaf community begin to emerge.

The new deaf education programs triggered a significant change for deaf Nicaraguans. During the 1980s, friendships that developed among deaf students at CEEM were maintained even after those students completed the sixth grade, the highest grade offered in the programs. Many of these students continued with vocational training at Villa Libertad, where they learned a variety of skills such as hairstyling and beauty care, carpentry and basic cabinetry, baking, and bicycle repair. As they entered their teens, deaf teenagers also began dating. According to Kegl's recollections (R. J. Senghas and Kegl 1994), one of the significant topics of conversation at Villa Libertad in the mid- to late-1980s concerned who was dating whom. Certain homes and one ice cream shop in particular became important gathering spots where people would gather to be with other people who were deaf.

In 1986, the Asociación Pro-Integración y Ayuda al Sordos (Association for the Integration of and Aid to the Deaf, APRIAS) was founded. This association was the first formal organization for deaf Nicaraguans. With assistance from Sveriges Dövas Riksförbund (the Swedish Federation of the Deaf, SDR), a house was purchased in Managua that became a center for Deaf activities. In 1994, APRIAS officially adopted the new name Asociación Nacional de Sordos de Nicaragua (ANSNIC) to reflect that the organization was an entirely Deaf organization, run by and for Deaf members.[12] It also clarified the organization's intended role as the primary political and social organization for deaf Nicaraguans at national and international levels.

THE DEVELOPMENT OF DEAF INDIVIDUALS AND A DEAF COMMUNITY IN NICARAGUA

Over the past 20 years, the language, culture, and identity associated with deaf people in Nicaragua has changed significantly from both hearing and Deaf perspectives. We can see changes in terms of individual development: Nicaraguan children who are deaf now acquire a language at an early age, which allows them to develop normal linguistic capacities. We can also see changes at the group level: A new community has emerged and continues to develop, and the language that this community uses has also changed and expanded. Furthermore, the development of the Nicaraguan Deaf community is clearly affected by the changes in the development of its individuals, on the one hand, and the development of social relations at the global level, on the other hand. If we do not recognize these various levels of development as interrelated, we fail to properly understand the development at any given level.

However, we must remember that not all deaf Nicaraguans are equally involved in the emerging linguistic community of ISN signers, nor are all deaf Nicaraguans identified with the developing social community. Interconnectedness must not be conflated with homogeneity, uniformity, or universality. We may seek the universal in the particular, but we must not lose the particular when we abstract the universal.

CHILDHOOD LANGUAGE ACQUISITION, GRAMMAR, AND COMMUNITY-LEVEL EFFECTS

If we examine the language acquisition of individuals, we can see that individual development can introduce changes at the community level. Childhood language acquisition is one of the most thoroughly studied aspects of human development. Psycholinguists have seen the emergence of the new sign language in Nicaragua as a unique opportunity to analyze how children's built-in ability to learn their first language may also contribute to the creation of new languages.

This case appears to be the first time that a new language, whether spoken or signed, has been documented firsthand by scientific observers during its early phases of emergence. With other languages, including ASL and several other signed languages, the early histories have been difficult to reconstruct, often resulting in competing theories rather than any clear consensus (see Kegl and Mc-Whorter 1997; see also the topic of monogenesis in pidgin and creole studies as discussed by John Holm 1988, 44–52). In the Nicaraguan case, however, we have direct evidence of linguistic forms and historical records. The first language cohorts are still alive and active within their community, and they are still relatively young.[13]

New languages and their formation are the central topics of linguists who study pidgin and creole languages (see Holm 1988, 1989). Pidgins and creoles are languages that emerge when speakers of different languages come in contact with one another. Pidgins are spoken by people who use another language as their first language (or mother tongue); creoles are languages that have been acquired by children as their first or primary language. These languages have specific patterns that have been studied by creolists as they describe how human languages develop the structure we call grammar. Many creole theories identify social, historical, and other environmental factors in language development; others highlight innate, or "universal," factors.

Derek Bickerton (1984) proposed a theory of creolization based on the psycholinguistic theories of Noam Chomsky (see 1986). Chomsky's notion of Universal Grammar, that is, innate human predispositions to learn languages with certain kinds of grammatical structures, suggested to Bickerton that new languages would form quickly. If children were predisposed to learn certain patterns, they would quickly introduce regularity to newly emerging languages such as creoles that might not already show clearly established grammatical patterns. Therefore, Bickerton claimed, a new grammar should form within just a generation or two. He coined the term *abrupt creolization*, in contrast to more conventional ideas of languages creolizing over longer spans of time, to emphasize the rapidity of this process.

Kegl (Kegl and Iwata 1989; Kegl and McWhorter 1997) has focused on the Nicaraguan sign language case as a demonstration of abrupt creolization. The relatively rapid formation of this new sign language rather than a development that spans generations is consistent with Bickerton's projection that creoles should form rapidly if children have linguistic predispositions consistent with a Universal Grammar paradigm. Once Kegl identified the new sign language, other researchers also began studying the language.

Ann Senghas (1995; Senghas et al. 1997) has conducted quantitative analyses of the language use of deaf Nicaraguans. She identifies some new forms that have been emerging in the Nicaraguan case and identifies who introduces these forms. Her findings suggest that signers entering the signing community at a younger age are more likely to acquire complex linguistic forms and that the new sign language has indeed become measurably richer over the last two decades. An unusual result of these two factors is that the most proficient signers in this particular community are its youngest and newest members. How did she identify these changes?

Her first study (Senghas 1995) involves 25 participants classified according to two criteria: age at entry into the deaf signing community and historical time of entry into that community. Age at entry is classified into three subcategories: young, medium, and old. Time of entry is classified into two subcategories: before and after 1983. She examines the grammatical complexity of the participants' signing by determining the proportion of verbs that support at least two arguments (a subject and an object) and the number of inflections per verb (temporal information or links with other sentence elements such as agreement between verb and object). The results of her study show that those participants who were exposed to Nicaraguan signing at a young age can indicate more arguments with their verbs than signers who were first exposed to the language when they were older. The results also indicate that young and medium age-of-entry groups of signers use twice as many inflections per verb and that this difference is even greater in the signers who entered the signing community after 1983. A similar pattern holds for verbal inflections that specifically indicate agreement.

Ann Senghas's later study (Senghas et al. 1997) focuses on eight Nicaraguan signers, all of whom entered the signing community before the age of six years. Four signers entered the signing community before 1985 and four after. The study examines grammatical structures in the participants' language by analyzing the order of words used and possible verbal agreement as indicated by direction of movement. Although spoken languages often use word endings to indicate, for example, the subjects and objects in a sentence, signed languages often use space and movement to indicate these relationships. Again, Senghas presents evidence suggesting a change in the sign language toward more grammatically complex forms and that such grammatical complexity is introduced by children in a lin- guistically impoverished environment during the acquisition of their first lan- guage.

If the Nicaraguan signing community has indeed been as linguistically iso- lated as claimed by researchers so far, the studies just summarized demonstrate that deaf Nicaraguan children have indeed contributed to the structure of their newly forming language. Because language itself is a cultural form, deaf Nicara- guan children have provided one source of new cultural forms as a side effect of their individual, linguistic development.

Consider other effects of individual language development on the develop- ment of the community at large. The emerging grammatical complexity of ISN allows for finer distinctions in the ways that sentence elements relate to one an- other. If a language's grammar facilitates the association of subjects, verbs, and objects, and especially any causative relationships among these, it would stand to reason that notions of capability would develop. Ideologies of personhood are involved. Instead of people spending a great deal of time during a conversation clarifying who was involved and what seems to have happened, they could quickly focus the conversation on the implications of that event. For example, the question of who might deserve credit or blame (if anyone) for an event could be more easily "said" and discussed.

The establishment of conventional forms and constraints of language raises issues that are familiar to anthropologists who have considered habitual uses of speech patterns and how they relate to habitual ways of thinking within commu- nities (see also Lucy 1994, 1995; Hoijer 1995; Whorf 1995). If conventionalized ways of indicating relationships become established, then inevitably, other ways of conceiving the relationships become more infrequent and, possibly, become more marked because of their less frequent use.

Another way that individual language development can have a significant effect on the community involves literacy. Children acquiring a language have the possibility of becoming literate. The ability of using written language then facili- tates the creation of social or political organizations, recording events for later consideration, and communicating with others over distances and spans of time. The legal status of ANSNIC, the Nicaraguan Deaf Association, would be impossi- ble without written legal documents. The more control Deaf people have over the use of written language in such documents means the greater control Deaf people have over their organization's structure and processes. Literacy also allows greater participation with media forms that Benedict Anderson (1991) cites as key to national identities.

Furthermore, literacy would allow an individual to pursue higher education or to participate in professions that depend on literacy. The roles in society that would open to deaf individuals would change significantly. Public attitudes about deafness would be affected, and over time, deafness might not be considered a major impediment to intellectual development.

Sociocultural Developments and Individual-Level Effects

Let us now consider how community and society levels of development can have significant effects on individual development. I stated in my introduction that ideologies of personhood also involve ideas about language and its use. For instance, even if a person is capable of using language, whether or not that use is recognized by society can have as much impact on the individual's life as actually having the capacity itself. Imagine that an infant says something that sounds exactly like an obscenity. Do we laugh, politely ignore it, or discipline the infant? As we look at the Nicaraguan case, we should ask this question: What significant effects do changes in ideas about language have on the development of individuals?

The anthropologist Grace Harris considers language as the critical, universal characteristic that marks a "normal" human being (1989, 601–2). Nicaraguan history bears out Harris's assertion that society must attribute the capacity for language to an individual before that individual will be considered a normal human person. Once Nicaraguans recognized that deaf children had the capacity for language, attitudes and policies changed significantly. The Ministry of Education now separates deaf children into classes specifically for deaf students; before, dyslexic and mildly retarded hearing children had often been mixed in with deaf students in special education classes. Also, by 1993, the ministry officially adopted sign language as a medium of instruction whereas, previously, it had been considered simply *mimicas* and discouraged in favor of oralist pedagogy.[14] Although, formerly, Nicaraguans had seen deaf children as "eternally dependent" (Polich 1996, 1998) and, therefore, had often kept them in relative isolation, in 1995, I heard Nicaraguan families describe their deaf children as *normal y inteligente* (normal and intelligent). A Managuan taxi driver used both these terms in a conversation with me when he expressed concern that his child was not going to get the education that he rightly deserved.

Nicaraguan legal recognition of deaf people quite clearly reflects its roots in the legal history of Spain. A distinction has long been made between those who can speak but are deaf *ex accidente* and those who are deaf and have never been able to speak. Speaking has been considered the litmus test for linguistic competence; if a deaf individual can speak intelligibly, then legal personhood may be acknowledged. The second category of individuals, who have often been referred to in Spanish as *sordomudo* (deaf-mute), have typically been denied legal personhood. As Susan Plann (1997) sets the context for her history of deaf education in Spain from 1550 through 1835, she traces the legal status of deaf people even further back. She notes King Alfonso X's denial in the 13th century of deaf people's right to bear witness, make a will, or inherit a feudal estate, even though he did allow deaf people to marry if they could signal consent (Plann 1997, 18). Later exceptions, including deaf individuals being admitted into the Roman Catholic priesthood, usually highlighted literacy as a demonstration of the individual's linguistic competence.

In contemporary practice, Deaf Nicaraguans themselves make a distinction between deaf individuals who can use language and those who cannot, even if these distinctions are not made in academic terms. One day while I was spending time at ANSNIC's center in Managua, I learned a sign that Deaf Nicaraguans use to identify someone who cannot sign, which they gloss as NO-SABE ("doesn't know" or "know-nothing").[15] NO-SABES are welcomed at ANSNIC but are given limited roles in activities. When I was first spending time at ANSNIC, certain members made sure that I understood when I was conversing with NO-SABES, apparently in an effort to clarify why I might be having trouble communicating (that is, that our communication problems might be due to the NO-SABE's limited capacities, rather than my own limited competence in ISN).

NO-SABES either (a) do not use (sign) language yet, even if they seem to have normal mental functions or (b) do not seem capable of acquiring language, even after long exposure. The first category includes children and usually young adults who have not yet been exposed to sign language at the time they first encounter the Deaf community. As these individuals begin showing competence in sign language, they are re-categorized and are no longer considered to be NO-SABES. The second category, those who seem unable to acquire language, includes those individuals who are mentally retarded or have other cognitive disabilities. Some adults who were not exposed to language during their critical period of language acquisition in childhood are permanently limited in their language capacity, sometimes extremely so (see Newport 1990).

Deaf Nicaraguans hold very similar ideologies of personhood to those held by hearing Nicaraguans, especially with respect to the role of language in determining personhood. Although Deaf Nicaraguans recognize ISN as a language and although some hearing Nicaraguans still do not, Deaf and hearing Nicaraguans alike see the capacity for language as a prerequisite for being treated as an accountable adult. Both consider proper language use and even literacy as marks of intelligence and responsibility. But what counts as proper language use is sometimes open for debate. In 1993, I witnessed one argument in a region south of Managua. A Deaf man who had been attending sign language seminars at APRIAS chastised a Deaf woman for using an older, "ugly" sign for a bank rather than the "new" one approved by the APRIAS seminar organizers. The woman indicated that, as far as she was concerned, the older signs were perfectly fine and that it did not matter what the folks from Managua had to say about it. The issue of using proper signs remains an important topic at ANSNIC today and is one motivating factor behind continuing the dictionary project there.

ANSNIC is so concerned with language issues that it has made significant efforts specifically addressing language. To increase the legitimacy of ISN, ANS-NIC has produced an ISN/Spanish dictionary (1997) and continues to work on a second volume. ANSNIC also provides language classes for parents and other family members of deaf Nicaraguans and emphasizes that, if more hearing people would learn sign language, more opportunities would be available to Nicaraguans who are deaf.

ANSNIC officers are also keenly aware that literacy is crucial to the socioeconomic security of deaf adults. Deaf adults who cannot read or write are often the first workers considered for layoffs when businesses are short on funds, which is a frequent condition in Nicaragua. Similarly, if deaf adults cannot read or write, they have a harder time determining whether the compensation they receive for their work is typical or fair. Because literacy is seen as such an important element of linguistic competence, sign language classes at ANSNIC are actually a combination of lessons in ISN and written Spanish.

The point about literacy as an element in ideologies of personhood bears further attention. As the cumulative effect from several factors, deaf Nicaraguan adults have unintentionally been prevented from becoming teachers in public deaf education programs. Deaf students attending special education programs have not developed sufficient reading and writing skills to enable them to advance through high school and university.[16] At the same time, few hearing special education teachers have developed a sufficient competence in ISN to teach in it, in part, because lower pay, a higher workload, and inadequate training all contribute toward a high turnover within the teaching staff. As a result, Deaf students receive a limited education at best. For the most part, they have been allowed neither to develop literacy nor to receive the content of other disciplines such as history or science whose teaching pedagogies assume literacy. Because Deaf adults are prevented from completing secondary- and university-level schooling, they are unable to earn teaching credentials, and so, they are not allowed to teach, even though they are the ones most capable of communicating with deaf children. The situation remains a vicious circle.

The future holds hope, however. In 1999, I saw some signing Deaf adults serving as teachers' aides in classrooms at CEEM. This kind of opportunity may provide the opening necessary to advance the education of deaf children and prepare them to succeed at higher levels than before. With their greater experience and more developed skills, these Deaf adults are more likely to understand what the hearing teachers are trying to teach. They can then use their own fluency in sign language to explain the concepts in ways that the children find more understandable. The Deaf adults also provide models to the children, both linguistically and socially.

The changing expectations of Deaf adults and of parents for their deaf children, as well as the shift in deaf pedagogy to include sign language as a central component have all fostered new learning opportunities. These opportunities include school programs and the ANSNIC center where deaf children may interact with other children and adults, which thereby create relatively normal situations in which language acquisition may occur. The point should be clear by now that changes at the social level have had radical effects on the development of individual deaf children.

BEING NICARAGUAN: DEAF ISOLATION OR INTEGRATION?

An outsider to the Nicaraguan Deaf community, whether Deaf or hearing, cannot help but notice how Nicaraguan its members are, as seen especially in what clothes they choose to wear, their goals and aspirations, what and who they talk about, and how they talk about them. My observations of Deaf Managuans, in particular, repeatedly highlight Deaf Nicaraguans as culturally competent actors drawing upon typical Managuan paradigms as they live and participate in Managuan society (R. J. Senghas 1997). I stress this point to counter an inadvertent side effect of the psycholinguistic literature addressing the Nicaraguan case, especially some of the popular accounts based on them. Several accounts conflate linguistic isolation with social and cultural isolation. Noam Chomsky, for example, described the situation during an interview with the BBC:

> The Nicaraguan case appears to be a very rich example, the richest yet known, of a natural experiment in which a language-like system, maybe an actual human language, was developed on the basis of *no external input as far as we know*, and that's intriguing. (Chomsky 1997, emphasis added)

Chomsky's characterization seems extreme. It is clear that facial and other gestures of hearing Nicaraguans have been incorporated as part of the grammatical structure of the new sign language. The nose-wrinkle that hearing Nicaraguans often make when they have a question has been adopted into ISN, not unlike the lowered eyebrows used in ASL to mark questions such as who, what, when, where, and why. Deaf Nicaraguans have interacted with hearing Nicaraguans, Deaf foreigners, and foreign researchers, and consequently, normal language contact effects now occur, including the borrowing of signs from foreign signed languages. (These borrowed signs are often modified to better fit the "rules" of ISN.) Still, language socialization and other related linguistic studies that highlight sociocultural context (such as pragmatics) hover at the margins of "formal" linguistics and remain underrepresented in linguistic research, so far. (No doubt, in part, because of the difficulty and complexity of such studies.)

For the most part, however, the Nicaraguan Deaf community has indeed been one of the most linguistically isolated new linguistic communities ever documented. For psycholinguists, a key aspect of this case is that the first cohort of deaf signers had no adults or older peers around to act as fluent models of a natural sign language. As a result, the deaf children filled this vacuum with their own signing, which quickly became structured with its own grammar. Consistent with the priorities of their discipline, the psycholinguistic researchers' emphasis has been on language acquisition and language change.[17]

Proper socialization, however, is closely intertwined with language acquisition. Ochs (1988) and Schieffelin (1990) have shown that, as part of childhood language acquisition, children learn about the different kinds of persons in their respective societies, including the kind of language use such persons can sensibly employ. In some communities, young children are encouraged to stand up for themselves and directly challenge others who might take their toys or food. Other communities teach them that children must go seek an authority figure to mediate such a conflict, that it is improper for a child to directly confront a social "superior," even if the offender is another child. Even social space affects language choice and can determine which linguistic forms are used to say "here" or "there" (see Hanks 1990).

Although deaf Nicaraguans may have experienced a fair amount of linguistic isolation, they are not culturally isolated. Certainly, not having easy access to spoken Spanish has a noticeable effect on their experiences, but by looking at day-to-day situations and actions involving deaf Managuans, we can see that they use and understand much of the cultural forms of Managuan life. These deaf people are like most people throughout the world: They learn to observe and participate in their encompassing societies. They may develop their own particular perspectives, but they are certainly socially involved.

Seemingly mundane observations emphasize this point. Most Deaf Managuans dress and act much like most other Managuans, especially those from similar socioeconomic backgrounds. In fact, their dress usually goes unnoticed. Divisions of labor among Deaf Managuans follow the same gender patterns seen in the general Managuan society. Deaf men seek work outside the home; deaf women tend to fulfill domestic duties. Deaf Managuans understand kinship. They know what brothers, sisters, mothers, fathers, aunts, uncles, cousins, and grandparents are, and they know who most of their own relatives are, even if they do not live with them. Deaf people grow up living in the very same houses with their hearing families and constantly interact with them. They go to the same churches, hang out in the same streets, and participate in weddings and funerals with their families. Deaf Nicaraguans are now marrying and having their own children. The explanations Deaf Managuans give me about Managuan social life and practices are also quite consistent with those I observe among hearing Managuans.

Most aspirations of Deaf Nicaraguans are typical of Nicaraguans in general. At times, these aspirations reflect both the desires to acquire traits or possessions attainable by most hearing adult Nicaraguans and explicit understandings that language has an important role in attaining those goals. For example, Deaf Nicaraguans have lobbied the National Assembly so the civil code might be changed to allow deaf Nicaraguans to hold titled property. Currently, deaf adults may vote in national elections, but the civil code allows them neither to own houses or cars nor to sign contracts as a person with the legal standing of a typical adult. These restrictions are holdovers from the legal history discussed previously. Many Deaf adults have told me that, until they could be legally recognized as the head of a household, they would always be relegated to a second-class status.

At many levels, multiple sociocultural processes such as language socialization and political movements operate concurrently and are constantly affecting one another. Much of local cultural knowledge is learned through other channels besides just language. For this reason, Nicaraguans who are deaf still become socialized in ways consistent with the surrounding cultural forms. The issues of language, however, do limit their options within their local society.

Being Deaf in Nicaragua

Some of the identity issues for Deaf Nicaraguans are specific to being deaf and are relevant primarily in a local frame of reference. Many of these issues involve language, both directly and indirectly. At times, members of the Nicaraguan Deaf community use language or other cultural forms to mark themselves in contrast to the encompassing hearing society. At other times, members even identify themselves as distinct from other subgroups within the Deaf community itself (for example, groups involved in APRIAS/ANSNIC or the special schools). In some instances, I have observed community members distinguishing themselves from other deaf Nicaraguans who are not seen as part of their Deaf community. These patterns are familiar and have been associated with the maintenance of ethnic groups and boundaries as discussed by Fredrik Barth (1969), among others.

Previously, I have documented that, at ANSNIC's center in Managua, Deaf Nicaraguans have established a Deaf place apart from the dominant hearing society (R. J. Senghas 1997). Like Deaf clubs in other parts of the world, sign language is the preferred medium of communication at ANSNIC, and an act of excluding Deaf people by not using sign language can produce immediate and heated censure (R. J. Senghas 1997, 7–10). A growing number of ANSNIC affiliate organizations are being established throughout Nicaragua, and opening day celebrations for each of these affiliates emphasize that these new centers are Deaf places. Speeches given by ANSNIC national and local affiliate officers during these ceremonies invariably mention that each new center is another special place where deaf people can come together freely and use sign language. A point frequently made is that, in these Deaf centers, deaf people are not "disabled" (*descapacitados*).

Opening celebrations for these affiliates include activities and performances that have become common at Deaf fiestas. A body of traditional stories, skits, and dances has emerged to become a central element in Deaf social life in Nicaragua. Some of these performances include deaf characters, others include humor that highlights deafness, and others are simply presented in mime or sign language in ways particularly appreciated by Deaf audiences (for example, Peréz Castellón 1995). One popular skit involves two signers, one standing behind the other. The person in front hides both arms behind his or her back while the person hiding behind reaches around the person in front to provide the arms for signing. The trick is to carefully coordinate the hand and arm movements with the facial gestures and body movement, as if the two people were really just one. Deaf people laugh at the errors sometimes produced (especially when a hand squashes the front person's face or inadvertently tickles the front person), but they also delight in particularly complicated utterances that are performed flawlessly. Certain Deaf individuals have become well known for their acts, and their performances are in demand at Deaf fiestas.

In addition to providing a social environment for Deaf people, ANSNIC and its affiliate organizations are pushing for political and legal changes that affect deaf people in particular. Recall, for example, that the Deaf association has helped coordinate appeals to the National Assembly to change the legal status of deaf Nicaraguan adults, especially with regard to contracts and property rights. ANSNIC often allies itself with other organizations to increase political pressure for change or to heighten awareness of Deaf people and their opinions among the hearing society.

Another organization in Nicaragua that also deals with deafness is Los Pipitos (The Little Darlings), an organization of parents with children of various disabilities. Los Pipitos has an oralist orientation, does audiological screening of children, and directs them toward speech pathologists and other professionals but away from ANSNIC. Los Pipitos officials and staff members are often professionally trained and certified, so they claim a professional competence unattained by current ANSNIC members or officers. I have found that parents of deaf children who have received assistance from Los Pipitos often are never informed that ANSNIC exists, even if the children show no promise of acquiring spoken language through traditional oralist methods. In 1995, I met one mother of a deaf 10-year-old who had been fitted with two hearing aids. The child still showed no indication of any hearing, and his language skills were extremely limited. Though we met just a few blocks from ANSNIC's center, the mother had never heard of ANSNIC.

Indeed, it is important to realize that not all deaf Nicaraguans are even aware of ANSNIC's existence let alone choose to identify with or reject it. I have also heard members of ANSNIC and Los Pipitos speak suspiciously of one another's organizations. ANSNIC members emphasize that they are autonomous, and therefore, as Deaf individuals speaking for themselves, they are a more authentic voice for the needs and opinions of deaf Nicaraguans than Los Pipitos. They also point out that, because Los Pipitos deals with many different types of disabilities and medical conditions, the organization often does not place a priority on deaf issues. But to their credit, I have seen both organizations participate together in public events in efforts to raise public awareness of the need for more resources for deaf individuals.

Certainly, it is important to recognize that not all deaf Nicaraguans who sign and even consider themselves part of Deaf social networks are necessarily aligned with ANSNIC or its members. Some deaf individuals consciously stay away from ANSNIC for political or personal reasons. Others find that work or domestic obligations prevent them from participating in ANSNIC activities, so they become peripheral to the ANSNIC community. Many of these individuals are mothers of young children. At times, some deaf individuals are discouraged from participating in ANSNIC events or visiting the ANSNIC center by ANSNIC officers or members. Individuals with drinking problems or people who have been violent or disruptive are sometimes excluded. Some deaf individuals have indicated that they have been excluded for seemingly political reasons. Those not welcomed at ANSNIC have sometimes been referred to as *malcriados* (spoiled or ill-mannered). Individuals who consort with *malcriados* risk being labeled as such themselves.

Within the Nicaraguan Deaf community, I have observed distinctions that indicate internal social categories. These distinctions include identification with ANSNIC specifically or identification with the Managuan community instead of communities from other regions of Nicaragua. The examples are not limited to the NO-SABE and *malcriado* categories mentioned above. Current ANSNIC officers have expressed their worry that, if Nicaraguans do not all use the same signs, confusion and disorder will result. Recall the argument over the proper sign for *bank*; that example was one manifestation of local identity issues played out through language use. ANSNIC officers have also indicated that, if foreign visitors do not see the Nicaraguans using a standardized vocabulary, they will assume that the Nicaraguan Deaf community is uneducated. These worries show that Deaf Nicaraguans see themselves as members of communities, sometimes at the local level and sometimes even at the national level.

Global Factors and Deaf Identity

As part of the international Deaf Pride or Deaf Way movement that emerged during the 1980s, we see communities from around the world taking pride in their own signed languages and community identities (Erting et al. 1994). In some cases, there is a nationalist tinge to this pride, especially when local Deaf communities see themselves as resisting the linguistic imperialism of "foreign" languages. Those foreign languages are most frequently spoken languages but, sometimes, are even other sign languages such as American Sign Language. These issues are important in Nicaragua. Deaf Nicaraguans are proud of their language and see it as one characteristic that distinguishes them as civilized humans. Their language also distinguishes them from Deaf communities in the United States and Europe and from Deaf communities in neighboring Central American countries. The Nicaraguan national Deaf association and their dictionary of Nicaraguan Sign Language are both cultural forms that simultaneously unite Deaf Nicaraguans with Deaf communities around the world while also marking the Nicaraguans as distinct and autonomous. They are not simply Deaf; they are Deaf Nicaraguans.

However, foreign cultural influences can be seen when observing the Managuan Deaf community, especially if we focus our attention on ANSNIC. Certain examples from the Nicaraguan case support Ulf Hannerz's (1992) metaphor of a "global cultural flow," that is, the way cultural forms move all over the world as part of normal human interactions. The timing related to the development of this community is important to consider. APRIAS was originally organized in the mid- to late-1980s when the Deaf Way movement was drawing international attention.[18] Thus, one is not surprised to hear accounts from both hearing and Deaf Nicaraguans of a Deaf Swede named Anders Andersen who visited Nicaragua in 1990 and discussed Deaf identity, language, and community with APRIAS members. The Swedish Federation of the Deaf (SDR) provided funding to APRIAS to buy a house for a Deaf center and to pay salaries for its officers. Also, in 1994, one very central member of APRIAS was hosted by SDR in Sweden for nine or ten months.[19] During his visit, this member had considerable contact with Deaf people and organizations of Sweden. While there, he learned some Swedish Sign Language (a poster of the Swedish Sign Language alphabet hangs in his office) and was exposed to one of the most well-organized associations of Deaf people in the world.

Significant foreign influences include the fact that SDR has continued to assist Deaf Nicaraguans in establishing an autonomous Deaf community. Also, early special education programs brought deaf students to international athletic competitions in neighboring Central American countries. During these events, some deaf Nicaraguan athletes saw sign language in use. Over the past decade, representatives of ANSNIC have attended several international meetings of Central American Deaf associations. The Nicaraguan Sign Language Dictionary Project also reflects international influences: ANSNIC had copies of sign language dictionaries from several different countries and was documenting Nicaraguan sign language forms according to language paradigms familiar in other countries.[20]

More indirectly but perhaps as significant, the current legal and constitutional structure of the current Nicaraguan government is the result of historical international relations. The recent revolutionary period drew inspiration from sources around the globe, including both democratic and socialist governments. It is by and through the national Nicaraguan government that ANSNIC has its legal status as a recognized organization. ANSNIC must therefore follow the government's guidelines that assume certain paradigms of organization. These include concepts of voting, accountability, and tax-exempt status.[21] ANSNIC has adopted certain structures, roles, and offices, and these certainly have social implications within the Deaf community. As one example, the layout of the ANSNIC facilities and the differential access to these facilities (for example, most people need permission to use or enter certain offices) marks certain individuals as being more influential. Also, a few individuals in particular, for example, the president and vice president of the organization, regularly represent the association in affairs external to ANSNIC.

Arguably, the most significant difference between the history of Deaf communities in the United States and Nicaragua is that no established sign language was acting as a major influence on the newly emerging Nicaraguan language. A second important difference is that the Nicaraguan Deaf community has emerged during an era of modern electronic telecommunications. Many communication devices today do not depend on voice or hearing and are, therefore, particularly useful for deaf people: consumer products such as fax machines, computers and e-mail, TTYs, and—most importantly—video cameras and video cassette recorders. I recall one deaf boy who was obsessed with Rambo; every time I saw him, he wanted to talk about Rambo. Sometimes he carried Rambo videotapes to school inside his shirt.

Modern technologies create amazing bridges between Deaf people and communities in far-flung regions of the globe. Often, a Deaf person in Managua can communicate more easily with a Deaf person in the United States or Sweden than with a Deaf person in another part of Nicaragua. We should not underestimate the importance of Deaf people being able to "write" in their native sign languages through videotaped letters or histories. Thus, the patterns of social interactions of the late–20th century add complexities and opportunities not seen during the formation of Deaf communities in the United States or Europe in previous centuries.

Because of the key role that APRIAS/ANSNIC has had in the development of the Nicaraguan Deaf community, significant influences on this organization will, in turn, clearly affect the community. These influences have included foreign sources, global movements such as the Deaf Way, and the international assistance provided by SDR. Individuals traveling internationally, including researchers studying the Nicaraguan case, also influenced the community. Finally, telecommunications and consumer electronics have global influences that reach quite literally into the homes of deaf Nicaraguans.

Concluding Comments

Psycholinguists have been and are continuing to demonstrate that this Nicaraguan case reveals innate and learned human capacities to generate new languages, given a certain social environment. Drawing on their work, we can see that unconscious but significant linguistic developments contribute to processes of social identity and agency. Therefore, we must continue anthropological efforts that search for universal aspects of human cognition and action, including symbolic and linguistic practices. But we must simultaneously consider the wide range of more general sociocultural processes involved in the interactions of humans, especially in a world where technology has radically transformed how and with whom we can communicate.

I hope I have successfully shown an approach that accounts for interplay between individual developmental and social factors, and have produced a useful description of the development of a community and its individual members. Language change and group identity development at all levels are affected by events that involve individuals as they develop and act within larger social systems. Language, culture, and identity are dependent on several innate and environmental factors, including individual developmental and larger sociocultural processes. Clearly, individuals by themselves should not be seen as the sources of linguistic and social change. Rather, the acting and developing of individuals—within developing social systems—are what bring about new or changing forms at all levels.

The case in Nicaragua is worth comparing with the history of deafness and sign languages in the United States or Europe. Each of these three regions has experienced disputes over deaf individuals' status in its society. In most debates, the role of language has been a central factor. In all three regions, wherever sign language has been recognized as "true" language, the potential personhood of deaf individuals has significantly changed. Yet the Nicaraguan case is unique because the sign language there is indeed new. A second unique characteristic of the Nicaraguan situation is that the oldest signers are just entering their early forties, and the more fluent signers are even younger. The oldest Nicaraguan signers did not have the same rich linguistic environment that is available to the young deaf children today. These older signing adults are exploring new roles and possibilities as they set the stage (and act as models) for their younger community members. In other countries, older signers can use language to hand down their experiences, effectively fulfilling positions as elders in their communities. Unlike the Nicaraguans, those older signers have been able to draw on a wide range of sources and traditions, many of them specific to their Deaf communities.

Ironically, the uniqueness of this case draws attention to characteristics that are nevertheless still shared. Interestingly, many of the very same ideological issues about language that affect other linguistic minorities—including those of both spoken and signed languages—have arisen in the Nicaraguan case. These issues include language standardization, the choice of language for schooling (whether the dominant spoken language or a minority language), language as a marker of identity, and language authority as a reflection of other social authority.

Let us now look ahead. To date, there is still no record of any other case where a new language has emerged that does not derive directly from one or more previously existing languages. Although the sociohistorical situation of the Nicaraguan case is different from North American and European historical patterns, it may be only one example of perhaps several similar cases in other regions of the globe—cases waiting to be documented. Any place where deaf people have historically been isolated from one another has the potential to repeat the pattern seen in Nicaragua. If new programs in such places begin bringing together many deaf children, an eye should be kept open for the creation of yet another new sign language.

It is unlikely that a similar case could occur involving spoken languages, however, because the linguistic isolation required would probably not be possible.

Yet, the findings from studies of situations involving signed language should not be considered irrelevant to those who study spoken languages and hearing people. The fact that these multiple levels of development, from individual to community levels, are all interrelated in the Nicaraguan case suggests that similar processes might be occurring elsewhere. Ideologies of personhood allow one area of focus that highlights such interrelationships, and these ideologies certainly occur in hearing situations, too. Societies' various expectations of linguistic competence, for instance, affect the lives of children everywhere. When we hold beliefs that define the "normal" process of language acquisition by children, such beliefs affect the roles and opportunities we allow these children during their development. If our schooling and parenting paradigms permit only a very narrow range of variation in children's developmental processes, larger numbers of children must then be socialized as "special" or "abnormal" cases, which has lasting effects on not only the individuals themselves but also the communities of which they are members.

Acknowledgments

My work in Nicaragua would not be possible without the cooperation and assistance of so many people, especially the Deaf community there. My sister, Ann Senghas, has been crucial to my research and my ongoing education. In an applied way, my wife, Tina Poles, and daughter, Ursula, have been equally instructive in issues of social relations and child development, and of loving tolerance. Funding for my research and subsequent documentation has been generously sponsored by a Fulbright Fellowship, a Spencer Foundation Dissertation Fellowship, and a Sonoma State University faculty RSCAP Mini-Grant and a RSCAP summer stipend. I thank the many Nicaraguans who have helped me in my efforts and my fellow researchers of this case who have proved invaluable in the field and back at home. Thanks, too, to the members of my faculty writing group at Sonoma State who suffered through earlier versions: Kathy Charmaz (our esteemed leader), Dolly Freidel, Virginia Lea, Elaine McHugh, Lisa Nakamura, and Adam Hill. Last minute stylistic suggestions by Wade Tarzia and Joan Malerba-Foran have made this chapter easier for us all to read and understand. Any remaining blame falls squarely on my own shoulders. Finally, I applaud the efforts of Leila Monaghan for her initiative and her editorial duties for this volume, and I value her continuing friendship.

Notes

1. I follow the convention of using the uncapitalized term *deaf* to indicate the audiological characteristic of limited or no hearing and the capitalized term *Deaf* to indicate a cultural identity regardless of actual audiological capacity.

2. Although other names have been used by various researchers to identify Nicaraguan Sign Language, throughout this chapter, I use ISN, because it is the name that ANSNIC, the Nicaraguan National Deaf Association, has chosen in its recently published dictionary.

3. These researchers include Judy Kegl who first identified signing in Nicaragua as a language, Ann Senghas, Jill Morford, Marie Coppola, Laura Polich, Gayle Iwata, John McWhorter, Gary Morgan, among others. At times, several of these researchers have infor-

mally and formally worked together as part of the Nicaraguan Sign Language Project (NSLP). NSLP has since been incorporated and is now directed by Judy Kegl.

4.   I have no reason to suspect that these rates would be any lower in Nicaragua. If anything, they might be higher, whether attributable to the use of infection-fighting antibiotics that are known as ototoxins or to the lack of timely treatment of infections, which results in permanent damage (see Polich 1998).

5.   The population of greater Managua is estimated at three million, roughly three-fourths of the population of Nicaragua.

6.   The Ministry of Education has been merged with other ministries and is now referred to as the Ministry of Education, Culture, and Sports (*Ministerio de Educación, Cultura, y Deportes*, MECD).

7.   Before the late 1970s, there were some few small special education schools, most of which espoused basically oralist pedagogies. With one exception, there have been no residential schools for deaf children in Nicaragua. That one exception is a remote school that, at this point, does not seem to have had a significant role in the emergence of sign language or a Deaf community.

8.   The first special education school to receive governmental support was founded by Dr. Apolonio Berrios, who ran this school from 1946 until shortly before his death in 1974. It was closed when a larger school was opened in Barrio San Judas.

9.   The Villa Libertad school has since closed. It was operating during my field session of 1993 but was closed by my 1995 field session.

10.   In this respect, the lives of deaf Nicaraguans in past decades seem similar to the lives of deaf people on Providence Island as described by Washabaugh (1986).

11.   Polich (1998) questions the completeness of Schein's theory itself, indicating that Schein does not fully account for all necessary factors.

12.   Eventually, the officers of this organization received salaries. The organization received funding from a Swedish Deaf organization and also sold products made by members in its workshops.

13.   Previously, the literature addressing sign language emergence in Nicaragua has used the term *generation* to denote what I term a *cohort*.

14.   According to one education official, this policy was in part a response to the failure of the oralist policy to effectively promote literacy among its deaf students.

15.   Words written in small capitals are glosses for signs. Although a rough translation may thus be linked to the glossed sign, one must remember that glosses are shorthand and are not true translations; nor do they adequately show grammatical structure.

16.   Compounding this problem is the fact that ISN interpreters are still not generally available in Nicaragua.

17.   Ann Senghas's work (described above) demonstrates certain aspects of this very process quantitatively. It is important to emphasize, though, that Ann Senghas's position is that, without the proper social environment, these language capacities will not be activated. Innate capacities are never isolated from social factors; the two go hand in hand.

18.   During several years in the 1980s, the U.S. government imposed a trade embargo on Nicaragua. Although other Central American countries may have been directly influenced by the Deaf Way movement and its followers at Gallaudet University in Washington, D.C., Nicaraguan Deaf history may have taken a different trajectory because of the political and economic isolation from the United States. This possibility also may account for why the Swedish influence was so strong while influence from Gallaudet was significantly less so.

19.   A parent with a deaf son was also hosted for a shorter visit.

20.   Kegl, a North American psycholinguist, wrote its prologue (ANSNIC 1997, ix–xi)—yet another example of foreign influence, this time involving researchers.

21.   Ironically, according to the Nicaraguan Civil Code, deaf Nicaraguans are legally

prevented from holding titled property, but as a legally recognized organization, ANSNIC can hold property—even though all its members are deaf!

REFERENCES

Anderson, Benedict. 1991. *Imagined communities: Reflections on the origin and spread of nationalism.* 2d ed. New York: Verso.

ANSNIC (Asociación Nacional de Sordos de Nicaragua). 1997. *Diccionario del Idioma de Señas de Nicaragua.* Managua: ANSNIC.

Barth, Fredrik, ed. 1969. *Ethnic groups and boundaries.* Oslo: Universitetsforlaget.

Bickerton, Derek. 1984. The language bioprogram hypothesis. *Behavioral and Brain Sciences* 7:173–221.

Chomsky, Noam. 1986. *Knowledge of language: Its nature, origin, and use.* New York: Praeger.

———. 1997. Interview. *Horizon: Silent children, new language.* BBC Two, 3 April. Program and interview transcript available on the Internet at http://www.bbc.co.uk/horizon/silent.shtml.

Erting, Carol J., Robert C. Johnson, Dorothy L. Smith, and Bruce D. Snider, eds. 1994. *The Deaf Way: Perspectives from the International Conference on Deaf Culture.* Washington, D.C.: Gallaudet University Press.

Hanks, William F. 1990. *Referential practice: Language and lived space among the Maya.* Chicago: University of Chicago Press.

Hannerz, Ulf. 1992. *Cultural complexity: Studies in the social organization of meaning.* New York: Columbia University Press.

Harris, Grace. 1989. Concepts of individual, self, and person in description and analysis. *American Anthropologist* 91(3):599–612.

Hoijer, Harry. 1995. The Sapir-Whorf hypothesis. In *Language, culture, and society: A book of readings,* ed. Ben G. Blount, 113–24. 2d ed. Prospect Heights, Ill.: Waveland Press. Originally published in Harry Hoijer, ed., *Language in culture* (Chicago: University of Chicago Press, 1954).

Holm, John A. 1988. *Pidgins and creoles.* Vol. 1, *Theory and structure.* Cambridge: Cambridge University Press.

———. 1989. *Pidgins and creoles.* Vol. 2, *Reference survey.* Cambridge: Cambridge University Press.

Kegl, Judy, and Gayla Iwata. 1989. Lenguaje de Signos Nicaragüense: A pidgin sheds light on the "creole?" ASL. In *Proceedings of the Fourth Annual Meeting of the Pacific Linguistics Conference, University of Oregon, Eugene,* ed. R. Carlson, R. S. DeLancey, S. Gildea, D. Payne, and A. Saxena, 266–94. Eugene: University of Oregon.

Kegl, Judy, and John McWhorter. 1997. Perspectives on an emerging language. In *Proceedings of the Twenty-Eighth Annual Stanford Child Language Research Forum,* ed. Eve V. Clark, 15–36. Palo Alto: CSLI.

Lucy, John A. 1994. *Grammatical categories and cognition: A case study of the linguistic relativity hypothesis.* Cambridge: Cambridge University Press.

———. 1995. Whorf's view of linguistic mediation of thought. In *Language, culture and society: A book of readings,* ed. Ben G. Blount, 415–38. 2d ed. Prospect Heights, Ill.: Waveland Press. Originally published in Elizabeth Mertz and Richard Parmentier, eds., *Semiotic mediation* (Orlando, Fla.: Academic Press, 1985).

Morford, Jill. 1996. Insights to language from the study of gesture: A review of research on the gestural communication of non-signing deaf people. *Language and Communication* 16 (2):165–78.

Newport, Elissa. 1990. Maturational constraints on language learning. *Cognitive Science* 14:11–48.

Ochs, Elinor. 1988. *Culture and language development: Language acquisition and language socialization in a Samoan village.* Cambridge: Cambridge University Press.

Peréz Castellón, Adrián Martín. 1995. The Panama Canal Story. Segment in *A lesson in geography.* Produced by Nicaraguan Sign Language Projects, Inc. Summit, N.J.; Asociación Nacional de Sordos de Nicaragua, Managua. Videocassette.

Plann, Susan. 1997. *A silent minority: Deaf education in Spain 1550–1835.* Berkeley: University of California Press.

Polich, Laura Gail. 1996. Constructions of deafness: The case study of Nicaragua. University of Texas, Austin. Typescript.

———. 1998. Social agency and deaf communities: A Nicaraguan case study. Ph.D. diss., University of Texas, Austin.

Schein, Jerome. 1992. *At home among strangers.* Washington, D.C.: Gallaudet University Press.

Schieffelin, Bambi. 1990. *The give and take of everyday life: Language socialization of Kaluli children.* Cambridge: Cambridge University Press.

Senghas, Ann. 1995. Children's contribution to the birth of Nicaraguan Sign Language. Ph.D. diss., Massachusetts Institute of Technology.

Senghas, Ann, Marie Coppola, Elissa Newport, and Ted Supalla. 1997. Argument structure in Nicaraguan Sign Language: The emergence of grammatical devices. In *Proceedings of the 21st Annual Boston University Conference on Language Development*, ed. E. Hughes, M. Hughes, and A. Greenhill, Vol. 2, 550–61. Somerville, Mass.: Cascadilla Press.

Senghas, Richard J. 1997. An 'unspeakable, unwriteable' language: Deaf identity, language and personhood among the first cohorts of Nicaraguan signers. Ph.D. diss., University of Rochester.

Senghas, Richard J., and Judy Kegl. 1994. Social considerations in the emergence of Idioma de Signos Nicaragüense (Nicaraguan Sign Language). *Signpost* 7 (1):40–45.

Senghas, Richard J., Judy Kegl, and Ann Senghas. 1994. Creation through contact: The emergence of a Nicaraguan deaf community. Paper presented at the 2nd International Conference on Deaf History, October, in Hamburg, Germany.

Smith, Hazel. 1993. *Nicaragua: Self-determination and survival.* London: Pluto Press.

Wallin, Lars. 1994. The study of sign language in society: Part two. In *The Deaf Way: Perspectives from the International Conference on Deaf Culture*, ed. C. J. Erting, R. C. Johnson, D. L. Smith, and B. D. Snider, 318–30. Washington, D.C.: Gallaudet University Press.

Washabaugh, William. 1986. *Five fingers for survival.* Ann Arbor: Karoma Publishers.

Whorf, Benjamin Lee. 1995. The relation of habitual thought and behavior to language. In *Language, culture and society: A book of readings*, ed. Ben G. Blount, 64–84. 2d ed. Prospect Heights, Ill.: Waveland Press. Originally published in Leslie Spier, A. Irving Hallowell, and Stanley S. Newman, eds., *Language, culture, and personality: Essays in memory of Sapir.* Menasha, Wis.: Sapir Memorial Publication Fund, 1941.

15 Sign Languages and Deaf Identities in Thailand and Viet Nam

James Woodward

Recent research (Woodward 1996, 1997, 2000, forthcoming) has revealed the existence of at least seven distinct sign languages in Thailand and in Viet Nam. This research has also shown that these seven languages belong to three different language families. Some rather unexpected, surprising relationships have been found among the sign languages, however, that need to be explained. Before attempting this explanation, it is useful to review the sources of comparative data for sign language varieties in Thailand and Viet Nam and summarize the findings of previous comparative lexical research on sign language varieties in those countries.

SOURCES OF DATA

THE TYPE OF LINGUISTIC DATA COLLECTED

The amount of data available on the language varieties determines the historical-comparative technique that should be used to analyze the data. Standard books on historical linguistics (including Crowley 1992; Lehmann 1992) point out that lexicostatistics is often used for determining relationships across unwritten languages that are underdescribed or undescribed and for which relatively limited amounts of data are available. Because all seven sign languages examined in this chapter are unwritten and are either underdescribed or undescribed and because data on six out of the seven languages are limited, lexicostatistics was chosen as the appropriate historical-linguistic technique for analysis.

> Lexicostatistics . . . allows us to determine the degree of relationship between two languages, simply by comparing the [core or basic] vocabularies of the languages and determining the degree of similarity between them. . . . [C]ore vocabulary includes items such as pronouns, numerals, body parts, geographical features, basic actions, and basic states. (Crowley 1992, 168–69)

Although the original 200-word Swadesh list is commonly used to compare for cognates in basic vocabulary across spoken languages (Crowley 1992, 170–71), using the same list for sign language research is not desirable because that use may result in slight overestimation of the relationship of closely related sign languages, moderate overestimation of the relationship of loosely related sign languages, and great overestimation of the relationship of historically unrelated sign languages (Woodward 1993a). The original 200-word Swadesh list contains many items such as body parts and pronouns that are represented indexically (often, simply by pointing) in many sign languages. The comparison of these indexic signs (NOSE, EYE, ME) results in a number of false potential cognates.

To avoid these problems of overestimation, a special vocabulary list (see table 15.1) has been used for comparisons of sign language varieties within Thailand (Woodward 1996, 1997), within Viet Nam (Woodward forthcoming), and between Thailand and Viet Nam (Woodward 2000). The list in table 15.1 that removes typically indexic signs is a modification of the 200-word Swadesh list and has proven useful in earlier comparisons of sign languages (Woodward 1978, 1991, 1992a, 1993a, 1993b).

TABLE 15.1   **Special Modified Swadesh Vocabulary List for Sign Languages**

1. all	26. grass	51. other	76. warm
2. animal	27. green	52. person	77. water
3. bad	28. heavy	53. play	78. wet
4. because	29. how	54. rain	79. what
5. bird	30. hunt	55. red	80. when
6. black	31. husband	56. right/correct	81. where
7. blood	32. ice	57. river	82. white
8. child	33. if	58. rope	83. who
9. count	34. kill	59. salt	84. wide
10. day	35. laugh	60. sea	85. wife
11. die	36. leaf	61. sharp	86. wind
12. dirty	37. lie	62. short	87. with
13. dog	38. live	63. sing	88. woman
14. dry	39. long	64. sit	89. wood
15. dull	40. louse	65. smooth	90. worm
16. dust	41. man	66. snake	91. year
17. earth	42. meat	67. snow	92. yellow
18. egg	43. mother	68. stand	93. full
19. fat/grease	44. mountain	69. star	94. moon
20. father	45. name	70. stone	95. brother
21. feather	46. narrow	71. sun	96. cat
22. fire	47. new	72. tail	97. dance
23. fish	48. night	73. thin	98. pig
24. flower	49. not	74. tree	99. sister
25. good	50. old	75. vomit	100. work

THE BACKGROUND OF THE DEAF CONSULTANTS

Sign translations of the basic vocabulary list in table 15.1 were collected from fluent deaf signers in four signing communities in Thailand and three signing communities in Viet Nam. The locations of these communities are shown on the map in figure 15.1, and the distances between the communities are shown in table 15.2.

The four signing communities in Thailand include (1) the Ban Khor signing

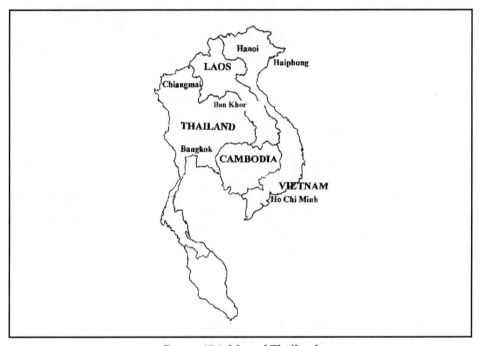

FIGURE 15.1 Map of Thailand

TABLE 15.2   Distances in Miles between the Seven Signing Communities

	Ban Khor	Original Chiangmai	Original Bangkok	Hai Phong	Ha Noi	Ho Chi Minh	Modern Thai
Ban Khor	0	394	381	268	260	474	12*
Original Chiangmai		0	364	519	472	757	364**
Original Bangkok			0	637	615	467	0**
Hai Phong				0	54	695	256*
Ha Noi					0	710	248*
Ho Chi Minh						0	462*
Modern Thai							0

*Nakornpanom City
**Bangkok

community, (2) the original Chiangmai signing community, (3) the original Bang-kok signing community, and (4) the modern Thai signing community.

The three signing communities in Viet Nam include (1) the Hai Phong signing community, (2) the Ha Noi signing community, and (3) the Ho Chi Minh City signing community. See table 15.3 for specific information with respect to data collection.

Previous research has compared for cognates in basic vocabulary across the four signing communities in Thailand (Woodward 1996, 1997), across the three signing communities in Viet Nam (Woodward forthcoming), and between each of the signing communities in Viet Nam and each of the sign signing communities in Thailand (Woodward 2000). Table 15.4 shows a summary of the results of the cognate comparisons of the sign language varieties used in the seven communi-ties.

According to standard lexicostatistical guidelines (Crowley 1992; Lehmann 1992), if language varieties have 80% or fewer cognates in basic vocabulary, they should be classified as separate languages. The percentages of cognates in table 15.4 indicate that the seven sign language varieties should be classified as seven separate languages.

Having determined that the seven sign language varieties are seven separate languages, we can now ask which of these seven languages should be classified as belonging to the same language family and which should be classified as be-longing to different language families. According to standard lexicostatistical guidelines (Crowley 1992; Lehmann 1992), if languages have from 36% to 80% cognates, they should be classified as belonging to the same language family. Thus, retaining the percentages above 35%, we see the language family relation-ships shown in table 15.5.

We can summarize the language family relationships in table 15.5 as follows:

1. The seven sign languages in Thailand and in Viet Nam can be classified into three language families.
2. The first language family includes Ban Khor Sign Language. Ban Khor Sign Language is the only known member of this sign language family.
3. The second language family includes Original Chiangmai Sign Language, Old Bangkok Sign Language, and Hai Phong Sign Language.
4. The third language family includes Modern Thai Sign Language, Ha Noi Sign Language, Ho Chi Minh Sign Language, and Hai Phong Sign Language.

PROBLEMS IN USING PREVIOUSLY PUBLISHED INFORMATION TO EXPLAIN THE FAMILY RELATIONSHIPS

Normally, we would expect to be able to explain these language family relation-ships by referring to previously published information about relationships be-tween language and nationality, language and geographical proximity, and language and ethnic identity in the communities studied. However, when we at-tempt to explain findings 2, 3, and 4 in terms of what is already published about language in relation to nationality, geographic proximity, and ethnic identity, we immediately run into problems.

First, traditional notions of nationality, geographical proximity, and ethnic

TABLE 15.3   Summary of Information about the Seven Signing Communities

Signing Community	Location	Age of Community Members	Source of Signs	Year Signs Were Collected
Ban Khor	Certain rice farming Villages in Ban Khor, Northeastern Thailand	All ages	9 females, 5 males (with ages ranging from 13 to 60)	1996
Original Chiangmai	Metro Chiangmai, Northern Thailand	Certain signers above 45	1 male (late forties)	1996
Original Bangkok	Metro Bangkok, Central Thailand	Certain signers above 45	1 male (late fifties) 1 female (late forties)	1996
Modern Thai	Urban areas in Thailand	Under 40, certain signers Above 40	Bangkok: 2 males & 2 females (under 40) Nakornpanom City: 2 males & 2 females (under 40)	1996
Hai Phong	Metro Hai Phong, Northern Viet Nam	All ages	2 females (late twenties) 1 male (early twenties)	1996
Ha Noi	Metro Ha Noi, Northern Viet Nam	All ages	1 male (late twenties)	1997
Ho Chi Minh City	Metro Ho Chi Minh City, Southern Viet Nam	All ages	2 females (early twenties)	1997

TABLE 15.4   Percentages of Cognates across Seven Sign Language Varieties

	Ban Khor	Original Chiangmai	Original Bangkok	Hai Phong	Ha Noi	Ho Chi Minh	Modern Thai
Ban Khor	>81%	34%	33%	26%	19%	18%	24%
Original Chiangmai		>81%	65%	46%	33%	23%	29%
Original Bangkok			>81%	48%	31%	25%	26%
Hai Phong				>81%	54%	54%	40%
Ha Noi					>81%	58%	45%
Ho Chi Minh						>81%	39%
Modern Thai							>81%

TABLE 15.5   Language Family Relationships of Sign Languages in Viet Nam and Sign Languages in Thailand

		Ban Khor	Original Chiangmai	Original Bangkok	Hai Phong	Ha Noi	Ho Chi Minh	Modern Thai
Family 1	Ban Khor	>81%						
Family 2	Original Chiang-mai		>81%	65%	46%			
	Original Bangkok			>81%	48%			
	Hai Phong				>81%			
Family 3	Hai Phong				>81%	54%	54%	40%
	Ha Noi					>81%	58%	45%
	Ho Chi Minh						>81%	39%
	Modern Thai							>81%

identity cannot explain finding 2. Hearing people living in Ban Khor share the same Thai nationality, speak the same language, and belong to the same ethnic group as hearing people living in Nakornpanom City, only 12 miles away from Ban Khor. Yet deaf people in Ban Khor use a completely different sign language in a completely different language family from that used by deaf people in Nakornpanom City, less than 12 miles from Ban Khor.

Second, traditional notions of nationality, geographical proximity, and ethnic identity cannot explain finding 3. Young hearing people living in Hai Phong do not share the same nationality, speak the same language, or share the same ethnic identity as older hearing people living in either Chiangmai or Bangkok. Yet younger deaf people in Hai Phong use a language that belongs to the same language family as that used by older deaf people in Chiangmai and in Bangkok. (Note also that, even though Ha Noi is only 54 miles from Hai Phong, Ha Noi Sign Language does not show the same relationship to Original Chiangmai Sign Language and Original Bangkok Sign Language as Hai Phong Sign Language does.)

Finally, traditional notions of nationality, geographical proximity, and ethnic identity cannot explain finding 4. Young hearing people living in Bangkok do not share the same nationality, speak the same language, or share the same ethnic identity as younger hearing people living in Hai Phong, Ha Noi, or Ho Chi Minh City. Yet younger deaf people in Bangkok use a language that belongs to the same language family as that used by younger deaf people in Hai Phong, Ha Noi, and Ho Chi Minh City. (Note also that, even though Bangkok is closer to Chiangmai (364 miles) than it is to Ho Chi Minh City (467 miles), Ha Noi (615 miles), and Hai Phong (637 miles), Modern Thai Sign Language belongs not to the same language family as Original Chiangmai Sign Language but to the same family as Hai Phong Sign Language, Ha Noi Sign Language, and Ho Chi Minh City Sign Language.)

After having examined traditional notions of nationality, geographic proximity, and ethnic identity from previously published information, we still have not been able to explain the following:

1. Why doesn't Ban Khor Sign Language, which is used in Thailand, belong to a language family that includes other Thai sign languages? Why is it separate from all the other sign languages examined?
2. Why doesn't Modern Thai Sign Language belong to a language family that includes other Thai sign languages? Why does it belong to a language family that appears to be made up mostly of sign languages used in Viet Nam?
3. How can Hai Phong Sign Language, which is used in Viet Nam, belong to two separate language families, especially when one of these language families appears to include only original Thai sign languages?

It is useful at this point to consider the hypothesis that the explanations for the linguistic findings in this chapter can be found in unique events in Deaf histories in Thailand and Viet Nam.

ASPECTS OF DEAF HISTORIES IN THAILAND AND VIET NAM THAT CAN EXPLAIN THE LINGUISTIC RELATIONSHIPS AMONG THE SEVEN SIGN LANGUAGES

BAN KHOR

Ban Khor Sign Language has developed over the last 80 years as a unique response to a substantial increase in the number of deaf villagers. Some villages in Ban Khor such as Mu 2 and Mu 10 have more than one deaf person per 100 people, which is from five to ten times the expected population of one to two in every 1,000 and from five to ten times the actual percentage of deaf people in the other six communities. Deaf and hearing people in Ban Khor have chosen to respond to this increase in ways that are similar to responses of other small communities found in many parts of the world with similarly large proportions of deaf people: the South Pacific (Kuschel 1973), the Caribbean (Washabaugh, Woodward, and De Santis 1978), North America (Groce 1985), Africa (Frishberg 1987), and South America (Johnson 1991; Woodward 1992b). The great majority of hearing people in Ban Khor have adopted either neutral or positive attitudes toward deaf people. As a result of these attitudes, hearing people and deaf people have developed a purely indigenous sign language for use in the local area—a sign language that developed without any significant outside contact and that is maintained without outside contact and influence. This sign language is used by the overwhelming majority of deaf people in Ban Khor as their first and only language and by the large majority of hearing people bilingually. Ethnographic field observations would suggest that, although both hearing and deaf people are aware of other sign languages in Thailand, they have no desire to change or replace their indigenous sign language for one that did not develop inside their own local community.

In summary, Ban Khor Sign Language patterns differently from other sign languages in Thailand because the history of deaf people in Ban Khor is not shared by Thai deaf people who use Original Chiangmai Sign Language, by Thai deaf people who use Original Bangkok Sign Language, or even by Thai deaf people 12 miles away in Nakornpanom City who use Modern Thai Sign Language.

Modern Thai Sign Language

Modern Thai Sign Language has developed over the last 50 years as a unique response to the introduction of an almost exclusively hearing-controlled centralized system of formal education for Thai deaf people (see Reilly 1995). During the development of this centralized system, several highly influential Thai hearing people introduced American Sign Language (ASL) vocabulary into the emergent educational system. This introduction of ASL vocabulary into a school deaf population almost totally lacking in deaf children of deaf parents has resulted in a 52% absorption rate of ASL cognates into basic vocabulary in Modern Thai Sign Language in the last 50 years (Woodward 1996).

Given the great amount of foreign contact and borrowing that has influenced Modern Thai Sign Language's development and use and the lack of this contact and borrowing in other sign languages in Thailand, little doubt should remain as to why Modern Thai Sign Language is not closely related to any other sign language in Thailand and why it belongs to a language family separate from any other sign language in Thailand. But why then does Modern Thai Sign Language appear to belong to the same family as sign languages in Vietnam?

The relationship of Modern Thai Sign Language to sign languages in Vietnam in fact is not a result of direct contact but of indirect contact. Ha Noi Sign Language, Ho Chi Minh Sign Language, and Hai Phong Sign Language all show very strong influences from French Sign Language, which was introduced into Vietnamese schools for the deaf. French Sign Language and American Sign Language have a 61% rate of shared cognates in basic vocabulary and, therefore, belong to the same language family (Woodward 1978). Thus, the influence of ASL on Modern Thai Sign Language and the influence of French Sign Language on Ha Noi Sign Language, Ho Chi Minh Sign Language, and Hai Phong Sign Language result in a large number of shared cognates between Modern Thai Sign Language and sign languages in Vietnam.

In summary, Modern Thai Sign Language patterns differently from other sign languages in Thailand because the history of deaf people who use Modern Thai Sign Language is not shared by Thai deaf people who use Original Chiangmai Sign Language or by those who use Original Bangkok Sign Language or Ban Khor Sign Language. At the same time, Modern Thai Sign Language patterns similarly to Ha Noi Sign Language, Hai Phong Sign Language, and Ho Chi Minh Sign Language because all of these sign languages have been strongly influenced by one or more sign languages from the French Sign Language family.

Hai Phong Sign Language

Ha Noi Sign Language, Ho Chi Minh Sign Language, and Hai Phong Sign Language have all three been influenced by French Sign Language. However, Hai Phong signers, perhaps because of their relative isolation from Ha Noi and Ho Chi Minh City, have managed to preserve more original Southeast Asian signs than the other signers in Ha Noi and Ho Chi Minh City.

Even when Hai Phong has borrowed a French sign for a vocabulary item, Hai Phong signers sometimes keep the original Southeast Asian sign along with the French sign. This practice has resulted in pairs of cognates for a number of words. One sign in the cognate pair is cognate with original sign languages in Thailand and one with French Sign Language. Examples of this pairing can be found in signs for WIFE, HUSBAND, and PIG, among others. Because of these pairs, Hai Phong Sign Language shows strong similarities to Southeast Asian sign languages that have not been influenced by French Sign Language or ASL (Original Chiangmai Sign Language and Original Bangkok Sign Language) and also shows strong similarities to Southeast Asian sign languages that have been influenced by French Sign Language or ASL (Ha Noi Sign Language, Ho Chi Minh Sign Language, and Modern Thai Sign Language). When we put all of these facts together, an interesting picture of linguistic relationships emerges. This picture is graphically represented in figure 15.2.

Types of Sign Languages in Thailand and Viet Nam

Figure 15.2 suggests that four types of sign languages are found in Thailand and Viet Nam: "indigenous," "original," "link," and "modern." Each of these types results from differences in the history of deaf people in the signing community, especially in relation to the amount and type of outside contact the signing communities have had.

Indigenous sign languages like Ban Khor Sign Language developed independently of contact with other Southeast Asian Sign Languages and independently of contact with Western sign languages such as French or American sign lan-

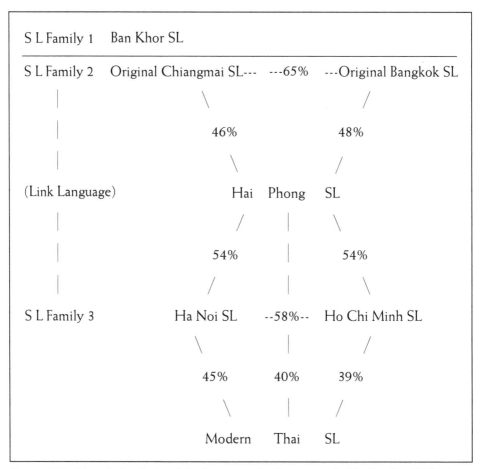

FIGURE 15.2. **Linguistic relationships between sign languages in Thailand and Viet Nam**

guages. Therefore, indigenous sign languages will belong to different language families from original, link, and modern sign languages.

Original sign languages like Original Chiangmai Sign Language and Original Bangkok Sign Language developed out of contact with other Southeast Asian sign languages and independently of contact with Western sign languages. Therefore, original sign languages will belong to different language families from indigenous and modern sign languages and will probably be grouped with link sign languages.

Link sign languages like Hai Phong Sign Language developed out of contact with other Southeast Asian sign languages and Western sign languages. Link sign languages show strong relationships to both original sign languages and modern sign languages and will probably appear to belong to an original sign language family and to a modern sign language family. Thus, link languages can be viewed as linking two separate language families and showing a continuum of historical relationship between the two families.

Modern sign languages like Ha Noi Sign Language, Ho Chi Minh Sign Language, and Modern Thai Sign Language developed out of contact with other Southeast Asian sign languages and Western sign languages. Modern sign languages, however, show less relationship to original sign languages than they do to Western sign languages and will belong to different language families from indigenous and original sign languages.

DIFFERENCES IN THE LINGUISTIC AND SOCIAL IDENTITIES OF DEAF PEOPLE IN THAILAND AND VIET NAM WHO USE DIFFERENT TYPES OF SIGN LANGUAGES

Deaf people who use the four types of sign languages in Thailand and in Viet Nam display clear differences in linguistic and social identity. Major differences can be summarized by asking and answering four questions.

First, do deaf people maintain a separate linguistic identity by using a (sign) language that the majority of hearing people in the community do not know?

For six of the seven situations, the answer is yes. In only one case, Ban Khor, where an indigenous sign language is used, is the answer no. Deaf people in Ban Khor do not maintain a separate linguistic identity from that of hearing people in the area because the great majority of hearing people in Ban Khor know and use Ban Khor Sign Language.

Second, do deaf people maintain a separate social identity by creating, maintaining, or participating in deaf social institutions such as deaf schools, deaf clubs, or deaf associations?

For four of the seven situations (all of the link and modern sign languages) the answer is yes because deaf people in these four situations attend special schools for the deaf and maintain deaf clubs. For the other three situations (all of the indigenous and original sign languages), the answer is no. Specifically, in the case of the indigenous sign language situation, deaf people in Ban Khor simply do not have and do not want to have a culturally Deaf social identity. Deaf people in Ban Khor have traveled to nearby Nakornpanom City and to Bangkok; have met culturally Deaf Thai adults who use Modern Thai Sign Language; and have had the opportunity to learn Modern Thai Sign Language, to attend special schools for deaf people, and to enter the national Thai Deaf Community. However, deaf people in Ban Khor have expressed in ethnographic interviews that they do not identify with and do not want to identify with culturally Deaf people in Thailand and that they have no desire to form a social, cultural, or linguistic group that is distinct from hearing people in Ban Khor. In the case of the original sign language situations (Original Chiangmai Sign Language and Original Bangkok Sign Language), deaf people did not attend deaf schools because no special schools for deaf people existed in Thailand at that time (approximately 50 years ago). Users of original sign languages in Thailand also did not establish and maintain deaf clubs or other formal deaf organizations.

Third, do deaf people organize "Deaf-only" social events where the norm is for hearing people, especially nonsigners, to be excluded?

For three of the seven situations (all of the modern sign languages) the answer is yes because deaf clubs in these three situations organize many of their events exclusively for their deaf membership. For the other four situations (all of the indigenous, original, and link sign languages) the answer is no. In the case of Ban

Khor, an indigenous sign language, all social events include hearing and deaf people on an equal basis. At these events, deaf and hearing people converse and socialize freely and on an equal basis in Ban Khor Sign Language.

In the case of the original sign languages, it is clear that deaf people and hearing people attended many of the same social functions. Because this interaction occurred approximately 50 years ago, it is somewhat difficult to determine the type and extent of interaction of hearing and deaf people. However, because relatively few hearing people signed, deaf and hearing people probably did not often converse at these events but, rather, interacted in other ways.

In the case of Hai Phong Sign Language, a link language, I was able to attend a typical meeting of the Hai Phong Deaf Club, which shows a particularly interesting inclusion of hearing people. At this evening meeting, about 60 deaf people and about 15 hearing people, most of whom could not sign, were present. The first half was a business meeting conducted in Hai Phong Sign Language by deaf people. During this time, most of the hearing people sat in the back of the room and talked quietly to each other. After the business meeting, the deaf and hearing people took part in group and individual dancing for the rest of the evening. No one was left out of any dance, everyone was expected to participate, and even reluctant dancers such as myself were gently pulled out on the dance floor by small groups of deaf people. There was little conversation and little need for conversation, but deaf people and hearing people in Hai Phong truly seemed to enjoy this type of intergroup interaction.

Finally, we consider the fourth question, do deaf people have a national sense of deaf identity?

For one of the seven situations (Modern Thai Sign Language) the answer is yes because Modern Thai Sign Language is the only national sign language of the seven languages and because it is the only community associated with a national association of deaf people, the National Association of the Deaf in Thailand (see Suwanarat et al. 1986; Suwanarat et al. 1990). For the other six sign languages, the answer is currently no.

At this point, it will be helpful to summarize the differences in linguistic and social identity in chart form. Table 15.6 shows answers to the four questions in a graphic format. The table shows that the answers to the four questions fit into an implicational scale. This implicational scale can be explained as follows:

- The existence of a separate national identity implies the existence of separate Deaf-only events (Modern Thai Sign Language), but not vice versa (other modern sign languages).

- The existence of separate Deaf-only events implies the existence of separate Deaf institutions (all the modern sign languages), but not vice versa (link sign languages).

- The existence of separate Deaf institutions implies the existence of a separate linguistic identity for Deaf people (link and modern sign languages), but not vice versa (original sign languages).

- Finally, the implicational scale shows that the existence of a sign language does not imply the existence of a separate Deaf linguistic identity (Ban Khor Sign Language).

TABLE 15.6   Summary of Differences in Linguistic and Social Identity

Language Name	Language Type	Q1 Separate Deaf Linguistic Identity	Q2 Separate Deaf Social Identity With Deaf Social Institutions	Q3 Separate Deaf Only Events	Q4 National Deaf Identity
Ban Khor	Indigenous	No	No	No	No
Original Chiangmai	Original	Yes	No	No	No
Original Bangkok	Original	Yes	No	No	No
Hai Phong	Link	Yes	Yes	No	No
Ha Noi	Modern	Yes	Yes	Yes	No
Ho Chi Minh	Modern	Yes	Yes	Yes	No
Modern Thai	Modern	Yes	Yes	Yes	Yes

SUMMARY AND DISCUSSION

In summary, this chapter has shown the following:

1. The sign language family relationships in Thailand and in Viet Nam differ from the spoken language family relationships in the same communities.
2. The sign language family relationships are not explainable from what is known about language in relation to the nationality, geographic proximity, and ethnic identity of hearing people in Thailand and in Viet Nam.
3. The sign language family relationships are explainable from what is known about unique aspects of Deaf histories in Thailand and in Viet Nam.
4. A separate sign language is a necessary condition for the development of separate Deaf linguistic and social identities (all original, link, and modern sign languages).
5. A separate sign language is not a sufficient condition for the development of separate Deaf linguistic and social identities (indigenous sign languages such as Ban Khor).
6. A separate Deaf linguistic identity can develop without formal social institutions (such as schools and clubs) for deaf people (original sign languages such as Original Chiangmai Sign Language and Original Bangkok Sign Language).
7. The existence of formal social organizations of deaf people is a necessary condition for the existence of "Deaf-only" events and the general exclusion of hearing people, especially nonsigning hearing people, from these events (all modern sign languages such as Ha Noi Sign Language, Ho Chi Minh Sign Language, and Modern Thai Sign Language).

8. The existence of formal social organizations of deaf people is not a sufficient condition for the existence of "Deaf-only" events and the general exclusion of hearing people, especially nonsigning hearing people, from these events (link sign languages such as Hai Phong Sign Language).

In addition to the eight findings discussed above, the linguistic and ethnographic data on these communities suggest the following additional trends for the four types of sign languages.

Indigenous sign languages tend to occur in relatively small village communities where there is a larger proportion of deaf people than expected and where a large proportion of hearing people have contact with deaf people and learn the signing that naturally developed. In indigenous signing communities, deaf people are well integrated into the village community. Most people in the village have similar occupations (farmers, fishermen, etc.), and deaf people have equal access to these occupations. Most deaf people do not attend special schools for deaf people.

Most deaf people do not participate in formal associations of deaf people. Most deaf people in the village do not want to form or belong to a separate deaf community. Because of their full participation in village life, they do not see themselves as intrinsically different from hearing people in the village. Thus, it is the norm for deaf people who use an indigenous sign language not to form a separate community or to have a linguistic and social identity that is intrinsically different from that of hearing people in the same community.

Original sign languages tend to occur in larger, more urban areas where few hearing people learn to use the signing that is used by deaf people in the area. Thus, it tends to be the norm for deaf people who use an original sign language to have a linguistic identity that differs in important ways from the linguistic identity of hearing people in the same urban area. Original sign languages and the linguistic identities associated with them tend to be regionally limited. Although some contact may occur among signers from different regions in the country (or between neighboring countries) and although this contact may result in closely related sign languages and linguistic identities, this contact is not extensive enough to result in deaf people having the same language and linguistic identity. In addition, it appears that these kinds of regional communities do not consider systematic contact with other deaf communities—nationally or internationally—to be a high priority. In original sign language communities, there have been no reported efforts to establish formal separate institutions of or for deaf people, including special schools, regional associations of deaf people, a national association of deaf people, or to establish a national Deaf identity or sign language. When schools or organizations are established with link or modern sign languages, deaf users of original sign languages tend to gradually give up their original sign language and linguistic identity for a new identity based on a link sign language or on a modern sign language introduced into the school system.

Link sign languages, which are partial mixtures of original sign languages with foreign sign languages (typically French Sign Language, American Sign Language, or both), have been introduced in schools in relatively isolated urban areas such as Hai Phong. Link languages preserve many older forms that still connect sign languages in modern sign language families with certain sign languages in original sign language families. Although link languages are associated with schools for deaf people and with the formation of local and regional deaf clubs and associations, users of link sign languages may still retain a significant amount of deaf-hearing interaction in their social events.

Modern sign languages, like link sign languages, have resulted in the mixing of original sign languages with foreign sign languages, typically French Sign Language, American Sign Language, or both. In most situations, modern sign languages have replaced original sign languages and have endangered the existence of original sign languages. Modern sign languages are often promoted through schools for deaf people in Southeast Asia (Reilly 1995), and in general, modern sign languages tend to be used in somewhat wider regions than original sign languages. Users of modern sign languages tend to establish formal social institutions that promote contact and interaction with other deaf associations. These associations often start at the local level through schools and ultimately open the door for the establishment of a national Deaf identity and a national sign language.

It is important to note that a national identity for deaf people most probably would not have developed in Thailand or would not be in the process of developing in Viet Nam without the establishment of a national association of deaf people, and the establishment of a national association of deaf people would most likely not have developed in Thailand or in Viet Nam without international contact with other national or international associations of deaf people.

In Thailand, the formation of local associations led rather quickly to contact with national associations of deaf people outside of Thailand and with the World Federation of the Deaf. This contact was fostered by foreign experts working in Thailand. The contact, in turn, led to the establishment of the National Association of the Deaf in Thailand and to the development of a national linguistic and social identity for Deaf people in Thailand. While the linguistic and social shift to a national Deaf identity has provided a nationally unifying force for empowerment of Deaf people in Thailand, ironically, it has endangered at the same time an important part of Thai Deaf history and culture—the original sign languages in Thailand that developed internally in Thailand with little, if any, outside influence.

The movement toward a national association of deaf people in Vietnam and toward the development of a national Deaf identity in Vietnam has moved at a slower pace. However, Vietnam is now poised to establish a national association of deaf people, which can be attributed in large part to recent contact with the Japanese Federation of the Deaf (the Asia Pacific regional representative for the World Federation of the Deaf) and the National Association of the Deaf in Thailand. This contact was fostered through a meeting in Ha Noi that was sponsored in part by the United Nations Economic and Social Commission for Asia and the Pacific (UNESCAP).

In fact, the sign language data from Hai Phong were collected at that meeting in Ha Noi. It was not surprising to find Deaf people from Viet Nam arguing for "standardization" of regional sign languages into one national sign language. It was also not surprising to find hearing people in Viet Nam suggesting importation of vocabulary from Western sign languages, including American Sign Language. Nevertheless, it was refreshing to note that all international participants (deaf and hearing) at the conference strongly recommended intensive study and documentation of sign languages in Viet Nam before any formal language policy be considered.

After discussion, participants from Viet Nam and international participants were able to unanimously agree on strategy. In the report of the meeting in Viet Nam, they resolved to do the following:

(8) Encourage the documentation and description of Vietnamese sign language(s), (and) the development of reference materials related to Vietnamese sign language(s), including dictionaries, grammatical handbooks and sign language instructional materials, and the formal training of Vietnamese sign language interpreters. (UNESCAP 1996, 1–3)

The formal documentation and description of sign languages in Viet Nam began in early 1999. Linguistic work related to sign languages in Viet Nam will include formal training in basic sign language linguistic research for deaf people as part of the process of documentation and description of sign languages in Viet Nam. The linguistic research will have two primary foci. One primary focus will be the study of any remaining original sign languages in Viet Nam. The second primary focus will be the study of modern "link" sign languages such as Hai Phong Sign Language, which preserve older forms and which still link certain sign languages in modern sign language families with certain sign languages in original sign language families.

At this point, it remains uncertain what effect the establishment of a national association of deaf people in Viet Nam will have on distinct sign languages in Vietnam such as Hai Phong Sign Language, Ha Noi Sign Language and Ho Chi Minh Sign Language. Researchers hope that the training in sign language linguistics provided to Deaf people in Viet Nam will help lessen or eliminate potential negative effects on these sign languages.

In conclusion, although we have gained some knowledge about the relationships of linguistic and social identities of deaf people in Southeast Asia, a great deal of work remains. Other related indigenous sign languages may be found in other small villages with large deaf populations in the same general region as Ban Khor in Northeast Thailand. For example, the villages of Pla Bag and Bang Na, which are relatively close to Ban Khor, also appear to have larger deaf populations than expected, and Pla Bag and Bang Na may have sign language varieties related to Ban Khor. In addition, other indigenous sign language families may be found in Thailand, in Viet Nam, or in both countries. Researchers also will probably find other sign language families of the indigenous type spread throughout Southeast Asia. For example, Miller (forthcoming) reports an indigenous sign language community in Bali, Indonesia.

In relation to original sign languages, it is likely that there are original sign languages in the northeastern and in the southern parts of Thailand in addition to those found in Chiangmai and Bangkok. In addition, an Original Hai Phong Sign Language, an Original Ha Noi Sign Language, and an Original Saigon (Ho Chi Minh City) Sign Language most likely were in use before French Sign Language had an effect on sign languages in Viet Nam. Other original sign languages have also probably been used in other parts of Southeast Asia. Some of these original sign languages may still exist among older signers. Some probably have already died out. These original sign languages may belong to the same original sign language family as those in Thailand and Viet Nam or to another original sign language family or families.

With respect to link sign languages, the possibility exists that, in addition to Hai Phong Sign Language, other link languages will be found in relatively isolated deaf communities in Viet Nam. Other link sign languages may also be found in other countries in Southeast Asia. These link languages are very important because they provide important clues about the history of sign languages and Deaf identities in Southeast Asia.

Gaps also remain in our knowledge of modern sign languages, but these gaps are not so crucial at the present time. Modern sign languages are mixtures, probably creolizations, of original sign languages with French Sign Language, American Sign Language, or both. Modern sign languages have already replaced original sign languages among younger signers in Thailand and in Viet Nam as well as in Malaysia, Singapore, and the Philippines and have endangered the continued existence of original sign languages. Within 50 years, the likelihood is high that all original sign languages in Southeast Asia will be extinct, dying out with the users who still remember them.

What is needed at this point is a large-scale, in-depth sociolinguistic study of sign languages in Southeast Asia combined with an extensive ethnographic study of Deaf identities in Southeast Asia. The combined study must look at a large number of deaf people who have competence in one or more sign languages in Southeast Asia. These deaf people must be selected from various stratified age groups and various regions of Southeast Asia, and these deaf people should represent various deaf and Deaf social identities in Southeast Asia. This research needs to include communities using original, indigenous, and modern sign languages and needs to focus primarily on communities where sign languages are most endangered and where link languages are used. Link languages, which preserve older forms and which still link certain sign languages in modern sign language families with certain sign languages in original sign language families, provide important clues about the history of sign languages and deaf identities in Southeast Asia.

At this point, we know that the great majority of users of original sign languages in most countries in Southeast Asia are approximately 50 years old. If the documentation of these original sign languages is not completed in one generation, these sign languages quite likely will be lost to linguistic study forever because we currently have no records of these sign languages.

If original sign languages in Southeast Asia die before they can be properly documented and described, Deaf people in Southeast Asia will lose a valuable part of their history, all Southeast Asian people will lose a valuable part of their national or regional heritage, and the rest of us will lose one of the important keys to understanding the history of sign languages and deaf identities in Southeast Asia.

ACKNOWLEDGMENTS

Research on which this chapter is based was supported in part by the Research Department at Ratchasuda College; by an internal Mahidol University Grant, "A

Preliminary Study of Deaf Identity and Deaf Culture in the Bangkok Metropolitan Area"; by an external grant from the Thai government, "A Study of the Grammar of Thai Sign Language and of Thai Deaf Culture"; by a grant from Ratchasuda Foundation, "A Pilot Study of Sign Language Varieties in Ban Khor, Nakornpanom"; and by Sign Language Research, Inc. Parts of this chapter were presented at the 1997 annual meeting of the American Anthropological Association, Washington, D.C., in the panel "Ethnically Deaf: Identity, Culture, and the Making of Sign Language Communities," organized by Karen Nakamura and Leila Monaghan. I would like to thank Angela M. Nonaka and Leila Monaghan for their comments and suggestions on various drafts of this chapter. I would also like to thank Phornthip Saksirisamphun for her help in producing the map used in this chapter.

REFERENCES

Crowley, Terry. 1992. *An introduction to historical linguistics.* Oxford: Oxford University Press.

Frishberg, Nancy. 1987. Ghanaian Sign Language. In *Gallaudet encyclopedia of deaf people and deafness,* ed. John V. Van Cleve, 778–79. New York: McGraw Hill.

Groce, Nora. 1985. *Everyone here spoke sign language.* Cambridge, Mass.: Harvard University Press.

Johnson, Robert. 1991. Sign language, culture, and community in a Yucatec-Mayan village. *Sign Language Studies* 73:461–74.

Kuschel, Rolf. 1973. The silent inventor: The creation of a sign language by the only deaf-mute on a Polynesian island. *Sign Language Studies* 3:1–27.

Lehmann, Winifred. 1992. *Historical linguistics: An introduction.* New York: Routledge.

Miller, Don. Forthcoming. Sign languages of Bali. In *Proceedings of the First Australasian Deaf Studies Conference,* ed. Jan Branson and Don Miller. Melbourne: Khiros Press.

Reilly, Charles. 1995. A Deaf way of education: Interaction among children in a Thai boarding school. Ph.D. diss., University of Maryland.

Suwanarat, Manfa, Anucha Ratanasint, Vilaiporn Rungsrithong, Lloyd Anderson, and Owen Wrigley. 1990. *The Thai Sign Language dictionary: Revised and expanded edition.* Bangkok: The National Association of the Deaf in Thailand.

Suwanarat, Manfa, Anucha Ratanasint, Vilaiporn Rungsrithong, Waruunee Buathong, Charles Reilly, Lloyd Anderson, Soontorn Yen-Klao, and Owen Wrigley. 1986. *The Thai Sign Language dictionary: Book one.* Bangkok: The National Association of the Deaf in Thailand.

UNESCAP. 1996. *Resolutions of the Workshop on the Promotion of Self-Help Initiatives of People with Disabilities in Viet Nam, 28–31 October 1996, Ha Noi.* Bangkok: UNESCAP.

Washabaugh, William, James Woodward, and Susan De Santis. 1978. Providence Island Sign Language: A context-dependent language. *Anthropological Linguistics* 20 (3):95–109.

Woodward, James. 1978. Historical bases of American Sign Language. In *Understanding language through sign language research,* ed. Patricia Siple, 333–48. New York: Academic Press.

———. 1991. Sign language varieties in Costa Rica. *Sign Language Studies* 73:329–46.

———. 1992a. Historical bases of New Costa Rican Sign Language. *Revista de Filología y Lingüística de la Universidad de Costa Rica* 18 (1):127–32.

———. 1992b. A preliminary examination of Brunca Sign Language in Costa Rica. *Estudios de Lingüística Chibcha* 11:1–7.

———. 1993a. Lexical evidence for the existence of South Asian and East Asian sign language families. *Journal of Asian Pacific Communication* 4 (2):91–106.

———. 1993b. The relationship of sign language varieties in India, Pakistan, and Nepal. *Sign Language Studies* 78:15–22.

———. 1996. Modern Standard Thai Sign Language, influence from ASL, and its relationship to original sign language in Thailand. *Sign Language Studies* 92:227–52.

———. 1997. A preliminary examination of Ban Khor Sign Language. Research Department, Ratchasuda College, Mahidol University at Salaya. Typescript.

———. 2000. Sign languages and sign language families in Thailand and Viet Nam. In *The signs of language revisited: An anthology in honor of Ursula Bellugi and Edward Klima*, ed. Karen Emmorey and Harlan Lane, 23–47. Mahwah, N.J.: Erlbaum.

———. Forthcoming. Sign language varieties in Viet Nam. In *Proceedings of the First Australasian Deaf Studies Conference*, ed. Jan Branson and Don Miller. Melbourne: Khiros Press.

16 | A for Apple: The Impact
of Western Education and
ASL on the Deaf
Community in Kano State,
Northern Nigeria

Constanze Schmaling

Nigeria, with its approximately 100 million inhabitants, is the most populated country in Africa. Hausa is the majority language of much of northern Nigeria and the southern parts of the Republic of Niger. There are an estimated 50 million Hausa speakers of which up to 40 million live in northern Nigeria and up to four million live in Niger (Wolff 1993, 1–2). Colonies of Hausa settlers can also be found in other parts of West Africa. Approximately 80%–90% of the estimated 25 million people whose mother tongue is Hausa live in northern Nigeria. The Hausa-speaking heartlands include the areas of Kano, Katsina, and Sokoto. This chapter focuses on the deaf community in Kano State and is based on ethnographic data collected during 18 months of fieldwork in northern Nigeria between 1994 and 1998. The state capital, Kano City, with its approximately two and a half million inhabitants, is the largest and most important Hausa city.

Deaf people in Hausaland are highly socially integrated and play a full part in the everyday life of the community. Hausa society is a predominantly rural and relatively egalitarian society. Productivity is much the same for all members. Most Hausa are part-time farmers and part-time specialists in various craft occupations, and most are also involved in small-scale business or trading. This also includes deaf people. Most people live in large compounds with the extended family. People, whether deaf or hearing, are always seen in the context of their family and relatives, their village, and the wider society (see also Devlieger 1994).

While living in Kano, the author used Hausa Sign Language when interacting with deaf people and Hausa when interacting with hearing people.

Social life takes place as much on the streets as in houses or compounds, and deaf people are part of it just like everybody else.

The integration of deaf people within Hausa society is also furthered by the fact that many people become deaf, whether because of an accident or a sickness, after they have already found their place within a certain social setting. Their social status does not change after they become deaf, and their family, friends, and neighbors treat them the same way as they had before. Religion also plays an important role in this context; the majority of the Hausa are Muslim, and they hold a strong belief that everything comes from God, including deafness.[1]

This society has always accepted that deaf people use sign language for communication. Spoken language has never been forced on deaf people either at home or at school. On the contrary, hearing people exhibit a willingness to use signs or sign language to communicate with deaf people, and many hearing people are able to converse freely and effectively with deaf people through signs (or gestures) and sign language, at least on a basic level (see also Last 1991, 3). Hearing people are not ashamed of "talking" with their hands. In Hausaland, the hands are used much more often for communication even among hearing people, and many common gestures occur frequently in daily conversation, either as a substitute or complement to spoken language.[2] The same practice seems to be true for other West African countries. The fact that people are used to a multilingual environment may also contribute to the readiness for improvisation. Many hearing people have acquired their sign language knowledge through contact with the deaf community. This informal way of learning may also contribute to the integration of deaf people within the larger Hausa society.

The Deaf Community in Kano State

Deaf people in Kano State also come together as a community of their own. They have established a wide network and share a sense of common identity. One rarely finds deaf people who live in isolation and have never associated themselves with the deaf community. Deaf people have places in the towns and villages where they come together in the afternoons or in the evenings to share information and experiences, just as hearing people do. At Gidan Shattima, for example, near the Central Mosque in Kano's Old City, mainly younger deaf people meet daily. Members of the deaf community all share a common language, Hausa Sign Language. No records exist on the history of Hausa Sign Language, but as far back as people can remember, deaf people have always used *maganar hannu* "the language of the hands." Deaf people generally do not acquire Hausa Sign Language through formal instruction but learn it from other deaf people.

The social structure of the deaf community in Kano State reflects that of the larger Hausa society. There are and always have been lines of division between different groups, with respect to, for example, age (*tsoffi* "old people" as opposed to *yara* "children, young people") or place of residence (*'yan birni* "city people" as opposed to *'yan k'auye* "villagers"). Some of these differences are also reflected in the language. Some signs are preferred by older deaf people whereas other signs are used only by younger deaf people. Likewise, some signs are normally used by village people and other signs are exclusively used in the city.

The type or extent of deafness has never led to any group division. Members of the deaf community may be native signers or may have acquired sign language later in life because of postlingual deafness. Whether somebody has some residual hearing or is profoundly deaf is without significance because little corrective technology is available; there are no hearing aids and only a few audiometers in the whole area. Differences between deaf and hard of hearing people (*bebaye* as opposed to *kurame*)[3] are, however, evident in the usage of certain signs and also in the structure of signed sentences. Some late-deafened people regularly resort to a kind of signed Hausa, using signs from Hausa Sign Language but following the word order of spoken Hausa.

Deaf people have also been organizing themselves over the past years. The Kano State Association of the Deaf (*K'ungiyar Bebaye ta Jihar Kano*), or the KSAD, was founded approximately 15 years ago. Until the mid-1990s, the KSAD was the largest and most important association of the deaf in Kano State. It was initially composed mainly of younger deaf people who had had access to formal education. Its activities included weekly meetings to discuss current issues, including how to find jobs for their members, and biweekly meetings with Qur'anic teachers. In late 1994, the Kano State government merged the KSAD and another deaf organization that had mostly older, "illiterate" members. As a result of this merger, most projects of the KSAD were cancelled, and many "literate" members left the organization. However, in 2001, eight new deaf associations were established within Kano State, including one in Kano Municipal that has resumed some of the original activities. There are also several deaf soccer clubs (soccer is a favorite sport). At Rumfa College, for example, deaf students have soccer training every afternoon.

The Introduction of Formal Education

The first school for the deaf in Nigeria, the Wesley School for the Deaf, was established in Lagos in 1958 (Ojile 1994).[4] It was initially run by the Society for the Care of the Deaf (founded by a group of philanthropic Nigerians) and the British Methodist Mission. In 1960, Andrew Foster, a deaf African American missionary, opened a school for the deaf in Ibadan, and in the following years, other schools were opened, mainly in the southern parts of the country. Under the Education Act of 1977, the first and only school for the deaf in Kano State, Tudun Maliki School for the Deaf and the Blind, was opened. This opening occurred during the oil-boom years, a time when Nigeria could afford to invest money in special education.

Tudun Maliki is still the only school for the deaf in Kano State and one of the few in the northern part of the country. Initially, the school had eight students who were deaf and six who were blind. The school now has approximately 250 students, almost all in the deaf section. Students are educated for nine years, six years in the Primary Section and three years in the Junior Secondary Section. Afterward, they are integrated into Senior Secondary Schools or Technical Colleges. Some Tudun Maliki students have gone on to university, where most of them have obtained a diploma in special education.

Just as the system of formal education for the deaf was imported to Nigeria, so the communication method of the exporting country was also acquired. In the Wesley School, deaf children were taught orally. In 1960, Foster introduced the manual method and American Sign Language (ASL), a foreign sign language. In the following years, the use of the manual method and of ASL for teaching was further encouraged by deaf "pioneers" who had been trained by Foster and who helped with establishing other schools for the deaf. Theoretically, Total Communication, based on signs from ASL, is used today as the language of instruction at most Nigerian schools for the deaf. In practice, however, it is a kind of Signed English that is based on signs from ASL but that follows syntax and idiomatic expressions of spoken Nigerian English.

At Tudun Maliki School, ASL-based signing was introduced in the 1977–1978 school year. The arrival of Western education and—more importantly—the introduction of ASL have resulted in structural changes in the deaf community and have divided the Kano State deaf community between deaf people who attended school—'yan makaranta (students)—and those who did not—jahilai (illiterates). Until the late 1970s, deaf children in Kano State had been either co-educated or mainstreamed or had not undergone any formal education at all. It is important to note, however, that many hearing people also had (and still have) no access to formal Western education. In fact, the illiteracy rate is still very high even among hearing people. Undoubtedly, the introduction of formal education for the deaf was a step in the right direction. However, there is a danger in transferring certain educational concepts and ideas from one society to another. The problem of choosing a language for teaching is most crucial in this context.

A FOR APPLE—PROBLEMS WITH ASL

Choosing a language for teaching has been a vital issue in Africa since the early days of colonialism. The common argument was that the indigenous languages, the so-called "local African dialects" or "local idioms," were insufficient for use in schools and that the only solution was to use one of the "more developed" (i.e., colonial) languages.[5] The examples of Hausa and Swahili, among many others, show that African languages can, of course, be systematically developed for use in any context. The multilingual situation in countries such as Nigeria, with an estimated 400 different languages, has also been cited as an argument against the use of African languages for teaching. Various researchers have, however, shown the importance of the mother tongue in education (Bamgbose 1976; Boadi 1976).

Just as African languages are often treated as local dialects, sign languages in Africa are frequently referred to as "local signs" or "local gestures" and not as developed languages. Some have argued that choosing a language for teaching deaf students in a multilingual country like Nigeria is a difficult task and that—if sign language is used for instruction—it should be one of the "more developed" sign languages, namely, a European sign language or ASL (see also Okombo 1991, 1992). In the 1970s, the Nigerian Sign Language Working Group was established with the goal to adopt and modify ASL signs to fit the Nigerian context. This group has not met for a considerable amount of time, and its work has never been published.[6] African sign languages can, of course, be systematically developed to function in any communicative situation—just as ASL and some European sign languages have been.

The process to transfer signs developed in one country to another country is not only difficult but also problematic. To date, no research has been done on the effects of teaching deaf children in a foreign sign language. Nigeria is only one of many African countries using a foreign sign language in deaf education. Depending on the kind of foreign aid programs, different European sign languages and ASL have been imported to different African countries. Some countries have been exposed to a number of foreign sign languages (in Botswana, ASL, Danish Sign Language, and German Sign Language have been introduced; in Ethiopia, Swedish Sign Language, ASL, and Finnish Sign Language; in Gambia, Dutch and British Sign Language; in Mali, ASL and French Sign Language; in Tanzania, ASL and several European sign languages, including Swedish and Finnish Sign Language).[7] Some of the problems with using foreign sign languages in Africa have been described by Akach (1993) and Okombo (1991, 1992).

Tudun Maliki School provides examples of other problems that can arise when using ASL: Teachers at Tudun Maliki School teach in a language that they themselves often only know inadequately. They are neither mother-tongue speakers of English nor native ASL signers. On the contrary, most teachers have a very limited knowledge of spoken English—and American English and Nigerian English differ from each other in many ways. In Nigerian English, for example, meanings of existing words are extended or restricted, and single words are used in a different way; loan words are introduced from different Nigerian languages, and there are local coinages of new words or expressions.[8]

The teachers know even less ASL, and only a few have learned ASL systematically. In the late 1970s to early 1980s, some teachers went to the United States or to Britain for courses in deaf education and came back with some knowledge of either ASL or British Sign Language. ASL is now taught at a number of Nigerian universities. It is, however, taught by people (both deaf and hearing) who themselves are not native ASL signers, and only a few teachers at Tudun Maliki School have undergone these courses. Most often, the teachers use some kind of Total Communication for teaching, based on signs from both ASL and Hausa Sign Language. If they lack the proper signs, they resort to gesture and pantomime, speechreading, and fingerspelling.

The students, therefore, learn only single signs of ASL and leave school with a limited vocabulary; ASL grammar is not taught at all. This fact becomes visible when they use ASL for communication. ASL signs are sometimes used inaccurately. In addition, some loan signs have been altered in the way they are performed, and others have undergone some semantic alteration or have received an additional meaning. Students also have a limited knowledge of Hausa Sign Language, which is widened, however, as soon as they participate in meetings of the deaf community outside the school. Most often, students mix the various languages: Hausa Sign Language signs appear regularly in sentences that are signed, spoken, or both in ASL or English, and ASL signs appear in Hausa Sign Language sentences.[9]

Many ASL signs do not fit the Nigerian context. One of the first words or signs students learn at school when they are taught the manual alphabet is "apple" as in "A for apple." Until recently, apples were not commonly known in Kano. Conversely, there is no sign in ASL for the "guava" fruit. In fact, ASL has no signs for basically the entire Hausa cultural vocabulary, including words for foods and drinks, clothes, plants and trees, crafts, and religious terms.

Finally, students will learn signs that are of little use outside the school context except when they get together with other students or former students of Tudun Maliki because other deaf people do not commonly understand ASL signs. This situation also applies to initialized signs and to fingerspelling, which students use frequently and which theoretically can be understood only by people who have learned the American one-handed manual alphabet. Some initialized signs are one-off, ad hoc inventions whereas others have become lexicalized and are now widely used within the deaf community, even by those people who never learned the manual alphabet. These lexicalized signs include some of the signs for Nigerian towns and states. Fingerspelling, however, can be used and understood only by people who have at least some basic reading and writing competence.

The introduction of ASL has also led to a change in the Hausa Sign Language's lexicon, especially among younger deaf people. Some ASL signs have been introduced by the students when they participate in meetings of the deaf community outside the school and are now also used among "illiterate" deaf people. Most of these signs are basic vocabulary, and some of them slowly seem to be replacing the original Hausa Sign Language signs. These ASL signs are not easier to perform and often do not fit the sociocultural background. Many Hausa Sign Language signs have an obvious etymology, but ASL signs are among the first foreign signs the students learn at school. In ASL, SATURDAY is an initialized sign whereas the Hausa Sign Language sign ASABAR (Saturday) is the same as the sign KUD'I (money) because Saturday used to be the day when government workers got their weekly salary. The students' use of ASL differs, however, from that of deaf people outside the school whose knowledge of ASL is restricted to a small number of signs.

The introduction of ASL has influenced the attitude of deaf people—especially the younger generation—toward themselves, their deafness, and their place in society. The awareness of being different is rising. Most especially, deaf people have changed their attitude toward their own sign language. ASL is frequently regarded as being more prestigious because it is seen as being related to Western education. Many students, particularly younger ones, but also other members of the deaf community believe that ASL is a "proper" sign language as opposed to the "local signs" or "gestures" (Hausa Sign Language) they have been using all their lives. They believe that their own sign language does not have value because it has never been the focus of academic research and has not been systematically developed to function in any communicative situation the way ASL has been. Some people even believe that there is only one "real" sign language, ASL, which is used everywhere in the world.

This view is further supported by the lack of attention that special education departments at Nigerian universities give to the indigenous sign language or signed languages.[10] Deaf education has always centered on ASL and on American or European concepts and theories of deafness. Most of the Nigerian literature about deaf people and deaf education is based on findings from Europe and America that are simply transferred to the Nigerian context regardless of the different cultural, social, and religious background; the particular political and economic circumstances; and the different linguistic situation. Many of these Western theories are not applicable to the Nigerian setting and certainly need to be modified to fit the sociocultural framework of Hausa society. Important factors such as the predominance of Islam and its significance in daily life as well as the importance of the traditional concept of communal existence and education have to be taken into consideration.

Furthermore, students have gained access to information and publications such as the World Federation of the Deaf's journal, the *WFD News*, that come from the United States and from Europe. Western academic and political debates about deaf culture, deaf identity, and sign language have been imported to the deaf community. Whether these academic discourses are at all applicable to the deaf community in Hausaland is questionable. The students are confronted with "deaf issues" such as the lack of acceptance of sign language in many other countries, many of which do not apply to their own situation. Nevertheless, they feel that they have to adopt these concepts and ideas. For example, a KSAD member wrote an article for a Nigerian newspaper in which he advocated the acceptance of sign language and of teaching deaf children in sign, although this practice had never been objected to either by the teachers at Tudun Maliki school or by the ministry. The article was, in fact, almost a literal copy of an article in the *WFD News*.

CONCLUSION

Until recently, deafness was not considered as being something special or extraordinary and certainly not as being a handicap; rather, it was considered as being normal, both by deaf people themselves and by the wider hearing community. Deaf people in Hausaland have not been isolated but have always been integrated both within their families and within the wider society, and they have participated fully in the everyday life of the community. The society has always accepted that deaf people use sign language for communication, and many hearing people have some basic sign knowledge.

Deaf people are still fully integrated in these structures, especially at the rural level. This system of integration has, however, slowly begun to dissolve. Hausa society, with its cultural ideas and cultural framework, is changing, and so is the economic system. Individualization and urbanization has begun also in Africa. Thus, there is a danger that deaf people will be pushed aside, will be neglected and forgotten, and will slowly lose their rightful place in society. The introduction of formal deaf education has certainly played a part in this change. The attitude toward deafness and sign language is changing both within and outside the deaf community. The acceptance of sign language even outside the deaf community and the ready use of signs or sign language for communication with deaf people may gradually disappear as a result of these changes.

ACKNOWLEDGMENTS

I wish to express my gratitude to all those deaf (and hearing) people in Kano without whose help and hospitality I could not have written this chapter. *Allah ya saka muku da alheri.*

NOTES

1.   In the literature about deaf people in Nigeria, various authors mention prejudices against deaf people, sometimes resulting from religious or superstitious beliefs (e.g.,

Mba 1986, 1990; Ozoji 1993). These authors have almost exclusively collected their data in southern Nigeria. These prejudices generally cannot be found in Hausaland.

2.   These gestures are also used as part of Hausa Sign Language, for example ZO! (come!), TAFI! (go away!), TUBA (repent, be sorry), GARGAD'I (warning), BA-RUWANA (it's none of my business), UWAKA (damn you). Some of these gestures or signs are used by deaf people in a slightly modified way, for example, UWAKA is used as a directional sign and also may be glossed as ZAGA (abuse, insult).

3.   *Bebe* (pl. *bebaye*) usually refers to a person who uses little or no spoken language whereas *kurma* (pl. *kurame*) refers to a person who is able to articulate fairly well (and who has some residual hearing).

4.   In other sources, 1957 is given as the year of establishment.

5.   Phillipson and Skutnabb-Kangas (1995) even talk of an "active underdevelopment of African languages" (339).

6.   During the years I spent in Nigeria, I was unable to obtain any further information about this group. I met one of the founding members in 1997, but he was unable to give me any details about the group's initial work.

7.   See Schmaling (2001, 181) for a more extensive list.

8.   For an introduction to Nigerian English see Jowitt (1991).

9.   Some detailed examples of language mixing can be found in Schmaling (2001).

10.   With the data collected to date, it is impossible to decide whether one national sign language (i.e., Nigerian Sign Language) exists with Hausa Sign Language being one of its variants or whether a number of separate sign languages exist. Systematic sign language research is needed in other places within Nigeria.

REFERENCES

Akach, Philemon A. O. 1993. Barriers. *Signpost* 6 (1):2–4.

Bamgbose, Ayo. 1976. The changing role of the mother tongue in education. In *Mother tongue education: The West African experience*, ed. Ayo Bamgbose, 9–26. London: Hodder; Stoughton and Paris: Unesco Press.

Boadi, Lawrence. 1976. Mother tongue education in Ghana. In *Mother tongue education: The West African experience*, ed. Ayo Bamgbose, 83–112. London: Hodder; Stoughton and Paris: Unesco Press.

Devlieger, Patrick. 1994. Culture-based concepts and social life of disabled persons in sub-Saharan Africa: The case of the deaf. In *The Deaf Way: Perspectives from the International Conference on Deaf Culture*, ed. C. J. Erting, R. C. Johnson, D. L. Smith, and B. D. Snider, 85–93. Washington, D.C.: Gallaudet University Press.

Jowitt, David. 1991. *Nigerian English usage: An introduction*. Ikeja, Nigeria: Longman Nigeria.

Last, Murray. 1991. Adolescents in a Muslim city: The cultural context of danger and risk. In *Youth and health in Kano today*. Kano Studies (Special issue):1–21.

Mba, Peter O. 1986. Social integration—a new approach to the deaf. In *National Advisory Council for the Deaf: Conference papers (1982–1986)*, ed. Peter O. Mba, 39–46. Nigeria: NACD.

———. 1987. Nigeria. In *Gallaudet encyclopedia of deaf people and deafness*, ed. John V. Van Cleve, Vol. 2, 242–44. New York: McGraw-Hill.

———. 1990. The influence of attitudes on education of the deaf in developing countries. Paper presented at the International Congress on Education of the Deaf, Rochester, N.Y., July–August, 1990.

Ojile, Emmanuel. 1994. Education of the deaf in Nigeria: An historical perspective. In *The Deaf Way: Perspectives from the international conference on Deaf culture*, ed. C. J. Erting,

R. C. Johnson, D. L. Smith, and B. D. Snider, 268–74. Washington, D.C.: Gallaudet University Press.

Okombo, Okoth. 1991. Obstacles to the development of African sign languages. In *Equality and self-reliance: Proceedings of the XI World Congress of the WFD, Tokyo, Japan, July 2–11, 1991*, ed. WFD, 165–75. Tokyo: Japanese Federation of the Deaf.

———. 1992. African languages: Will sign languages have better luck? In *East African Sign Language Seminar, Debre Zeit, Ethiopia, Aug. 10–16, 1990*, ed. Finnish Association of the Deaf, 19–24. Helsinki: FAD.

Ozoji, Emeka. 1993. *Special education for the non-professional.* Jos, Nigeria: Fab Anieh.

Ozolins, Brigitta. 1991. Oppression of native sign language in Africa. In *Equality and self-reliance: Proceedings of the XI World Congress of the WFD, Tokyo, July 2–11, 1991*, ed. WFD, 705–6. Tokyo: Japanese Federation of the Deaf.

Phillipson, Robert, and Tove Skutnabb-Kangas. 1995. Language rights in postcolonial Africa. In *Linguistic human rights: Overcoming linguistic discrimination*, ed. Tove Skutnabb-Kangas and Robert Phillipson, 335–45. Berlin and New York: Mouton de Gruyter.

Schmaling, Constanze. 2001. ASL in northern Nigeria: Will Hausa Sign Language survive? In *Signed languages: Discoveries from international research*, ed. V. Dively, M. Metzger, S. Taub, and A. M. Baer, 180–93. Washington, D.C.: Gallaudet University Press.

Wolff, H. Ekkehard. 1993. *Referenzgrammatik des Hausa.* Münster and Hamburg: Lit.

Contributors

Debra Aarons
University of Stellenbosch
Matieland, South Africa

Jean Ann
State University of New York
Oswego, New York

Sangeeta Bagga-Gupta
Örebro University
Örebro, Sweden

Norine Berenz
Inter American University
San German, Puerto Rico
University of Witwatersrand
Johannesberg, South Africa

Penny Boyes Braem
Center for Sign Language Research
Basel, Switzerland

Benno Caramore
Sign Language Interpreter Training
*   Program*
Zürich, Switzerland

Lars-Åke Domfors
Örebro University
Örebro, Sweden

Franz Dotter
Universität Klagenfurt
Klagenfurt, Austria

Donald A. Grushkin
California State University, Sacramento
Sacramento, California

Patricia Shores Hermann
Sign Language Teacher Training Program
Zürich, Switzerland

Roland Hermann
Cultural Commission of the Swiss Deaf
*   Association*
Zürich, Switzerland

Anna Komarova
Centre for Deaf Studies and Bilingual
*   Education*
Moscow, Russia

Barbara LeMaster
California State University
Long Beach, California

Ceil Lucas
Gallaudet University
Washington, D.C.

Leila Monaghan
Indiana University
Bloomington, Indiana

Karen Nakamura
Macalester College
Saint Paul, Minnesota

Ingeborg Okorn
Klagenfurt, Austria

Michael Pursglove
University of Bath
Bath, England

Louise Reynolds
Deaf Community of Cape Town
Cape Town, South Africa

Susan Schatz
Gallaudet University
Washington, D.C.

Constanze Schmaling
Hamburg University
Hamburg, Germany

Richard J. Senghas
Sonoma State University
Rohnert Park, California

Rachel Sutton-Spence
University of Bristol
Bristol, England

James Woodward
Dong Nai Department of Education and
    Training
Bien Hoa, Dong Nai, Viet Nam

Index

Abadia, José Miguel Alea, 5
abortion, 11, 103
Abraham, E., 37–38
Abramov, Igor, 18, 249, 252–53
abrupt creolization, 267
activism: cochlear implants, protest against, 122; Deaf AIDS Project, 19; "Deaf President Now" (DPN), ix, 16, 121; "Deaf Shock," 223–24, 226; "Deaf Way," 121, 250, 275–77; D-groups, 223–24, 225; D-Pro, 223–24; exclusion of English by militant Deaf, 121–22; international issues and, 19; Kyoto School for the Deaf Student Strike, 219; militarism and rise of American Deaf community, 121–22; rejection of hearing values, 133; Russia, 251
African American identity, comparison to hard of hearing and deaf individuals, 126, 175
Ahlgren, Inger, 15, 68
AIDS/HIV, 19
Algerian nationalism movement, 226
alphabets, British, 25–48; Cistercian manual, 31; Dalgarno's manual, 34–35; Digiti Lingua (first known dactylogical manual alphabet), 31, 35; Druids and, 31; Norwegian manual, 27; Ogham manual, 31, 32; one-handed, American manual, 39, 307, —, British manual, 38–39; —, Irish manual, 26; 17th-century manual, 33–35; Spanish roots and, 2, 27, 40; two-handed, 27; unadopted manual, 36–38; Wilkin's arthrological manual, 31–33
Alves, João Carlos Carreria, 17, 178–79
American School for the Deaf, 4, 121

American Sign Language (ASL): African countries using, 16, 305–8; Deaf culture membership and, 153–54, 166; dictionary, 9; hard of hearing individuals and, 119, 120; Japanese Sign Language loan words, 223; mixture with other languages, 290–91, 296–97; Nigerian use of, 16, 305–8; oralism and unofficial use of, 9; recognition as full language, 68, 121; residential schools and, 142; Russian Sign Language and, 255; sociolinguistic dynamics in American Deaf communities, 141–52; Southeast Asian use of, 299; Swedish Sign Language and, 68; Swiss German sign for cochlear implant from, 106
Amman, Johann Conrad, 28
Andersen, Anders, 276
Anderson, Benedict, 211, 269
Andersson, Ronny, 78
Anschluss, 51–52
ANSNIC (Asociación Nacional de Sordos de Nicaragua), 263, 266, 268, 270–77. See also Nicaragua
anti-Deaf sentiment, 11–12
anti-Hearing sentiment, 121–22
apartheid, 18, 197, 200, 202–3
APRIAS (Association for the Integration of and Aid to the Deaf), 265–66, 270, 276. See also Nicaragua
Arnold, Thomas, 43
Arrowsmith, John Pauncefoot, 38
The Art of Reading, Spelling and Ciphering by the Fingers (Lucas), 37
ASL. *See* American Sign Language; Austrian Sign Language; Asociación

Lightning Source UK Ltd.
Milton Keynes UK
UKHW032035200123
415706UK00001B/29